Experimental Pharmacognosy

for Students of B Pharm and M Pharm

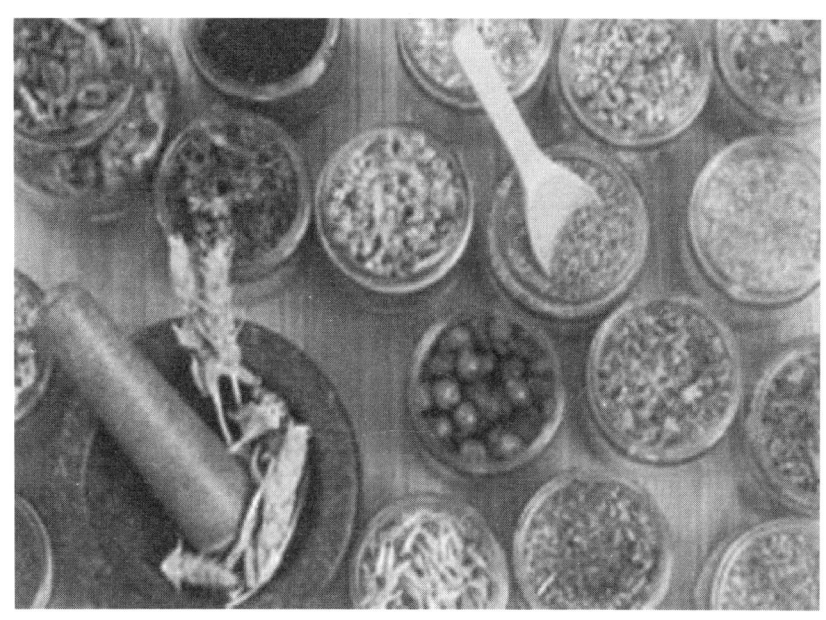

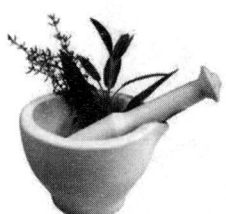

Experimental Pharmacognosy

for Students of B Pharm and M Pharm

Rajesh Kumar Nema
M Pharm, PhD, Ayurvedratna, FICC

Director
Lakshmi Narain College of Pharmacy (RCP)
Indore

CS Bhan
M Pharm, PhD

Principal
Akashdeep College of Pharmacy
Jaipur

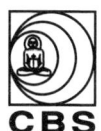

CBS Publishers & Distributors Pvt Ltd

New Delhi • Bengaluru • Chennai • Kochi • Kolkata • Mumbai
Bhopal • Bhubaneswar • Hyderabad • Jharkhand • Nagpur • Patna • Pune • Uttarakhand • Dhaka (Bangladesh)

Disclaimer

Science and technology are constantly changing fields. New research and experience broaden the scope of information and knowledge. The authors have tried their best in giving information available to them while preparing the material for this book. Although, all efforts have been made to ensure optimum accuracy of the material, yet it is quite possible some errors might have been left uncorrected. The publisher, the printer and the authors will not be held responsible for any inadvertent errors, omissions or inaccuracies.

Experimental Pharmacognosy
for Students of B Pharm and M Pharm

ISBN: 978-93-86217-53-0

Copyright © Authors and Publisher

First Edition: 2017
Reprint: 2019

All rights reserved. No part of this book may be reproduced or transmitted in any form or by any means, electronic or mechanical, including photocopying, recording, or any information storage and retrieval system without permission, in writing, from the authors and the publisher.

Published by Satish Kumar Jain and produced by Varun Jain for

CBS Publishers & Distributors Pvt Ltd
4819/XI Prahlad Street, 24 Ansari Road, Daryaganj, New Delhi 110 002, India.
Ph: 23289259, 23266861, 23266867   Website: www.cbspd.com
Fax: 011-23243014   e-mail: delhi@cbspd.com; cbspubs@airtelmail.in.

Corporate Office: 204 FIE, Industrial Area, Patparganj, Delhi 110 092
Ph: 4934 4934   Fax: 4934 4935   e-mail: publishing@cbspd.com; publicity@cbspd.com

Branches

- **Bengaluru:** Seema House 2975, 17th Cross, K.R. Road, Banasankari 2nd Stage, Bengaluru 560 070, Karnataka
  Ph: +91-80-26771678/79   Fax: +91-80-26771680   e-mail: bangalore@cbspd.com
- **Chennai:** 7, Subbaraya Street, Shenoy Nagar, Chennai 600 030, Tamil Nadu
  Ph: +91-44-26680620, 26681266   Fax: +91-44-42032115   e-mail: chennai@cbspd.com
- **Kochi:** 42/1325, 1326, Power House Road, Opposite KSEB Power House, Ernakulam 682 018, Kochi, Kerala
  Ph: +91-484-4059061-65   Fax: +91-484-4059065   e-mail: kochi@cbspd.com
- **Kolkata:** 6/B, Ground Floor, Rameswar Shaw Road, Kolkata-700 014, West Bengal
  Ph: +91-33-22891126, 22891127, 22891128   e-mail: kolkata@cbspd.com
- **Mumbai:** 83-C, Dr E Moses Road, Worli, Mumbai-400018, Maharashtra
  Ph: +91-22-24902340/41   Fax: +91-22-24902342   e-mail: mumbai@cbspd.com

Representatives

• Bhopal	0-8319310552	• Bhubaneswar	0-9911037372	• Hyderabad	0-9885175004
• Jharkhand	0-9811541605	• Nagpur	0-9421945513	• Patna	0-9334159340
• Pune	0-9623451994	• Uttarakhand	0-9716462459	• Dhaka (Bangladesh)	01912-003485

Printed at: Glorious Printers, Delhi, India

to
My Family

Preface

The book *Experimental Pharmacognosy* meets the pedagogic needs in the subject of pharmacognosy, and is being extensively used in pharmacy colleges and other institutions all over the country.

The book should prove to be of a great interest to B Pharm and M Pharm students in the experimental and pharmacognostical characteristic features of various drugs. It will elaborate to the students the divergent classification of crude drugs, basic concepts of pharmacognosy, basic techniques of pharmacognosy, methods of extraction, separation and identification, spectroscopic methods of analysis of herbal drugs, chemical tests for various classes of phytoconstituents, powder, morphological and microscopical studies, fibres, plant tissue culture, basic techniques of extraction, isolation, identification and estimation of phytoconstituents and preparation and standardization of Ayurvedic formulations. This book has been introduced as per the syllabi of various universities at the undergraduate and postgraduate levels of courses in pharmacy.

We are thankful to Dr (Mrs) Dhriti Nema for her valuable comments in updating the book. Thanks are due to the publishers, CBS Publishers & Distributors, New Delhi, for their cooperation and efforts in keeping the text free from any printing mistakes.

Rajesh Kumar Nema
CS Bhan

Contents

Preface *vii*

1. General Pharmacognostic Considerations 1–47

    I. Introduction 1
        History 1
        Scope and development of pharmacognosy 2
        Classification of crude drugs 3
        Evaluation of crude drugs 7
        Important definitions 19
    II. Basic Concepts of Pharmacognosy 21
        Unorganised drugs 22
        Organised drugs 22
    III. Basic Techniques of Pharmacognosy 22
        Macroscopical examination 22
        Microscopical examination 22
        Quantitative analytical microscopy 24
    IV. Methods of Extraction 25
        Maceration 26
        Percolation 26
        Hot continuous extraction 27
        Steam distillation 27
        Infusion 27
        Decoction 28
        Expression 28
        Filtration 28
        Vesication 28
        Pulverization 28
        Trituration 28
    V. Separation and Identification 28
        Thin layer chromatography (TLC) 29
        Paper chromatography 30
        High performance liquid chromatography (HPLC) 31

Gas liquid chromatography (GLC) 33
High performance thin layer chromatography (HPTLC) 33
VI. Spectroscopic Methods of Analysis of Herbal Drugs 34
Ultraviolet and visible spectroscopy (UV–visible spectra) 34
Infrared spectroscopy (IR spectra) 35
VII. Chemical Tests for Various Classes of Phytoconstituents 36
General tests 36
Alkaloids 36
Glycosides 36
Steroids and terpenoids 36
Tannins 37
Flavonoids 37
Oils and fats 38
Proteins and amino acids 38
Carbohydrates 38
Volatile oils 39
Amino acids 39
Lipids 39
Specific tests 45
Alkaloids 45
Glycosides 46
Resins 47

2. Powder: Morphological and Microscopical Studies 48–131

1. To study the simple and compound microscopes 48
2. To study the section cutting technique of stem, root and leaf, and staining and mounting of a section 49
3. To measure the length and breadth of fibres in the given sample 50
4. To measure the size of calcium oxalate crystals in the given powdered sample 51
5. To measure the diameter of starch grains in the given powdered sample 52
6. To determine the palisade ratio in the leaf sample 54
7. To determine the stomata number and stomata index of leaf 55
8. To determine the vein islet number and vein termination number of leaf 56
9. To determine the swelling index of the given sample drug 56
10. To determine the total ash, acid insoluble ash and water soluble ash of the given crude drug 57
11. To determine the extractive value of the given crude drug 58
12. To determine the moisture content of given crude drug by loss on drying method 58
13. To study the morphological, microscopical and powder characteristics of leaf of *Digitalis lanata* 59
14. To study the morphological, microscopical and powder characteristics of leaf of *Digitalis purpurea* 61

15. To study microscopical powder characteristics of Digitalis leaf 64
16. To study the morphological, microscopical and powder characteristics of Senna leaf 65
17. To study the morphological, microscopical and powder characteristics of Vinca leaf 68
18. To study the morphological, microscopical and powder characteristics of Vasaka leaf 70
19. To study the morphological, microscopical and powder characteristics of Datura leaf 73
20. To study microscopical powder characteristics of Hyoscyamus leaf 76
21. To study the morphological, microscopical and powder characteristics of Clove 77
22. To study the morphological, microscopical and powder characteristics of Ginger 80
23. To study the morphological, microscopical and powder characteristics of Coriander 82
24. To study the morphological, microscopical and powder characteristics of Rauwolfia 84
25. To study the morphological, microscopical and powder characteristics of Cinchona bark 86
26. To study the morphological, microscopical and powder characteristics of Cassia bark 88
27. To study the morphological, microscopical and powder characteristics of root of Liquorice 91
28. To study the morphological, microscopical and powder characteristics of Kurchi bark 95
29. To study the morphological, microscopical and powder characteristics of Ephedra (Ma-Huang) stem 97
30. To study the morphological, microscopical and powder characteristics of Ipecacuanha root 98
31. To study the morphological, microscopical and powder characteristics of Nux Vomica seed 101
32. To study powder characteristics of Rhubarb 104
33. To study powder characteristics of Indian Squill 106
34. To identify given unknown powder mixture (Senna and Squill) 107
35. To identify given unknown powder mixture (Vasaka and Ipecac) 108
36. To identify given unknown powder mixture (Digitalis and Liquorice) 109
37. To identify given unknown powder mixture (Cinchona and Vasaka) 109
38. To study morphology of given drugs: Ashoka bark, Arjuna bark, Tulsi, Bahera, Amla, Vasaka, Harad 111
39. To study morphology of given drug samples: Satavari, Giloi, Chhota Gokhru, Bada Gokhru, Rasna, Methi 116

40. To study morphology of given drugs: Majith, Guggal, Kantakari, Brahmi, Punarnava, Chitrak   120
41. To study morphology of given drugs: Turmeric, Ajowan, Black Catechu   125
42. To study morphology of given drugs: Neem, Aloe, Lemon grass, Nirgundi, Jatropha   127

3. Identification of Crude Drugs   133–150

I. Carbohydrates   133
  1. To identify the given sample of Jaguar gum   133
  2. To identify the given sample of Agar   133
  3. To identify the given sample of Acacia   134
  4. To identify the given sample of Pectin   134
  5. To identify the given sample of Honey   135
  6. To identify the given sample of Starch   136
  7. To identify the given sample of Tragacanth   136
  8. To identify the given sample of Sterculia gum   137
  9. To identify the given sample of Isapgol   137

II. Lipids   138
  10. To identify the given sample of lipids: Cod liver oil, Cocoa butter, Castor oil, Linseed, Rice bran oil, Hydrous wool fat, Lard, Shark liver oil, Sandalwood oil   138

III. Resin and Resin Combination   141
  11. To perform morphological and chemical tests of Asafoetida   141
  12. To perform morphological and chemical tests of Balsam of Tolu   141
  13. To perform morphological and chemical tests of Balsam of Peru   142
  14. To perform morphological and chemical tests of Benzoin   142
  15. To perform morphological and chemical tests of Colophony   143
  16. To perform morphological and chemical tests of Cannabis   143
  17. To perform morphological and chemical tests of Capsicum   144
  18. To perform morphological and chemical tests of Jalap   144
  19. To perform morphological and chemical tests of Ginger   145
  20. To perform morphological and chemical tests of Myrrh   145
  21. To perform morphological and chemical tests of Podophyllum   146
  22. To perform morphological and chemical tests of Turmeric   146

IV. Tannin and Tannin Containing Drugs   147
  23. To perform morphological and chemical tests of Black Catechu   147
  24. To perform morphological and chemical tests of Myrobalan   148

V. Chemical Evaluation of Powdered Drugs   148
  25. To perform chemical tests of Digitalis, Datura, Senna, Cinchona, Aloe, Rauwolfia, Nux Vomica   148

4.	**Fibres**	**151–158**

1. To identify the given samples of natural fibres (cotton and jute)   151
2. To identify the given samples of animal fibres (wool, silk)   153
3. To identify the given samples of artificial regenerated fibres (viscose rayon, acetate rayon)   154
4. To identify the given samples of artificial synthetic fibres (nylon, terylene)   155
5. To examine a fabric used as a surgical dressing (crepe bandage)   156
6. To examine surgical dressings   156
7. To determine crude fibres by Dutch method   157

5.	**Plant Tissue Culture**	**159–169**

General Procedures Involved in Plant Tissue Culture   159

1. To prepare and sterilize given tissue culture medium   163
2. To carry out aseptic germination of given seeds   165
3. To perform *in vitro* callus induction of aseptically germinated seedlings/given plant   166
4. To develop callus culture from carrot combine explants   166
5. To determine antimicrobial activity of crude drugs   167

6.	**Extraction, Isolation, Identification and Estimation of Phytoconstituents**	**170–212**

1. To carry out isolation of starch from potatoes   170
2. To carry out extraction of solanine from potatoes   171
3. To carry out isolation of citric acid from lemon   172
4. To isolate calcium citrate from lemon juice   173
5. To carry out extraction of pectin from fresh orange peels   173
6. To isolate hesperidin from orange peel   174
7. To prepare TLC plates   175
8. To isolate caffeine from tea leaves   176
9. To carry out isolation of nicotine picarate from Tobacco leaves   177
10. To carry out isolation of curcumin from *Curcuma longa*   178
11. To carry out isolation of calcium sennoside from Senna leaf powder   179
12. To carry out isolation of lawsone from Heena powder   180
13. To carry out isolation of vasicine in Vasaka leaf powder   181
14. To carry out isolation of diosgenin from Fenugreek seeds   182
15. To carry out isolation of aloin from Aloe powder   183
16. To carry out isolation of quinine sulphate from Cinchona bark powder   184
17. To carry out isolation of arteminin from *Artemisia annua*   186
18. To carry out isolation of vincristine from Vinca   186
19. To carry out extraction of strychnine and brucine from Nux Vomica seeds   186
20. To extract ammonium glycyrrhizinate from Glycyrrhiza powder and to carry out its TLC studies   188

21. To carry out isolation of glycyrrhetinic acid from Liquorice roots   189
22. To carry out extraction of *Withania somnifera*   189
23. To carry out extraction of resins from Jalap roots   190
24. To isolate piperine from Black Pepper and carry out its TLC studies   191
25. To isolate eugenol from Clove oil   192
26. To carry out isolation of eugenol from Cinnamon leaf oil   193
27. To isolate volatile oil from Fennel   194
28. To carry out isolation of lemon grass oil from Lemon grass   196
29. To determine volatile oil content in given sample of Eucalyptus leaves by hydrodistillation method   196
30. To determine volatile oil content in given sample of *Mentha piperita* leaves by hydrodistillation method   197
31. To prepare and submit TLC plate of given crude drug (Cinchona bark)   198
32. To carry out TLC study of Clove oil and Datura   198
33. To carry out TLC study of Rauwolfia, Cinchona and Black Pepper   199
34. To identify constituents of given herbal drug preparation by chromatographic methods   199
35. To identify constituents of given herbal drug preparation by circular paper chromatography   200
36. To identify the amino acids in given mixture by comparing their R_f values with reference standards   200
37. To perform paper chromatography of given known sample of protein   201
38. To identify alkaloids in cinchona bark extract by comparing their R_f values with reference standards   201
39. Estimation of vasaka alkaloids in *Adhatoda vasika* by titrimetry method and TLC   202
40. Estimation of total tannin in Harad powder   202
41. Estimation of sennoside from Senna powder by colorimetry (IP-1996)   203
42. Estimation of quinine in Cinchona bark powder as per BP-2000   203
43. To estimate vitamin C in Chayvanprash by colorimetry   204
44. To estimate citral in Lemon oil   204
45. To demonstrate the column chromatography   204
46. Pharmacognostical and phytochemical investigation of Tulsi plants   205
47. Determination of percentage purity of ginger in various samples by Wallis's lycopodium spore method   206
48. Determination of foaming index of given drug sample (Glycerrhiza and Shatavari)   208
49. Determination of swelling index of given drug sample (Isapgol and Methi)   209
50. To estimate sennoside B from Senna leaf powder   210
51. To determine barbaloin from *Aloe Vera*   211
52. To determine volatile oil content of Eucalyptus leaves   212

7. Preparation and Standardization of Ayurvedic Formulations 213–268

1. To perform phytochemical screening of crude drugs 215
2. To prepare and evaluate marketed formulation of churna (Hingastak churna and Trikatu churna) 220
3. Estimation of total tannin from Amla, Baheda, Harde by titrimetric method 222
4. To prepare and evalute Swarna Bhasma 224
5. To prepare and evalute Titoplodi churna 227
6. To prepare and evalute Triphala churna 228
7. Comparative TLC study of ellagic acid, gallic acid, curcumin in given marketed Pathayadi kwatha (Sadanga churna) 231
8. To determine the particle size of the given sample (nagod) by sieving method and optical microscopy 232
9. To prepare and evaluate Cahyavanparsh Avaleha 234
10. To prepare and evalute Dhatryaristha 236
11. To prepare and evalute Dashmularishtha 237
12. To prepare and evalute Mahavasava 240
13. To find out the antioxidant activity of kwath 241
14. Estimation of total flavonoids content of kwath 244
15. Estimation of total phenolic content of given compound 244
16. Determination of various leaf surface data (leaf constant of stomatal number and stomatal index) 246
17. To determine the total ash and acid insoluble ash of given drug (*Withania somnifera*/ Black Peppere) 248
18. To determine ash value of a given powdered crude drug (Liquorice) 248
19. To determine extractive value of a given powdered crude drug (Liquorice) 249
20. To determine the amount of ethanol present in the given sample of Asava or Arista 250
21. Estimation of total alkaloids 250
22. Preparation and evaluation of prepared herbal cream 251
23. To determine saponification value of the given sample of oil 253
24. Determination of leaf constant data (leaf constant of vein islet and vein let termination number) 254
25. To identify constituents of given herbal drug preparation by chromatographic method 254
26. To separate active principles of plant materials by column chromatography and high pressure liquid chromatography (HPLC) 255
27. To develope method in HPTLC and estimate sennoside B and glycerrhizin from capsule and simultaneous estimation of sennoside and glycerrhizin 260

8. Stains and Reagents for Microchemical Reactions 269–274

Suggested Readings 275
Index 277

Chapter 1

General Pharmacognostic Considerations

I. INTRODUCTION

The word 'pharmacognosy' is derived from the Greek word *Pharmakon:* drug and *gnosis*: knowledge. In a broadway, it is the study of medicines derived from natural and animal sources, relates with the scientific study of structural, physical, chemical and sensory characters of crude drugs of animal, vegetable and mineral origin and also includes their history, cultivation, collection and other particulars relating to the treatment they receive during their passage from producer to the distributor or pharmacist. In a broader sense, it embraces knowledge of the history, identification, distribution, cultivation, collection, selection, preparation, evaluation, preservation, commerce, and use of natural substances that affect the health of men and other animals.

HISTORY

The history of herbal medicine is as old as human civilization itself, when man in the quest for food learned to differentiate edible and nonedible. If the nonedible plant had a purgative action then it was used for that purpose, if found poisonous like *strophanthus*, they were used on arrows as arrow poison. Knowledge was empirical and obtained by trial and error method. Drugs were used as crude extracts, i.e. as infusions or decoctions. Documents of medicinal plants date back to antiquity, before the beginning of the Christian calendar.

In China, the use of medicinal plants dates back to 5000 BC. The oldest herbal document the *Pen T-Sao* written by emperor Shen Nung (3000 BC) contains 365 drugs, i.e. one for each day of the year.

In India, the Rigveda and the Atharvaveda (3500–1500 BC) describe the medicinal properties of plants and it is from which Ayurveda developed. In Ayurveda the ancient well-known treaties namely the Charaka and Sushrut Sanhitas deal with plants and surgery respectively.

In Egypt, people were familiar with the medicinal properties of plants and animals. They were familiar with human anatomy and knew how to embalm and preserve the dead bodies. The *Papyrus Ebers*, a scroll (60' long and 1' wide) dates back to the 1600 BC, the document text is dominated by more than 800 formulas and 700 different drugs. Drugs such as Acacia, Castor oil and Fennel are mentioned with reference to compounds like iron oxide, sodium chloride, sodium carbonate and sulfur.

Greek scientists hold a prominent place for their contribution to the knowledge of medicinal plants. Hippocrates (460–370 BC) is referred to as 'The father of medicine' and remembered for his famous oath till today.

Aristotle (384–322 BC), a student of Plato is known for his writings on the animal kingdom, which are considered authoritative even today.

Theophrastus (370–287 BC), a student of Aristotle, wrote about the plant kingdom.

Doiscorides (40–80 AD), described medicinal plants some of which like belladonna, ergot, opium and colchicum are used even today.

Pliny 'the Elder' wrote 37 volumes of natural history.

Galen, known as the first pharmacist devised methods of preparation of plant and animal drugs known as 'Galenicals' in his honour.

For the next few hundred years there was little change in the use of formulation of these medicaments.

The French scientist, Le'mercy (1645) described the use of alcohol for extraction.

Wilam Withering (1785), published the medicinal properties of foxglove, based on ten years of experimentation.

In 1803, the French pharmacist, Derosne isolated narcotine from opium and its role in alleviating pain was recognised. In the next few years, other phytoconstituents, viz. strychnine, emetine, brucine and piperine, quinine and colchicines were isolated. Other important discoveries during that period were isolation of nicotine from tobacco leaves, cocaine, pilocarpine, ephedrine and podophyllotoxin. The isolation of ergometrine, digoxin, reserpine, theophylline, quinidine, artemisin, camptothecin and taxol were some significant discoveries of the twentieth century.

The term pharmacognosy was used for the first time by the Australian physician Schmidt in 1811.

SCOPE AND DEVELOPMENT OF PHARMACOGNOSY

As an applied science, pharmacognosy has played a crucial role in the development of different disciplines of science. The knowledge of botany, plant taxonomy, plant breeding, plant pathology, and plant genetics is helpful in the development of cultivation technology for medicinal and aromatic plants. Plant chemistry (phytochemistry) has undergone significant development in recent years to become a distinct discipline on its own.

The technology involving extraction, purification and characterization of pharmaceuticals from natural sources is a significant contribution to natural and physical sciences. Knowledge of chemotaxonomy, biogenetic pathways for formulation of medicinally active primary and secondary metabolites, plant tissue culture and other fields is essential for complete understanding.

Pharmacognosy is an important link between *pharmacology* and *medicinal chemistry*. The rapid development of phytochemicals and pharmacological testing has been the reason for several plant materials finding their way into medicine as purified phytochemicals rather than traditional galenicals. Pharmacognosy is the source of several crude drugs that provide essential intermediates for synthesis of active compounds. *Phytopharmaceuticals* or synthetic drugs derived from phytochemicals have to be ultimately incorporated into suitable dosage form, which involves the knowledge of dispensing and preparative pharmacy, pharmaceuticals technology and analysis. In a nutshell, pharmacognosy is an important bridge between the pharmaceuticals and basic sciences. It is a vital link between the Ayurvedic and Allopathic systems of medicine. Active principles of crude drugs derived from natural origin can be formulated and manufactured in dosage forms which are acceptable to the allopathic system of medicine.

CLASSIFICATION OF CRUDE DRUGS

Crude Drugs: Drug which undergoes only two processes, i.e. collection and drying. It consists of entire plant or part of the plant/animal product. *Example*: senna leaves, cinchona bark, colophony, cantharides, agar, etc.

Organized Drugs: Crude drugs which have definite cellular structure are called as organized drug. *Example*: leaf, root, bark, etc.

Unorganized drug: Crude drugs which do not have definite cellular structure are called as unorganized drug. *Example*: gums, resins, juices, latex, wax, etc.

For any systematic study of drugs, they must be grouped according to the said classification. This not only helps in bringing out a correlation among them but also gives a better understanding. Several types of classification have been used with different purposes keeping in mind. Each of these systems has advantage and disadvantages.

Alphabetic Classification

In this system crude drugs are arranged according to the alphabetic order of their Latin or English name, e.g. IP, BP USP, EP, etc. *Example*: Acacia, balsam, cinchona, digitalis, etc.

Advantages: Easy to classify

Disadvantages: It does not reveal any taxonomical, morphological or chemical status.

Taxonomical Classification

Drugs are classified based on natural relationship among plants (phytogeny among plants). They are classified according to the plants or animals from which they are obtained in phylum, division, class, order, family, genus and species.

Example I:
 Phylum: Spermatophyta
 Division: Angiospermae
 Class: Dicotyledons
 Order: Tubiflorae
 Family: Solanaceae
 Genus: *Datura*
 Species: *stromonium*

Example II:
 Phylum: Spermatophyta
 Division: Angiospermae
 Class: Monocotyledons
 Order: Liliflorae
 Family: Lilliaceae
 Genus: *Asparagus*
 Species: *racemosus*

Advantages

A large number of plant families have certain distinguishing characteristics, thus it is, easy for identification and investigation of new sources of supply and related species.

Disadvantages

1. Fails to recognize organized and unorganized nature of crude drugs.
2. Fails to give an account of chemical nature of active constituents and their therapeutic significance.

Morphological Classification

Here crude drugs are grouped according to part of the plant/animal represented into organized and unorganized crude drugs.

Example I: Organized
 Seed: Nux-vomica, Isabgol
 Leaf: Senna, Digitalis,
 Bark: Cinchona, Cassia
 Wood: Quassia, Sandalwood,
 Root: Rauwolfia, Ipecac
 Rhizome: Zinger, Turmeric
 Flower bud: Clove, Pyrethrum
 Fruit: Cardamom, Coriander
 Entire plant: Chirata, Kalmegh

Example II: Unorganized
   Latex: Papain
   Resin: Asafoetida
   Dry juice: Aloe
   Gum: Acacia
   Extract: Catechu

Advantages
1. It gives morphological status of crude drug and useful when chemical nature of the drug is not understood.
2. To identify specific drug and to ascertain their adulterant.

Disadvantage
Therapeutic significance and chemical nature of active constituents are not given importance.

Pharmacological/Therapeutic Classification
This classification involves grouping of crude drugs according to their pharmacological action of the chief active constituents or their therapeutic use regardless of morphology, taxonomy and chemical nature. *Examples*:

Drugs Acting on GIT
   Bitters: Quassia, Gentian, Cinchona
   Carminative: Cardamom, Mentha, Fennel
   Emetics: Ipecac
   Antiamoebics: Kurchi bark
   Laxatives: Senna, Isabgol
   Antiulcer: Liquorice

Drugs Acting on Respiratory System
   Expectorant: Liquorice, Vasaka
   Antitussives: Opium
   Bronchodilators: Ephedra, Tea

Drugs Acting on Cardiovascular System
   Cardiotonics: Digitalis, Squill
   Cardiac depressants: Cinchona
   Antihypertensive: Rauwolfia

Drugs Acting on ANS
   Adrenergics: Ephedra
   Cholivergics: Pilocarpus
   Anticholinergics: Datura, Belladonna

Drugs Acting on CNS
   Stimulants: Coffee
   Depressants: Opium
   Hallucinogens: Cannabis
   Smooth muscles relaxants: Datura
   Skeletal muscle relaxants: Curare
   Anticancer: Vinca, Podophyllum
   Antirheumatics: Guggul, Colchicum
   Anthelmintics: Quassia, male fern

Drugs Acting on Skin
   Emollients: Olive oil, Wool fat
   Astringent: Catechu
   Antimalarial: Cinchona
   Local anesthetic: Coca

Advantages: Regardless of morphology, taxonomical status or chemical relationship.

Disadvantages: No importance given to the active chemical constituents of drugs.

Chemical Classification
Crude drugs are classified according to the chemical nature of their most important constituents. Since the activity and therapeutic uses of drugs are based on chemical constituents, it would appear that the chemical classification is a preferred method of study.

Examples:

1. Glycosides: Senna, Digitalis
2. Alkaloids: Datura, Cinchona
3. Tannins: Catechu, Ashoka
4. Volatile oils: Clove, Peppermint
5. Lipids: Castor oil, Bees wax
6. Carbohydrates: Acacia, Agar, Honey
7. Resins: Colophony, Benzoin

8. Vitamins: Amla, Shark liver oil
9. Hormones: Oxytocin, Insulin
10. Proteins: Gelatin
11. Enzymes: Papain, Bromelains

Advantages
1. Drugs classified regardless of morphology and taxonomy.
2. Since activity based on active constituents, it is a preferred method.

Disadvantages
1. Chemotaxonomical relation is not given importance.
2. It does not give any idea about its morphology or taxonomical and pharmacological activity.

Chemotaxonomy

It is the study of classification of crude drugs based on chemical and taxonomical characters or chemical evidences obtained from the plants. It is a comparative phytochemistry or biochemical systematics. In this system, equal importance is given to their taxonomy and biogenesis.

Definitions
1. Chemotaxonomy is defined as "a scientific investigation of the potentialities of chemical characters for the study of problems of plant taxonomy and phytogeny" (origins and races).
2. It is also a scientific discipline which attempts to utilize chemical facts to obtain a more exact understanding of biological evolution and natural relationship.

Type of Chemotaxonomy
1. Descriptive chemotaxonomy
2. Dynamic chemotaxonomy
3. Serotaxnomy
4. DNA hybridization

1. Descriptive Chemotaxonomy

Deals with study of chemical constituents and its comparison up to molecular level.

Secondary Constituents
1. Rare compounds
2. Intermediate
3. Common one

Example: Vinca alkaloids

Advantages
1. It involves isolation of compounds in the pure form.
2. Structural elucidation of these compounds can be done.

Disadvantages
1. It consumes more time.
2. Convergence and divergence.

Convergence: During evolution it may happen that the dissimilar plants may give rise to morphologically similar plants.

Divergence: Some time related plants may give rise to very dissimilar plants. Such phenomena cause considerable taxonomic difference.

Example: Xerophytes: Desert – more mucilage

Normal: Reduced mucilage content

2. Dynamic Chemotaxonomy

Classification is based on biosynthetic relationship. Different plants sometimes contain same constituents but are formed by different pathways. Such plants probably contain similar enzyme systems and the compound produce to indicate a relationship between the related plants.

Example: Benzoic acid in plants is formed by three ways (same compound formed by different pathways).

1. Shikimic acid pathway
2. By cyclization of acetate
3. Degradation of larger molecules

Different final compound may form by more or less similar pathways.

Example: Tryptophan–Quinoline alkaloids–Quinine.

Indole alkaloids: Reserpine

Advantage: Enzyme systems are closely related.

Disadvantages: Labeled precursors are required. Only assumption is possible.

3. *Serotaxonomy*

In this classification, comparison of protein mixture is done. Generally water soluble proteins are taken into consideration. The technique of serotaxonomy relies under immunological reactions shown by mammals, when they are invaded by foreign proteins.

The plant extract containing proteins (antigen) injected to mammals (usually rabbit). After some days, the recipient will form antibodies specific to the antigen. These antigens are extracted and can be used as a standard test against other plant extracts whose relationship has to be ascertained with the first plant and the amount of coagulation it causes measures similarity of species.

The protein extract of a plant whose relationship has to be ascertained is mixed with antibody of the first plant. If precipitate is formed even at higher dilution of the serum, indicates that two plants are closely related. If precipitate is not formed, it indicates they are not related.

Procedure: The antibody of specific antigen is placed in trough on a thin agar slab. After some time antigen and antibody components are diffused radialy from their position on the agar. When antigen meet antibody, precipitate occurs as an arc, which represent those proteins of the original plant.

Advantage: Very simple method, large number of samples can be tested.

Disadvantage: Only antigenic protein is tested but other enzymes may interfere partially.

4. DNA Hybridization

This classification is based on the similarity in the composition of the DNA molecules from different sources. It is possible to break a double helix DNA into two complimentary components (denaturing), the single strand consists of purine and pyrimidine bases (adinine, guanine, cytosine and thymine). Under suitable conditions two strands come together again and combined to form a complete molecule (reassociation or renaturing of DNA). Purine base adenine combines always with pyrimidine thymine and pyrimidine base cytosine combines with purine guanine.

Single strand DNA (unlabeled) in low concentration mixed with single strand of unknown DNA (labeled). Under suitable conditions, the two strands associate wherever they are common. The unpaired single strand removed by suitable means and radioactivity is measured. The amount of activity indicates the extent of hybridization.

Procedure: DNA exists as a double helix; the two complementary strands can be separated (disassociated) from each other by suitable heating and cooling.

For a known sample A (long single strands) DNA are immobilized on an agar plate. DNA from species whose relationship as to be ascertained is radio labeled and broken into short length by pressure. The short lengths of double helix are dissociated and reacted with immobilized single strands of species A. After a specific time, the unreacted short lengths of species B DNA are separated by suitable means.

The amount of labeled B DNA which as hybridized with spices A DNA is measured by difference in the radioactivity which will give the idea of extent of hybridization. If the DNA of the test and standard are similar, then no difference in radioactivity is seen if they are not similar then lot of difference in radioactivity is seen.

Advantage: Advanced easy method, classification can be done by comparing the DNA of a species.

Disadvantage: Complete DNA has to be studied.

Evaluation of Crude Drugs

Evaluation of crude drug means determination of identity and estimation of quality and purity.

Evaluate: First identify then determine quality and purity

Identity: Identification means collection of somple, Identified and matching from refrence

Comparison: Sample (authentic) or published description

Quality: Determination of the intrinsic value, i.e. amount of medicinal constituents present

Classification of Methods

i. Organoleptic evaluation
ii. Microscopic evaluation
iii. Physical evaluation
iv. Chemical evaluation
v. Biological evaluation

i. Organoleptic Evaluation

Organoleptic evaluation involves tests carried with the help of sensory organs.

Morphological characters: It includes an examination of visual appearance. It is possible when the drug is available in its entire form (entire plant or entire part of the plant, e.g. leaves, roots, barks, etc.)

Sensory characters: It includes an examination by means of sensory characters (colour, smell, taste and texture). These characters are felt by sensory organs.

For convenience of description, the macroscopic characters may include the following headings:

Macroscopic appearance (colour): Some drugs are green in colour when dried in shade but becomes pale and bleached when dried in sunlight.

Odour and taste: Some drugs have characteristic smell which helps in their easy identification (clove, cardamom and cinnamon have characteristic smell due to the presence of volatile oil). Some drugs can also be evaluated by taste (glycyrrhiza is sweet in taste, gentian and chirata are bitter while ginger and capsicum have a pungent taste).

Sound or Snap of Fracture

Feel of the drug to touch (texture): Drugs can be examined by their consistency, texture and nature of fracture, e.g. fracture of glycyrrhiza is fibrous, fracture of nux vomica is horny and fracture of nutmeg is oily.

Occurrence in the market: Various commercial forms are available as:

Entire: as seeds, flowers, fruits, leaves, roots and rhizomes

Cut, Broken, Sliced: Wood, barks, roots and few rhizomes

Matted: Chondrus

Powdered and moulded into forms: Rhubarb fingers

Periderm removed: roots (althea), rhizomes (ginger)

Underground plant parts: Rhizomes, roots, bulbs, corms, tubers?

Shape and Size

Shape	Example
Cylindrical	Sarsaparilla
Subcylindrical	Podophyllum
Conical	Aconite
Fusiform (*Ovoidor pyriform*)	Jalap
Terete	Stillingia
Disk shape	Nux vomica

Size: length and diameter in mm or cm of conical–wide and narrow parts.

External colour: White, yellow gray, yellow brown, reddish orange, to brownish black. Often grey due to clay dust.

External Markings

1. Furrows, ridges and valleys
2. Wrinkles, fine or delicate furrow

3. Annulations: transverse ring like markings
4. Fissures
5. Nodules
6. Projections: roots, stem base, buds
7. Scars: leaf, root, and bud, stem base scars

Fracture: The way by which plant part breaks when subjected to sufficient pressure.
1. Complete
2. Incomplete
3. Short
4. Fibrous
5. Splintery
6. Brittle
7. Tough
8. Weak

Fractured surface
1. Even
2. Uneven
3. Granular
4. Hard
5. Horny
6. Mealy
7. Resinous
8. Conchoidal
9. Waxy

Internal colour: Colour of the fractured surface.

Morphology of Plant Parts

Morphology of root

A typical growing root has four distinct regions. They are:
1. Root cap
2. Region of cell division
3. Region of elongation
4. Region of maturation

1. Root cap

The tip of the root is protected by a thimble like cap called root cap. It is composed of many layers of cells. It protects root meristem from friction of soil particle. As the result of continuous friction with the soil, the outer layers of the root cap get worn out and simultaneously new layers are formed within.

2. Region of cell division

This is the growing tip of the root which extends to a length of a few millimeters. The cells of this region are small, thin walled with dense protoplasm and undergo repeated division.

3. Region of elongation

Just above the meristematic region there is a region of elongation. The cells of this region undergo rapid elongation and enlargement. Hence the length of the root increases.

4. Region of maturation

The cells of this region undergo maturation and differentiation into various kinds of tissue. Lateral roots are produced here and the root also grows in thickness. There are two types of roots, i.e is tap and adventitious roots.

Table 1.1: Difference between tap root and adventitious roots

Sl.No.	Tap root	Adventitious root
1.	They are developed from the radicle of the embryo	They are developed from any part of the plant
2.	It is always underground	It can be underground or above the ground
3.	The main root is thick when compared to others	All the roots are fibrous
4.	Roots are differentiated in to primary, secondary and rootlets	No distinction of roots

Morphology of stem

Stem is the ascending organ of the plant. It is developed by the direct prolongation of plumule. It bears leaves, branches, flowers, and green in colour. Multicellular hairs are present in the stems. Stems have nodes and internodes, when the stem or branch end in vegetative bud, it will grow further, when end in floral bud, the growth ceases. Stems are of two types:

a. Aerial stem

b. Underground stem

Aerial Stem: Aerial stem are erect, rigid, strong upright or sometime weak.

1. Erect or strong stem

These stems are erect and cylindrical and consist of fallen leaves called caudex, e.g. palm

Jointed stem with solid nodes and hollow internodes are called culm, e.g. bamboo.

During flowering, underground stem produces erect unbranched aerial shoot with single or cluster of flowers, e.g. onion.

2. Weak stem

Weak stemmed plants cannot stand upright:

i. Stems which lies flat on the ground are called prostate, e.g. wood sorrel.

ii. Stems which after traveling for some distance lifts their head is called decumbent, e.g. tridax.

iii. Stems which are much branched and whose branches spread on all sides called diffuse, e.g. boerhavia

iv. Weak stems which creep on ground and have roots at nodes are called creepers, e.g. sweet potato.

v. Stems which bodily twines around a support without any special organ of attachment is called twinge, e.g. clitoria.

vi. Stems which attaches a to real support by some special pattern called climbing. climbers, rootless, hook, tendrils, twinees.

Underground stem: In many herbaceous plants, underground part of the stem stores food materials under favourable seasons. Underground stem is also called subterranean stem. The underground stem reproduced by as means of vegetative propagation. They have nodes and internodes; the underground stem is covered with the scaly leaves. The adventitious roots are arised from the underground stem. The buds develop from the axiles of the scaly leaves.

- Rhizome
- Corm
- Stem tuber
- Bulb

Rhizome: It is the prostate and dorsiventral underground stem. It groups horizontally beneath the soil surface. It is regularly branched and nodes bear the scaly leaves and the buds, e.g. banana.

Corm: It is a solid, condensed underground stem with definite shape and a prominent apical bud. The stem is swollen due to the storage of food materials, e.g. colocasia, amorphophallus.

Stem tuber: It is the swollen end of a special underground branches arising from the aril of a lower leaf, e.g. potato.

Bulb: It is a short and highly condensed underground stem. The stem is very much reduced to form a disc which serves to bear roots and scale leaves, e.g. onion.

Morphology of bark

Rhytidoma: Layers of dead phloem alternating with bands of cork frequently form somewhat massive external covering to a bark and composite dead tissue is termed rhytidoma. The presence of rhytidoma gives a scaly appearance, though this is often absent in bulks as quillaia because the outlet dead tissue are removed during the preparation of the bark. Commercial barks are then removed from the smaller branches and it becomes curved during drying owing to the unequal shrinkage of its constituent parts.

When only slightly concave on inside, the pieces are termed curved and if the concavity is on the outside, as occurs in rare instances, it is termed recurved. When the curvature on the inside is so great as to form a deep trough, the piece is said to be channeled. When still more curvature is present and one edge overlaps the other, a quill is formed, and if each edge is rolled independently into a quill the piece is a double quill. When quills are packed one inside the other, as is done with cinnamon and sometimes with cinchona, compound quills result.

Lenticles: When the cork is evenly developed, smooth surface results and this is frequently marked by lenticels which all commonly elongated and placed transversely to the long axis of the back, as cascara and wild cherry bark.

Cracks and Fissures: These are characteristic type arises in the outer surface owing to the lack of elasticity in the dead tissue and the continued increase in girth of the tree.

Wrinkles and Furrows: The shrinkage of bark during drying occurs chiefly transversely, because the longitudinally directed fibers tend to prevent the extensive shrinking in length and the greater shrinkage of the softer tissue results in the formation of wrinkles. If the trough between the wrinkles is very wide it is called furrows.

Fracture: The behaviour of barks when broken across transversely then the appearance of the exposed surface are known as the fracture, when all the fractured surface are smooth, the fracture is short, if the surface exhibit small rounded prominces it is granular, if jagged projecting points are formed the fracture is splintery, if fine fibrous threads extended from the broken surface it is fibrous and to the fractured region breaks into tangentially arranged layers, it is called laminated.

Morphology of wood

Annual Rings: These annual rings are found in plants which are present in temperate regions. They are not present in tropical plants.

Medullary rays: These are parenchymatic cells which extend throughout the vascular bundle. Medullary rays are right angled to the annual ring. In guaiacum medullary rays are uniseriate is one cell wide and in quassia these are multiserlate two or more cell wide.

Pores: In the substance of the wood between medullary rays small pores are present. A wood is said to be diffused porous, when the pores are occurs in small groups and are scattered uniformly throughout the wood, e.g. quiaum, quassia, log wood. If the wood is said to be ring porous this occurs chiefly in the spring wood and thus form well marked concentric rings, e.g: ashoka wood, oak wood.

Morphology of leaves

Leaf base (hypopodium): The basal part of the leaf that connects it with the stem is called leaf base. The small lateral outgrowths are developed on either side, called the stipules. A leaf with stipule is called stipulate. When the stipules are absent the leaf is said to be exstipulate. Stipules vary in form and size. In leguminous plant, the leaf base is swollen and called as pulvinus. Such leaves are called pulvinate. The pulvinus is responsible for sleep movements. The angle formed by a leaf with its stem is called the axil.

Petiole: The stalk of the leaf is called the petiole. A leaf having petiole is called petiolate. The leaf without petiole is called sessile. The main stalk of the compound leaf is known as the rachis. On the rachis, the leaflets are arranged. In some plants, the petiole is modified to perform various functions.

Lamina (epipodium): The green, expanded part of the leaf is called the lamina. The lamina varies in shape, size and form. The petiole enters the lamina as midrib. The midrib produces branches on its either side. They are called the veins. The tip of the leaf is called leaf apex. The edge of the lamina is known as the leaf margin. The lamina is the most important part of the leaf since it is the site for photosynthesis. There are simple as well as compound leaves depending upon the number of lamina. Simple leaves have a simple lamina and compound leaves have two or more lamina. In a compound leaf each lamina as known as the leaflet or pinna.

Leaves: Acicular, cordate, deltoid, elliptic, falcate, hastate, lanceolate, linear lyrate, obcordate, oblong, obovate, oval, reniform, spatulate, sagittate, runcinate spike, raceme, corymb.

Veins: Reniform, parallel, netlike

Shapes: Spear, round, neddle

Arrangement: Simple, compound

Edges: Smooth, toothed, lobed

Arrangement on the stem: Alternate, Opposite, Whorled.

Morphology of flower

Pedicel: A flower has a stalk. The stalk of the flower is known as the pedicel. The flower having pedicel is said to be pedicillate and without pedicel is called sessile.

Bracteole: The outgrowth of the pedicel is called bracteole. A flower having bracteole is called bracteolate, and without bactcole, is called ebracteolate. In some plants, bracteoles are modified below the calyx and are called epicalyx.

Thalamus: The swollen tip of the pedicel is called thalamus or receptacle. The floral parts are arranged on the thalamus. Thalamus has the nodes and internodes. A typical flower has 4 whorls of floral pacts: calyx, corolla, androecium and gynoecium.

Calyx: Calyx is the outermost whorl of a flower. It is composed of sepals. Sepals are green in colour. The role of the calyx is to protect the inner floral whorls during the bud formation.

Corolla: It is the second whorl of a flower inner to the calyx. It is composed of petals. The petals are brightly coloured and help in attracting the insects for pollination.

Androecium: It is the third inner whorl of a flower. It is composed of stamens. The stamen is the male reproductive part of a flower slender. Stalk of the stamen is called the filament which bears a two-lobed head called anther. The two lobes of the anther are connected by the sterile tissue called connective.

Gynoecium: It is the innermost whorl of a flower. It is the female reproductive organ of the flower. It is also called pistil. A gynoecium is composed of carpels. Each carpel has 3 parts. The basal swollen part of the carpel is called the ovary, the long or short middle portion is called style and the apical portion is the stigma.

Morphology of fruit

After fertilization, the ovary begins to grow and gradually matures into fruit. The fruit may, therefore, be regarded as a mature or ripened ovary. A fruit mainly consist of two portions, pericarp and seed.

Pericarp: It is developed from the wall of the ovary. The pericarp may be thick or thin, when thick, it may consist of two or three parts. The outer called epicarp, forms the skin of the fruit, the middle called mesocarp, is pulpy. The inner part is called endocarp is often very thin and membranous or it may be hard and stony. In many cases, however, the pericarp is not differentiated into these three regions.

Seed: Seed developed from the ovule of flower after fertilization. There are different type of fruits: simple fruits, aggregate fruits and multiple fruits. Simple fruits do not have any accessory parts.

Aggregate fruit: It is a collection of simple fruits and seen as clustered.

Multiple fruit: The flowers are crowded together and often fused with one another.

Morphology of seed

After fertilization, a series of changes takes place in the ovule as a result of which seed is formed. The seed mainly consist of seed coats, endosperms and cotyledons. In endosperm and cotyledons, after the food has been supplied to the growing axis, they gradually dry up and fall off. Therefore, they represents the present generation. Axis which establishes itself into a seedling during germination represents the future generation.

Embryo is the most important part of the seed. The embryo has a short axis and one or two cotyledons. The axis of the embryo is called tigellum. The basal part of the tigellum is called the radicle and the upper part of tigellum is called the plumule. The part of the axis just above the point of attachment of the cotyledons is known as the epicotyls and the part of the axis just below the point of attachment of the cotyledons is called hypocotyls. Actually epicotyl is present in between the plumule and cotyledon and hypocotyl in between the radical and cotyledons.

Seeds are divided into two types on the basis of the number of cotyledons. They are dicot seeds and monocot seeds. The dicot seeds are further divided into edospermous and nonendospermous.

Odour and taste

Distinct odour depends on volatile constituents. General terms to describe odour are aromatic, balsamic, spicy, alliaceous, camphoraceous, terebinthinate.

Taste

Substances may be classified according to taste into four following groups:

1. *Those possessing a true taste:*
   a. Acid
   b. Saline
   c. Saccharine
   d. Alkaline
   e. Bitter
2. *Those possessing no taste:* Tasteless and insipid
3. *Those possessing a characteristic odour which gives a name so called taste.* With which true taste may be associated:
   a. Aromatic
   b. Balsamic
   c. Spicy or disagreeable
   d. Alliaceous
   e. Camphoraceous
   f. Terebinthinate
4. *Those imparting distinctive sensation to tongue, exclusive of taste or touch. These sensations may or may not be associated with true taste.*
   a. Mucilaginous
   b. Oily
   c. Astringent
   d. Pungent
   e. Acrid
   f. Nauseous

A drug frequently gives more than one taste, the sensations observed in consecutive order.

ii. Microscopic Evaluation

The microscope is used to study of adulterants in powdered plant and animal drugs, and identification of pure powdered drugs. Drugs in a broken state or in a powdered form can be evaluated by microscopic characters. Histology and powder-microscopic appearance of drug in sectional view and powdered form can be classified as:

Histology: Character and arrangement of tissues present in the drug.

Histological thin sections (radial) TS or longitudinal sections (LS) mounted in stains, reagents or mounting media.

Microscopic linear measurements and quantitative microscopy: leaf constants

Palisade ratio: Defined as the average no of palisade cells beneath each epidermal cell.

Vein islet number: Number of vein islets per sq mm of the leaf surface midway between midrib and margin.

Vein termination: No. of veinlet terminations per sq mm of the leaf surface midway between midrib and margin.

Stomatal no: Average no. of stomata per sq mm of leaf surface of the epidermis.

Stomatal index: The percentage proportion of the ultimate divisions of the leaf which has been converted into stomata.

$$SI = \frac{S \times 100}{E + S}$$

Example: Senna varieties are distinguished by differing stomatal no and palisade ratio.

Diameter of starch grains in *Cinnamon cassia* is 10 mm hence useful for detecting adulterants.

No of sclerenchymatous cells per sq cm of cardamom helps to detect different varieties.

Other important features which can be detected by linear measurements include starch grains, length of fibres, pollen grain diameter, vessel diameter and length, etc.

Quantitative microscopy by lycopodium spore method

Important analytical technique for powder drugs when chemical and other methods of evaluation of crude drugs fail as accurate measure of quality.

Lycopodium spores: Exceptionally uniform in shape and size, i.e. 25 mm.

On average, 94,000 spores are present in each mg of powdered lycopodium. This technique is used if:

a. It contains well defined particles which can be counted, e.g. starch grains or pollen grains.
b. Single layered cells or tissues, area of which may be traced under suitable magnification and actual area calculated.
c. Objects of uniform thickness, length of which can be measured under suitable magnification and actual area calculated.

The % age purity of an authentic powdered ginger is calculated using the equation:

$$\% \text{ purity} = \frac{N \times W \times 94000 \times 100}{S \times M \times P}$$

N = no. of characteristic structures (e.g. starch grains) in 25 fields.

W = weight in mg of lycopodium taken.

S = no. of Lycopodium spores in the same 25 fields.

M = weight in mg of the sample, calc. on basis of sample dried at 105°C.

P = 2,86,000 in case of ginger starch powders

Lycopodium spore method can be used for evaluation of powdered clove, ginger, cardamom, nutmeg, umbelliferous fruits, etc. In case of a drug which contains definite cellular structur.

Microchemistry: Encompasses the study of constituents by application of chemical and physical methods to small quantities of drug in powder form or to histological sections of the drug.

Powdered drugs not less than 40 no. powder cells are mostly broken except those with lignified walls. Cell contents (starch, calcium oxalate crystals, aleurone, etc. to get scattered in the powder and become evident in the specimen. Phloroglucinol/HCl react with lignin – bast fibers, vessels, stone cells.

Mucilage–stained pink with ruthenium red Squill, Agar.

Chloral hydrate calcium oxalate, leaf epidermis, tissue, trichomes.

Cellulose swells and dissolves in cuoxam, N/50 iodine solution stains starch and hemicellulose blue (reagent colour).

iii. Physical Evaluation

Physical constants are rarely constant, the crude drugs but extensive to active principles of drugs such as alkaloids, volatile oils, fixed oils, etc. For crude drugs, some important physical evaluation methods include moisture content, specific gravity, optical rotation, refractive index, melting point, viscosity, solubility, ash values and extractives.

A. Moisture content

Percentage of active constituents is determined on air dried basis. Thus, moisture content should be determined and also controlled to prevent contamination and microbial decomposition. Excess moisture results in breakdown of important constituents by enzymatic activity and may also encourage the growth of yeasts and fungi during storage. Moisture content limits are stated in pharmacopoeial monographs, where no limit expressed (drug should be air-dried).

Determination of moisture content

a. *The loss on drying or gravimetric heating to constant weight:* 105° C in oven is only useful for compounds with no volatile constituents.
b. The *toluene distillation* method for those drugs containing volatile components (volumetric).

Azeotropic volumetric method

Principle: Toluene, benzene, xylene form a binary azeotropic mixture with water. If a moisture containing drug is heated with one of these solvents, water and solvent distil over as a mixture, composition of which depends on ratios of their molecular weight and vapour pressures.

The Deane Stark apparatus is used for azeotropic distillation. It allows the collected distillate to separate with water and solvent in a graduated receiver and water is (higher specific gravity) collected at bottom. When solvent level reaches side arm, it flows back to receiver.

A process of continuous distillation with same solvent volume, volume of water can be read directly from the graduated tube.

Titrimetric (Karl Fischer) method

Based on the stoichiometric reaction of a solution of sulfur dioxide and iodine in pyridine and methanol (Karl Fischer reagent) with water. The end point of the reaction is best determined by electrometrically estimations.

Crude drugs with moisture content limits.

Drug	Moisture Content (%w/w)
1. Aloes	Not more than 10%
2. Digitalis	Not more than 05%
3. Ergot	Not more than 08%
4. Acacia	Not more than 15%
5. Starch	Not more than 15%

B. Viscosity (Constant at a Given Temperature)

Used for standardizing liquid drugs index of composition, e.g. liquid paraffin-not less than 64 centistokes at 37.8°C. Pyroxylin-kinematics viscosity of about 1100–2450 centistokes.

C. Melting Point

Melting point judges purity of chemicals or phytochemicals.

Melting point range for few crude drugs

Colophony	75–85°C
Kokum butter	39–42°C
Cocoa butter	30–33°C
Bees wax	62–65°C
Wool fat	34–44°C

For pure compounds MP is important, e.g. cocaine at 96–98°C

D. Solubility

Presence of adulterant can be determined, e.g. castor oil is soluble only in 3 volumes of alcohol. Adulterated form may show good solubility, e.g. balsam of Peru is soluble in solution of chloral hydrate, colophony is freely soluble in light petroleum ether, asafoetida is soluble in carbon disulfide, Alkaloid bases in chloroform, alkaloidal salts in polar solvents, glycine-polar (alcohol and water), aglycone-non-polar (benzene and ether).

E. Optical Rotation

Rotate plane polarized light: dextrorotatory (right) or levorotatory (left), optical rotation determined at 25°C using sodium lamp as a source of light.

Optical rotation of few crude drugs

Caraway oil	70 to 80
Castor oil	3.5 to 6.0
Honey	3 to 15
Eucalyptus oil	0 to 10

F. Refractive Index (RI)

Depending upon purity, refractive is index for liquids is important particularly for fixed oils, and volatile oils. *Example*: The RI of peppermint oil is not less than 1.4590 and not more than 1.4650 at 20°C.

G. Specific Gravity

Particularly important for fats and volatile oils with crude drugs, which are occasionaly important, e.g. nut balls that do not sink in water.

Inferior jalap: specific gravity should be more than water, clove-lighter than water.

H. Ash Values

Helpful to determine quality and purity of crude drug especially in powder form, useful to detect low grade products exhausted drugs and excess of sandy or earthy matter.

Objective of ashing is to remove all traces of organic matter which may otherwise interfere in analytical determination. Residual matter or ash remaining after incineration consists of inorganic salts of carbonates phosphates and silicates of Na, K, Ca and Mg. These may naturally occur in drug or may be deliberately added as a form of adulteration.

Total ash, acid insoluble Ash, water soluble ash and sulfated ash are with different ash values.

Total Ash is useful to exclude drugs which have been coated with chalk, lime or calcium sulfate to improve the appearance, e.g. ginger or nutmeg.

Many drugs contain calcium oxide in varying amounts. Total ash is not useful when there is such a wide variation and will itself show wide variation, e.g. rhubarb-total ash content is 3–40%.

Acid insoluble ash, i.e. the ash insoluble dil. HCl is often more important than the total ash, because on incineration, the calcium oxide or calcium carbonate yielded by the oxalate is soluble in HCl. Thus acid insoluble ash is especially useful to provide evidence of excessive earthy matter like earth and sand-roots, rhizomes and densely pubescent leaves, e.g. foxglove are abundantly covered with trichomes secreting resin, e.g. henbane which retains earthy matter splashed on during heavy rainstroms.

Rhubarb

Total ash: 3–4%

Acid insoluble Ash: not more than one.

Water Soluble Ash is that part of the total ash which is soluble in water, and is used to detect the presence of materials exhausted by water.

Ginger	Total ash: 2.5–6%
	Water soluble Ash: 1.9–3%
Spent ginger (exhausted by water)	Total ash: 2–4%
	Water soluble Ash: 0.2–0.5%

Water soluble ash is subject to a much greater detail than total ash and thus is an indication of presence of exhausted material substituted.

Water soluble ash of ginger should not be less than 1.7%.

Tea	Total ash: 5–7%
	Water soluble ash: 3.2–4.2 %
Exhausted tea	Total ash: 4.4%
	Water soluble ash: 0.7 %

Water soluble ash of tea should not fall below 3.0%, for example tea-further check by detention. Alkalinity of water soluble ash expressed as potassium oxide (K_2O) should not be less than 1.3%

I. Extractives

Extracts obtained by exhausting crude drugs are indicative of measures of their chemical constants. Diversity in chemical nature of different solvent extractives are used.

a. Water soluble extractives (WSE)

Applied to drugs containing water soluble active constituents such as; tannins, sugars, plant acids, mucilage, glycosides, etc.

Drug	Water soluble Extractives (% w/w)
Aloe	> 25
Licorice	> 20
Ginger	> 10

b. Alcohol soluble extractive (ASE)

Solvent for extraction of chemicals like tannins resins, etc. generally 95% ethanol is used.

Determination of resin content-assay method for myrrh and asafoetida is used for determination or resin content.

Sometimes more dilute alcohol is used depending on the solubility of drug constituents.

c. Ether soluble extractives (ESE)

Soluble extractive values are volatile and nonvolatile. Volatile ether soluble extracts represent the volatile oil content of the drug, while the nonvolatile ether soluble extractives represent resin, fixed oil or colouring matter present in the drug.

e.g. Capsicum not more than 12.0% w/w

Male fern not more than 1.5% w/w

Linseed not more than 25.0% w/w

Some crude drugs are standardized on the basis of volatile oil content (% w/w)

Drug	Volatile oil content (% w/w)
Caraway	Not less than 2.5
Clove	Not less than 15.0
Fennel	Not less than 1.4

d. Chromatography

Different techniques like: Paper chromatography, thin layer chromatography, high performance thin layer chromatography, gas liquid chromatography, column chromatography, etc. are based on differential affinity between two immiscible phases–stationary and mobile phases.

TLC is useful in analysis of alkaloids, glycosides, sugars, etc. HPTLC is used for too many constituents, e.g. Berberine, quinine, opium alkaloid, etc. GLC is used for determination of volatile oil, alkaloid of opium.

e. Spectrophotometry

Ultraviolet, Infrared, fluorescence analysis is commonly used for the determination of active constituents in a drug by chemical method, e.g. cinchona under UV/fluorescent light shows numerous cell and a few light blue patches.

Rheum emodii: Brown

Rheum rhaponticum: Yellow

Emetine: Orange

Aconite: Light blue

f. Nuclear Magnetic Resonance (NMR), mass spectrometer and X-ray diffraction (Table 1.2)

Staining of chromosomes

Keep 5–6 bulbs of *Allium cepa* (garlic) in wet cotton for 2–3 days for the root formation. Dip these roots in HCl acid for 20 hours. Wash the roots thoroughly under running water. Stain these sections of roots with acetocarmine and view under the microscope.

iv. Chemical Evaluation

1. Chemical tests (qualitative and quantitative)
2. Chemical assays (titrimetric, gravimetric and spectrophotometric)

The principle techniques may be outlined as follows:

i. Isolation of constituents

A. By chemical solvents
   1. Microextraction
   2. Microfilteration
   3. Microcrystallization
B. By microsublimation

ii. Identification of constituents

A. By crystallography
B. By melting point determination

Phytochemical Tests

Table 1.2: Identification tests for cell wall components

Sl. No.	Experiment	Observation	Inference
1.	Treat the section or powder with chlor-Zn iodine reagent	a. Blue colour b. Yellow colour c. Yellow to brown colour	Cellular Pectic substances and lignin. Suberin of cutin
2.	Treat the section or powder in N/50 iodine solution	Blue colour	Hemicellulose
3.	Mount section or powder in N/50 iodine solution, remove excess of the reagent by blotting paper and then treat with a drop of 80% w/w H_2SO_4 acid	Blue colour	Cellulose
4.	Treat the powder with ammoniacal solution on copper oxide (cuoxam solution)	Walls dissolve	Cellulose
5.	Treat the section of powder with a few drops of phuroglucinol solution. After 2 min add a drop of concentrated HCl acid	Bright red colour	Lignin
6.	Mount section of powder in acid aniline sulphate solution.	Bright yellow	Lignin
7.	Mount material in 80% H_2SO_4 and warm slightly	1. Lignified walls dissolves 2. Suberin or cutin does not dissolve	Suberin or cutin
8.	Treat the powder or section with Sudan III, mount in glycerin and warm slightly	Red stain	Suberin or cutin
9.	Heat gently the material with potassium chlorate and HNO_3 on the slide	The outsided of cutinized walls change into droplets solution in organic solvents or in dilute potash	Suberin or cutin
10.	Mount materials in ruthenium red reagent and treat with a few drops of 10% lead acetate solution	Pink stain	Mucilaginous wall
11.	Mount material in corallin soda reagent and treat with a few drops of Na_2CO_3 solution	Pink stain	Mucilaginous wall

C. By confirmative tests
1. Chemical tests
2. Microchemical tests
3. Physical tests.

Chemical tests: These are used for isolation, purification, identification of active constituents in a drug by chemical method. These are two types:

i. *Quantitative chemical tests:* Acid value, Saponification value, Iodine value, Ester value, etc. are used for the identification of fixed oils and fats.

Some tests are useful for resins: Sulphated acid value for balsams, acid value, saponification value, ester value

Volatile oil: Aacetyl and ester values

Gums: Methoxy value and acidity (Volatile)

Preliminary phytochemical screening

ii. *Qualitative chemical tests:* These are used to detect adulteration, e.g. colophony-an adulterant of resins, balsams and waxes-detected by copper acetate test

Baudoins test: Used to detect sesame oil, when used to adulterate olive oil. In 2 ml oil add 1 ml HCl containing 1% sucrose and 2% furfuraldehyde; shake for half minutes. Aqueous layer should not become pink.

Halphen's test (Bevan's test): Used to detect cotton seed oil as an adulterant of olive oil. In 2ml oil add 1 ml amyl alcohol and 1 ml 1% solution of sulfur in carbon disulfide. Warm for 10 mins on water bath; no red colour should develop.

Specific chemical tests: e.g. Van Urk's test for Ergot (indole alkaloid)

Vitali test for tropane alkaloids

Murexide test for purine bases

Thalleoiquin test for quinolines (quinine alkaloid)

Specific chemical tests for drugs which represent active constituents of plants, e.g.

Reducing sugars: Molisch, Barfoed, Benedict, and Fehling

Alkaloids: Dragendorff, Wagner's, Hager's

Purity: by chemical assays

For example, convention titrimetric assays for estimation of alkaloids in crude drugs, ester and aldehyde content of volatile oil.

Gravimetric Methods: Alkaloidal drugs assayed for total alkaloid content and specific alkaloid, e.g.

Opium: Morphine

Belladonna: Atropine

Nux-vomica: Strychnine

Cinchona: Quinine

Rauwolfia: Reserpine

Volatile oils: For example, contents of balsamic acids, i.e. benzoic and cinnamic acid in balsam of Tolu, balsam of Peru and benzoin.

Glycosides: Chemical assay for anthraquinone and cardiac glycosides.

Microchemical tests: These tests are carried on slides, e.g. eugenol in clove oil is precipitated as needle shaped potassium euginate crystals by adding potassium hydroxide.

v. Biological Evaluations (Bioassays)

Biological evaluation is employed when the drug cannot be evaluated by any of the other methods. Biological assays are performed on living animals as well as intact or excised organs. In this method the response produced by the test drug on a living system is compared with that of the standard, e.g. cardiac glycosides like digitalis are evaluated by this method. Strength of drugs or their preparations are shown in terms of international units (IU).

The specific biological activity in each IU is:

Digitalis: 1 IU in 76 mg standard preparation.

Vitamin A: 1 IU in 0.344 mg standard preparation.

Vitamin D: 1 IU in 0.025 mg standard preparation.

Heparin: 1 IU in 7.7 mg standard preparation.

Bioassays

Bioassays are of three types:
a. Toxic
b. Symptomatic
c. Tissue

The following are the systems used for biological evaluation:

1. Intact animals, e.g. curare by head drop method in rabbits.
2. Isolated tissues, e.g. adrenaline in isolated rat uterus.
3. Microorganisms are used for bioassays, e.g. bacteria such as *Salmonella typhii* and *Micrococcus* are used to determine phenol coefficient or antiseptic evaluation of certain drugs (FDA)
4. Microbilogical assays used for antibiotic drugs, *Klebsiella pneumoniae*, *Micrococcus flavers*, penicillin on growth of *Bacillus subtilis*, etc.
5. Assay of digitalis using pigeons.
6. Cats for depressor activity and in assay of glucagon for injection.
7. Cat's or rabbit's eye for mydriatic drugs.
8. Guinea pigs for toxicity and antigenicity of certain biologics like diagnostic diptheria toxin and tetanus toxoid.

Before introduction of any new product in the market, it must prove safe in preliminary pharmacological tests on animals and finally clinical tests on humans.

Indications for biological evaluations:

1. When chemical nature of the drug is not known but it has a specific biological action.
2. When chemical methods are insensitive or not available.
3. When quantity of the drug is small and it cannot be evaluated chemically.
4. Drugs which have different chemical composition but same biological activity.

IMPORTANT DEFINITIONS

1. **Habit:** It is the characteristic form or bodily appearance of an organism.
2. **Habitat:** A habitat is an ecological or environmental area that is inhabited by a particular animal or plant species.
3. **Herb:** A plant with soft stem:annual, biennial or perennial whose aerial portion is relatively short lived, e.g. tulsi
4. **Shrub:** Perennial, woody plant of relatively low stature, typically with several stems arising from or near the ground; shrubs do not have a clear stem, e.g. rose
5. **Tree:** A perennial woody plant with a single trunk, e.g. neem
6. **Climber:** Plant with thin and long stems, with diffuse branches and special organs of attachment by means of it clings to the neighboring objects, e.g. giloy
7. **Epiphytes:** A plant that grows upon other plants, but does not absorb its food material from them as do the parasites.
8. **Parasite:** A plant that grows upon other living plants or animals and absorbs its food material from them.
9. **Root:** It is that portion of the axis of the plant body which grows down into the earth.
    a. Tap root: A stout, tapering main root arising from the radicle of the embryo and which persist throughout the life of plant and from which arises smaller lateral branches.
    b. Adventitious root: A root arising from any part of the plant except radical.
10. **Stem:** The stem is the aerial portion of the plant axis which bears leaf and flower and develops from the plumule portion of the embryo.
11. **Rhizome:** A horizontal underground stem, distinguished from the root by the presence of nodes and internodes and sometimes bud and scale leaves at the nodes, often thickened and containing accumulated food, e.g. ginger, turmeric.
12. **Stolon:** A slender, elongated, horizontal stem at or below the surface of the ground that gives rise to a new plant at its tip, e.g. colocasia.

13. **Leaf:** The leaf can be defined as a lateral outgrowth of the stem or an appendage developing upon a node and having a bud in its axils. Its main function is to carry on the process of photosynthesis.
14. **Phyllotaxy:** Arrangement of leaves on stem.
15. **Duration of leaf:**
    a. **Caducous:** Leaf sheds soon after the bud opens.
    b. **Deciduos:** Leaf lasts for one season only.
    c. **Persistant:** Leaf lasts for several seasons.
16. **Dorsiventral leaf:** The lamina is the stem with the flat surface more or less parallel to the ground and the upper surface of leaf receives more sunlight than the lower surface
17. **Isobillateral leaf:** The lamina is oriented upon the stem more or less vertically so that both the surfaces are equally illuminated.
18. **Simple leaf:** A leaf which may be entire or incised to any depth, but not down to the midrib or petiole, e.g. mango
19. **Compound leaf:** A leaf in which the leaf blade is incised upto the midrib or petiole, thus dividing it into two or more segments called leaflets.
20. **Venation:** The arrangement of vascular bundles or veins in a leaf.
21. **Reticulate venation:** The pattern of venation in which the veinlets are irregularly distributed, forming a network.
22. **Parallel venation:** The pattern of venation in which the veins run parallel to each other. In this type there are no veinlets and no network is formed.
23. **Inflorescence:** Arrangement of flowers on floral axis.
24. **Flower:** A metamorphosed shoot meant essentially for the reproduction of plant.
25. **Fruit:** Fruit is regarded as a mature or ripened ovary.
26. **Evaluation:** Evaluation of drug means confirmation of its identity and determination of its quality and purity.
27. **Adulteration:** It can be defined as admixture or substitution of genuine articles with spurious, inferior, defective or otherwise useless or harmful substances to the authenticity of the genuine drug.
28. **Standardization:** It is determination of quality and purity. It guarantees a consistent and appropriate level of plant medicinal elements within the product.
29. **Ethnopharmacology:** It can be defined as the scientific study of materials used by ethnic and cultural groups as medicines.
30. **Phytochemistry:** It is the study of phytochemicals. These are chemicals derived from plants. In a narrower sense the terms are often used to describe the large number of secondary metabolic compounds found in plants.
31. **Extraction:** The commonly employed technique for separation of active substances from crude drug.
32. **Phytoconstituents:** These are chemical constituents present in plants.
33. **Micrometers:** Two scales are required, a stage micrometer and an eyepiece micrometer. The stage micrometer is a glass slide 7.6 cm × 2.5 cm (3 × 1 inch) with a scale engraved on it. The scale is usually 1 or 1.1 mm. long and is divided into 0.1 and 0.01 parts of a millimeter. The eyepiece micrometer may be a linear scale or it may be ruled in squares.
34. **Stomata:** A stomata is a minute epidermal opening with a central pore and two kidney shaped similar cells containing chloroplasts known as guard cells and varying number of subsidiary cells covering the guard cells.
35. **Phytotherapy:** The use of plants or plant extracts for medicinal purposes (especially plants that are not part of the normal diet).

II. BASIC CONCEPTS OF PHARMACOGNOSY

Pharmacognosy can be defined as the study of drugs of natural origin. The term comes from two Greek words, *Pharmakon* meaning drugs or medicines *Genesis* meaning knowledge. The American Society of Pharmacognosy defines pharmacognosy as the study of the physical, chemical, biochemical and biological properties of drugs, drug substances or potential drugs or drug substances of natural origin as well as the search for new drugs from natural sources. The study of drugs from plants includes the subjects of botany, chemistry and pharmacology.

a. Botany includes the identification (taxonomy, macroscopy and microscopy), genetics and cultivation of plants.
b. Chemical characterization includes the isolation, identification and quantification of constituents in plant materials.
c. Pharmacology is the study of the biological effects of the chemical consitituents in the medicinal plants on cell cultures, animals and humans.

Pharmacognosy is interdisciplinary, drawing attention on a broad spectrum of biological and socioscientific subjects, including botany, ethnobotany, medical anthropology, marine biology, microbiology, herbal medicine, chemistry, biotechnology, phytochemistry, pharmacology and pharmaceutics. The information concerning any given drug falls naturally into sections, each relating to a separate department of knowledge and, in general, these sections are most conveniently taken in a definite sequence such as:

a. Biological sources
b. Geographical source
c. History
d. Cultivation, collection and processing
e. Macroscopical (morphological) and Microscopical characters
f. Chemical constituents
g. Chemical tests
h. Uses
i. Evaluation involving quantitative measurement
j. Adulterants
k. Substitutes/allied species

A typical protocol to isolate a pure chemical agent from natural origin in bioassay guided fractionation, meaning step by step separation of extracted components based on differences in their physicochemical properties, and assessing the biological activity followed by next round of separation and assaying.

i. Fractionating the crude extract (by solvent partitioning).
ii. Testing fractions thereby generated with *in vitro* assay.
iii. Isolation of pure active compounds (by chromatography).
iv. Structure determination of isolated compounds by using spectroscopic methods (NMR, mass spectroscopy).

The phytochemical investigation of a plant may thus involve the following:

i. Authentication and extraction of the plant material.
ii. Separation and isolation of the constituents of interest.
iii. Characterization of the isolated compounds.
iv. Investigation of the biosynthetic pathways to particular compounds and quantitative evaluations.

Parallel to this may be the pharmacological assessment of the separated components.

Crude Drugs

Crude drug: It is the unprocessed form of the drug obtained from the natural sources (plants, animals and minerals). Crude drugs can be classified into:

1. Unorganised drugs
2. Organised drugs

1. **Unorganised drugs** – As the name suggest, these do not have any specific structure.

   These are not composed of cells which built up into definite plants or animals members or organs.

   These are derived from parts of plants or animals by some process of extraction such as:

   Incision: e.g. opium

   Decoction: e.g. agar

   Expression: e.g. olive oil

   Natural secretions: e.g. myrrh, bees wax.

   These drugs are solid, semisolid or liquid in nature, e.g. oil, gums and balsams. Physical characters, solubility in common solvent and chemical tests are confirmatory tests for these drugs. These drugs can be classified based upon their origin and nature, such as:

   Latex: opium

   Extracts: catechu

   Resins: colophony

   Oleoresins: copaiba

   Oils and fats: castor oil, lard oil

   Volatile oil: clove oil

   Dried juice: aloe

   Gums: acacia

   Gum–resins: myrrh

   Waxes: beeswax

2. **Organised drugs** – These are organs of plants or animals made up of cells or definite structure. These are solid in nature. Macroscopy and microscopy are important criterias for the identification of these drugs. These can be classified depending upon the part used, e.g.

   Bark: Cinchona

   Leaves: Digitalis, senna

   Flowers: Clove, saffron, arnica

   Seeds: Ispaghula, nux vomica

   Fruits: Caraway, cardamom

   Roots: Ipecacuanha

   Rhizomes: Rhubarb

   Entire Drugs: Ephedra, ergot

III. BASIC TECHNIQUES OF PHARMACOGNOSY

To identify and authenticate the sample, sensory, macroscopic and microscopic characters are examined.

1. **Macroscopical examination:** It substantiates the results obtained after microscopical and physiochemical analysis. Shape, size, color, surface characteristics, texture, fracture characteristics and appearance of the crude drug is examined.

2. **Microscopical examination:** Microscopical examination reveals the structure of different cells, arrangement of tissues and the chemical nature of the cell contents.

   A. **Preparation of the crude drug sample**
   - For sectioning, dried materials are soften either by boiling with water (for roots and barks) or by exposing to moisture (for leaves and flowers). In case of stem/root/stolon direct sectioning can be done by holding vertically in between the first, second finger and the thumb. Cut transversely, using a sharp razor by moving back and forth from one end to the other to obtain thin sections. The thickness of the section depends upon the skill of the worker. Take sufficient number of sections.
   - In case of leaf, piece of leaf is cut which includes the midrib and small portion of lamina. Insert the leaf in a block of pith, similarly the section of leaf along with the pith.
   - Place the cut section in watch glass containing water.
   - Select the thin section and eject thick and oblique one.

- With the help of brush, place the section over a clean glass slide.
- If required, clear the section by heating with chloral hydrate solution (cleaning agent).
- Stain the section with staining solution. Each produces different reactions on different tissues.
  a. Phloroglucinol and concentrated HCl (1:1), stains lignified tissues pink or red
  b. Dilute iodine solution stains starch grains blue and aleurone grains yellow coloured.
  c. Sudan red III: Changes oil globules red
  d. Alcoholic picric acid : Aleurone grain yellow
  e. Safranin solution stains lignified tissues deep red
  f. Haematoxylin stains cellulose purplish violet
- Mount the stained section in glycerin continuously place the cleared cover slip with the help of forceps and needle to avoid the entrapment of the air bubbles.
- If any air bubbles are seen, slightly left the cover slip and add a drop of glycerin and replace the cover slip till the air bubble is removed.
- Wipe of the excess of glycerin present outside the cover slip. Observe the slide under microscope.

B. **Preparation of powdered sample**

Place 1–2 drops of water on a clean glass slide. Moisten the tip of needle and insert in the powdered sample. The powder adheres to the needle; add a drop of water over glass slide and spread. If required, heat the powder sample with cleaning agent chloral hydrate solution. Staining and mounting procedure is similar as mentioned above.

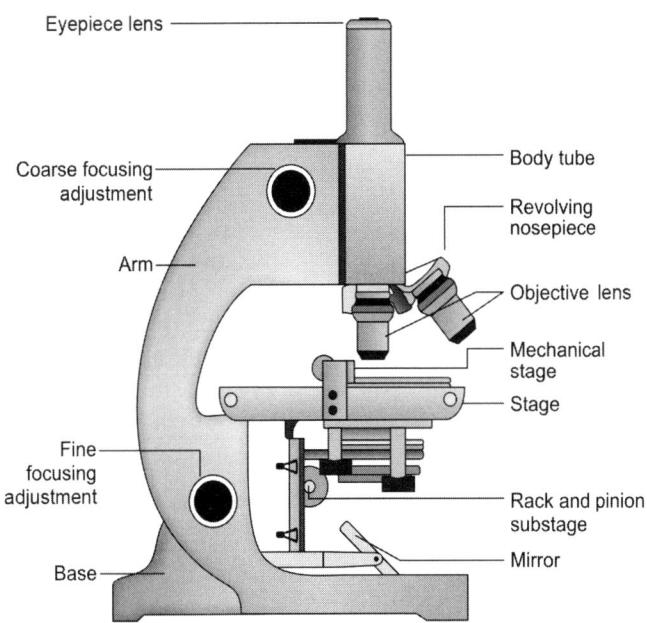

Fig. 1.1: Labelled diagram of a microscope

3. **Quantitative analytical microscopy:** Measurement of the dimension of the cells, cells contents or tissues provide valuable information in identifying the drugs or differentiating certain allied drugs or adulterants and form an integral part of the microscopic or histological evaluation of certain drugs both in entire and powdered forms (Fig. 1.1).

The dimension can be measured by using:
a. Micrometers
b. Camera lucida

a. **Micrometers:** The size of an object or part of it can be measured with the help of two types of micrometers.
 1. Stage micrometer
 2. Eye piece micrometer

 1. **Stage micrometer:** It is a glass slide which has a scale engraved on it.

    Two types of stage micrometers are available:
    i. Stage micrometer having 1 mm scale engraved on it and divided into 100 divisions. 1 division-1/100 = 0.01 mm or 10 µm.
    ii. Stage micrometer having 1 cm (10 mm) scale engraved on it and divided into 100 divisions. 1 division-10/100 = 0.1mm or 100µm.

 2. **Eye piece micrometer:** The eye piece micrometer is a small disc of glass with a linear scale of 10 mm divided into 100 divisions. The magnification of the scale changes with the optical system of the microscope. The scale is arbitrary and hence need standardization or calibration for each microscopic unit.

b. **Camera lucida:** Camera lucida is an instrument, used for tracing magnified image of the object under microscopic observation. The images can be traced on a black paper and its dimension can be determined. Abbe's and Swift Ive's camera lucida are commonly used.

 1. **Abbe's camera lucida:** It is fitted to the microscope and consists of a prism fitted over the eye piece of the microscope and side arm carrying a mirror, which is supported vertically over the tracing paper. Light from the drawing board is reflected by the plane mirror into the prism and further reflected into the observer's eye that can see the drawing paper and the pencil in the direction of the stage of the microscope. The prism has a small central opening through which the observer can also see the image of the object. The result is that both images appear superimposed to the observer who can conveniently trace the microscopic object.

 2. **Swift Ive's camera lucida:** Here the plane mirror of the Abbe's type is replaced by a right angled prism. It is small in size and can be conveniently fitted to the microscope. It is the most commonly used in tracing experiments (Fig. 1.2).

Calibration of Eye Piece Micrometer

Focus the scale of stage micrometer under low and high power. Introduce the eye piece micrometer into the piece of the microscope. Superimpose the scales and bring the 0th division of each to coincide. Note the next coinciding division of each.

Calculate the actual size of each division of eye piece micrometer by dividing the value of stage micrometer by the value eye piece micrometer.

For example:

10 divisions of eye piece micrometer = 4 divisions of stage micrometer

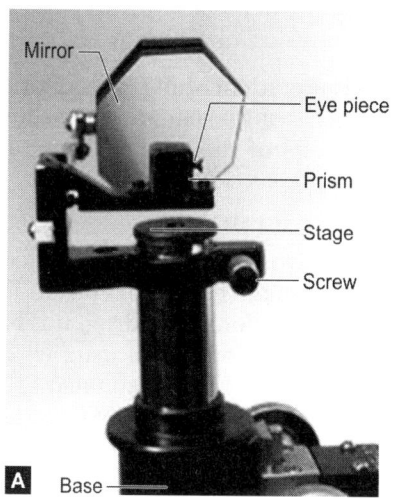

Fig. 1.2A: Abbe's camera lucida

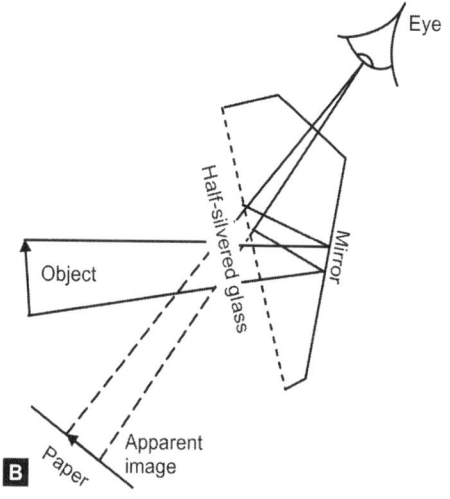

Fig. 1.2B: Refractive diagram of object vision in camera lucida

1 divisions of eye piece micrometer = 4/10 divisions of stage micrometer

1 divisions of eye piece micrometer = 0.4 mm divisions of stage micrometer

1 smallest division of stage micrometer is = 0.01 mm = 10 μ

Hence 1 division of eye piece micrometer = 0.4 mm of stage micrometer

$$= 0.4 \times 10 = 4 \text{ μm}$$

To measure the size of the object (starch grains, calcium oxalate crystals, pollen grains, etc.), count the number of divisions of eye piece micrometer covered by the object. Calculate the size in micrometer by multiplying the number of divisions with the calibrated value of eye piece micrometer.

Magnification power of the microscope

Set up the camera lucida and trace the divisions and for convenience mark 10, 20, 30, 40 divisions of stage micrometer. Calculate the magnification power of the microscope using the formula:

Magnification factor = magnified length/actual length

Replace the stage micrometer with the prepared slide and trace the outline of the object. Calculate the dimension of the object using the formula:

Actual length/breadth

$$= \frac{\text{magnified length/breadth} \times 1000}{\text{magnification factor}}$$

IV. METHODS OF EXTRACTION

Extraction – It is a process of the removal of soluble constituents from the insoluble residue by treating it with a liquid solvent. Water and alcohol are commonly used solvents. The entire process of drug extracts can summarily be divided into four essential steps:

1. Penetration of the solvent into the drug
2. Dissolution of constituents
3. Outward diffusion of the given solution from the cells
4. Separation of dissolved portion and exhausted drug.

Factors affecting choice of an extraction process:
1. Character of the drug
2. Therapeutic value of the drug
3. Stability of the drug
4. Cost of the drug
5. Solvent
6. Concentration of the product

The efficacy of drug extraction depends therefore upon the following:
1. Nature and properties of the drug and its extractable constituents
2. The particle size of powdered drug
3. The nature of solvent
4. The state of contact between the solvent and drug particles.

Various methods of extraction:

1. Maceration (to soak)

It is the most widely used method for extraction. Maceration is the process in which the drug is immersed in the solvent for several hours with frequent intermittent shakings until the cellular structure is softened and penetrated by the menstrum and the soluble constituents are dissolved. The fluid is then filtered off; the marc or solid portion pressed out, the fluid thus obtained being added to the filtrate and the marc rejected. It is employed in production of tincture, extracts, and concentrated infusions. The main disadvantage of this method is that it does not exhaustively extract the drug (Fig. 1.3).

Modified maceration: Modified maceration used for extracting unorganized drugs which have no cellular or tissue structure, e.g. gums, resins, gum-resins, oleo-gum resins.

Multiple maceration: Multiple maceration is aimed at achieving maximum extraction by using portions of the total volume of the menstruum for successive maceration.

2. Percolation (to strain)

In Greek, the word percolate, means "to pass through" or strain. This method results in the exhaustive extraction of the drug. It is based on the continuous contact of drug with the fresh solvent whereby the saturated solvent (with the soluble constituents) is constantly displaced by the fresh one. In this process the drug is packed in a conical vessel (a percolator) with a small outlet at its lower end and moistened with the solvent which is added from time to time, and allowed to run off slowly from the lower outlet until a certain quantity of solvent has passed through. The marc is usually pressed out and the fluid obtained added to the percolate (extractive). The marc or solid portion is not pressed out. Most drug extractions are performed by percolation. Percolation is carried out in equipment known as percolator which is conical in shape with a tap at the base (Fig. 1.4).

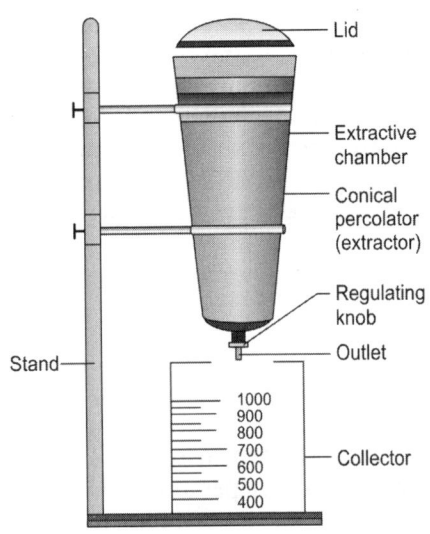

Fig. 1.4: Percolator

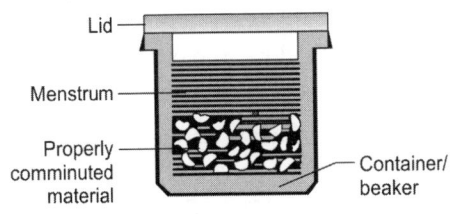

Fig.1.3: Maceration

3. Hot continuous extraction (soxhlation) / continuous hot percolation

This is carried out in Soxhlet apparatus where the drug is placed in the thimble in the central compartment. The solvent is placed in the lower compartment and the vapours of it passes through the side tube, goes up and condenses and finally falls upon the drug where the extraction takes place. In this process the drug is continuously comes in contact with the fresh solvent. As a result the liquid level rises in the siphoning tube attached to the central compartment and when the liquid reaches the top, siphoning occurs and all the contents extracted are transferred to the lower flask or compartment. Extraction by this method is fast and results into exhaustive extraction of drug.

In Soxhlet extraction similar to percolation, the plant material continuously flushed with fresh solvent. But the fresh solvent is formed by boiling the solvent containing extracted analytes. Thus, in contrast to percolation the total amount of solvent is limited. Inspite of what is sometimes; through a soxhlet extraction can be far from complete due to channeling or the presence of air in the semi-permeable thimble containing the plant material. Percolation is more useful for extracting loosely bound compound which occurs in high concentration and have low solubility in solvents. The soxhlet extraction method is useful for certain quantitative extraction of thermally stable compounds (Fig. 1.5).

4. Steam distillation

In this process, volatile substances are separated from nonvolatile or less volatile by the aid of heat. The volatile substances are passed over a cooled surface on which they condense and are collected. It is one of the most commonly used methods for the extraction of volatile oils from plant material. Distillation is the process of separation of one or more liquids which are miscible, partially miscible or immiscible with nonvolatile impurities by

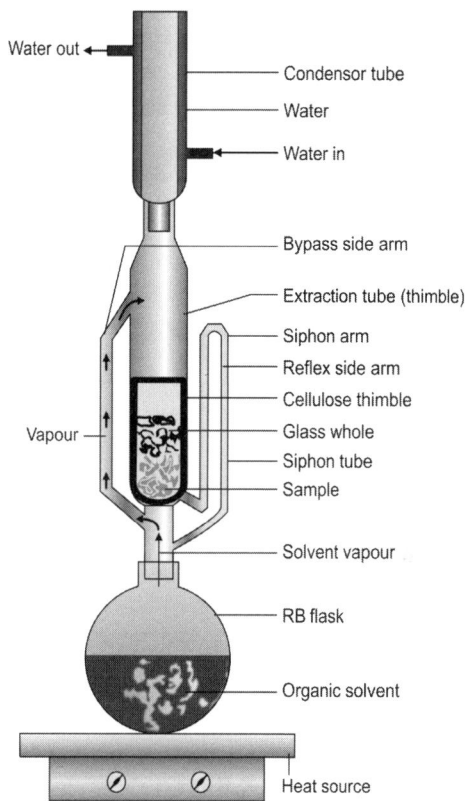

Fig. 1.5: Soxhlet apparatus

partial vaporization of the mixture and separate collection of the vapour (Fig. 1.6).

Steam distillation is carried out in 3 ways:

a. **Direct steam distillation** – In this method steam is directly passed through the plant material.
b. **Hydro steam distillation** – In this plant drug is placed in water and steam is allowed to pass through it. Here water is not boiled.
c. **Water distillation** – Here the plant drug is immersed in water and the water is continuously boiled. Steam is generated by boiling the water.

5. Infusion

In this process, a finally divided drug is treated with either hot or cold water for a certain length of time with or without shaking, after

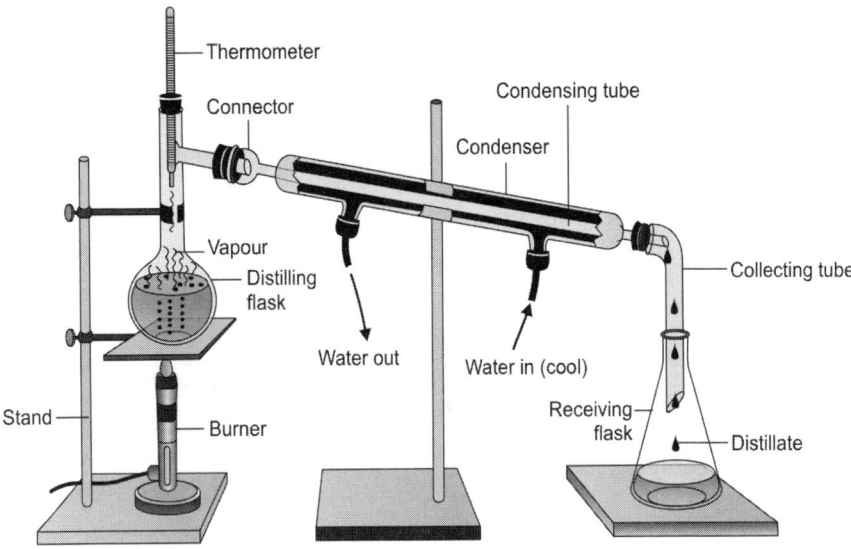

Fig. 1.6: Distillation unit

which the fluid portion is strained off and retained and the solid portion is rejected.

6. Decoction

In decoction process, the active principle is extracted by boiling in water.

7. Expression

In this process, the drug is subjected to pressure and thus its juices are obtained.

8. Filtration

In this process, solids are separated from fluids by allowing the latter to pass out through a porous diaphragm.

9. Vesication

In this process, the watery constituents of drugs are removed by the aid of currents of either hot or cold air.

10. Pulverization

By this process, the drug is reduced to a very finely divided condition (or powder). The degree of fineness is determined by the number of meshes to the linear inch of the finest sieve through which the powder can pass. The sieves used contain 20, 40, 60, 80, 100 meshes to an inch. The simplest method of pulverizing the drug is by means of a mortar and pestle but in large pharmaceutical houses this end is usually obtained by means of a mill.

11. Trituration

This term may be used as synonymous with pulverization, but more commonly refers to an intimate mixing and powdering of two drugs by means of a mortar and pestle or of a spatula.

V. SEPARATION AND IDENTIFICATION

Five chromatographic techniques are commonly used for the separation of phyto-constituents:

1. Thin layer chromatography (TLC)
2. Paper chromatography
3. High performance liquid chromatography (HPLC)
4. Gas liquid chromatography (GLC)
5. High performance thin layer chromatography (HPTLC)

Principle of Chromatography

Chromatography is a technique for separating mixtures that depends upon differential affinities of solutes between two immiscible phases. One of the phases is fixed bed of large surface area while other fluid, which flows through or over fixed phase. The fixed phase is called stationary phase and movable phase is called mobile phase. Those, solutes distributed preferentially in the mobile phase will move more rapidly through the system than those distributed preferentially in the stationary phase. Thus, solutes will elute in order of their increasing distribution coefficient with respect to the stationary phase. The stronger the forces between the solute molecules and those of stationary phase, greater will be the amount of solute held in the stationary phase under equilibrium conditions and vice versa. The choice of technique depends largely on the solubility properties and volatility of the compounds to be separated.

a. Thin layer chromatography

Definition

Chromatography is a separation process that is achieved by the distribution of substances between two phases, a stationary and mobile phase. The chromatographic principle was discovered first by a Russian Botanist, Michael Tswett (1906), who used a glass column containing calcium carbonate for separation of chlorophyll pigments from plants by using petroleum ether. The pigments according to their adsorption patterns resolved into various colored zones, then it separated and estimated.

Distribution coefficient

$$= \frac{\text{Concentration of component A in stationary phase}}{\text{Concentration of component A in mobile phase}}$$

Different affinity of these two components to stationary phase causes the separation.

- This technique is commonly used for qualitative analysis (due to nonhomogeneity in the packing structure density and surface structure of thin layer plates). This is used primarily for the identification of individual substance in a mixture, separating and also testing the purity. The identification of the substances is also done by matching the R_f value of the same with that of the reference substance. Separation by TLC is based on the principle of adsorption where the compound having strong affinity for the adsorbent is strongly adsorbed. In TLC, glass plate or other are used as support and adsorbent is applied over it, commonly silica gel is used. Others are aluminium oxide, polyamide, cellulose, sephadin, ion exchange resin. After application of adsorbent, plates are activated by heating in an oven at 100–110°C for 30 min. The substance to be identified is applied on the plate and further developed in suitable solvent (mobile phase). Detection is done visually or under UV light or by spraying with suitable detecting agents. For the isolation of compounds preparative TLC is used (Fig. 1.7).
- Preparative TLC is carried out on plates having adsorbent layer thickness of 2 mm.

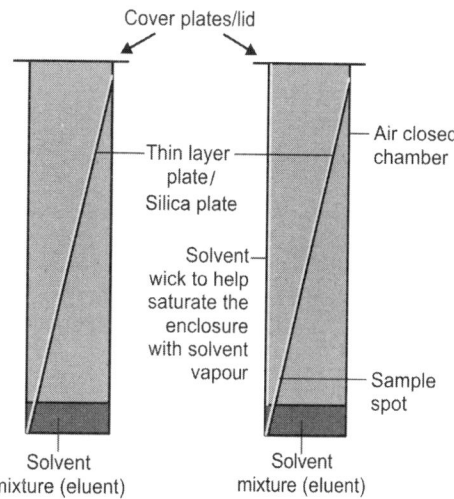

Fig. 1.7: Thin layer chromatography

Table 1.3: TLC of some herbal drugs

Drug	Constituent	Solvent	Detection	Rf value
Tribulus terrestris	Diosgenin	Toluene: Ethyl acetate (8:2)	Spraying with Anisaldehyde in sulfuric acid	Yellow green spot (0.30)
Amino acids	Glycine, Valine, Phenyl alanine, Aspartic acid	Phenol: Water (3:1) Phenol: Water (3:1) Phenol: Water (3:1) n-butanol: Acetic acid: Water (4:1:1)	Ninhydrin reagent Ninhydrin reagent Ninhydrin reagent Ninhydrin reagent	Red violet (0.24) Violet (0.40) Grey violet (0.55) Blue violet (0.17)
Alkaloids	Cinchona, alkaloid, Rauwolfia alkaloid	Chloroform: Diethyl amine (90:10) Ethyl acetate: Methanol: Water (100:13.5:10)	UV-365 nm/ Dragendorff UV-365 nm/ Dragendorff	
Essential oils		Toluene: Ethyl acetate (93:7)	UV-254 nm/ Anisaldehyde in sulfuric acid/Vanillin in sulphuric acid	
Flavonoids		Ethyl Acetate: Formic acid: Glacial acetic acid: Water (100:11:11:26) Universal detecting agent	UV-254 nm/UV-365 nm $FeCl_3$ Solution

Iodine vapours | |

- Separated constituents are removed by scrapping of the adsorbent at the appropriate layer on the developed plate, elluting the powder with a solvent such as ether.
- Quantitative analysis can be done over these recovered substances by dissolving the suitable solvent and determining by suitable analytical method.
- For quantitative analysis machine made precoated plates can be used.
- A new more efficient and superior technique to TLC is HPTLC (high performance thin layer chromatography) by which both the quantitative and qualitative analysis can be done.
- The increased efficiency is due to small particle size (3–5 µm).
- The characteristic feature of HPTLC is the finger print analysis which helps in correlating the botanical identity to the chemical constituent profile of the plant.
- TLC is useful in the analysis of alkaloids, glycosides, lipids, sugars and their derivatives, steroids.

b. Paper chromatography

- This technique involves either partition or adsorption chromatography.
- This is carried out on sheets of filter paper which serves both as the medium for separation and as the support (Fig. 1.8).
- The various types of filter papers used are Whatman paper no. 1, 3, 42, etc.
- Detection is done under visible light and UV light.
- Paper Chromatography (PC) is particularly applicable to water soluble plant constituents.

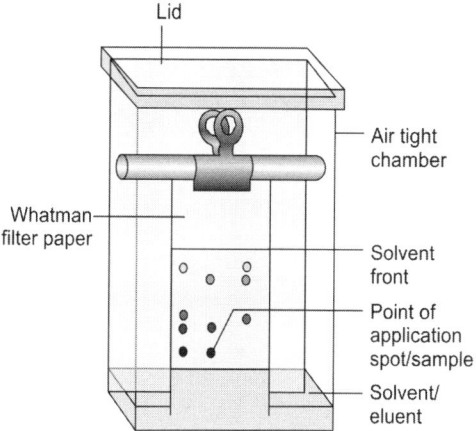

Fig. 1.8: Paper chromatography

- The main qualitative application is the identification of the compound by comparing the R_f value of particular compound of the sample to that of the standard.
- It is not much useful for the quantitative analysis.
- For example, flavanoids are best detected by paper chromatography. To separate flavanoids present in various samples, 2D paper chromatography is used with Benzene: Glacial acetic acid: water (4:1:5) solvent system.
- To achieve particular chromatography separation, filter papers are modified by various ways to reduce the polar properties of cellulose silicic acid or alumina is incorporated into the papers which makes suitable for separating lipids.

c. High performance liquid chromatography (HPLC)

HPLC is a method of chemical separation in which stationary phase contained in column and mobile phase in pumped at high pressure from one end. The pressure used here is about 5000 psi. In this method, separation of mixture from microgram to gram is done by passing the sample through a column of 5 mm diameter containing a stationary solid bed by means of pressurized flow of liquid mobile phase. The components of the mixture migrate through the column at different rates, and depending upon their solubility or molecular charge separation of the mixture occurs. This technique involves mass-transfer between stationary and mobile phases. HPLC utilizes a liquid mobile phase to separate the components of a mixture. These components (or analytes) are first dissolved in a solvent, and then forced to flow through a chromatographic column under a high pressure. In this column, the mixture is resolved into its components. The amount of resolution is important, and is dependent upon the extent of interaction between the solute components and the stationary phase. The stationary phase is defined as the immobile packing material in the column.

In this technique a liquid mobile phase is forced into the columns under high pressure either with **isocratic elution or gradient elution.** Normal flow rates of elute are 2 – 5 ml per minute but can be upto 10 ml/min, depending upon the diameter of the column and applied pressure (Fig. 1.9).

- HPLC is similar to GLC except that the former operates at ambient temperature.
- The apparatus required for HPLC includes:
  1. Column: Stainless steel column packed with silicon beads that separate the analyte from other compounds. Different types of stationary phase employed are:
     i. Silica
     ii. Alumina
     iii. Resins or polymers
     iv. Porous silica or polymers
     v. Chemically modified silica, polymers or porous graphite like C_{18} bonded phase, C_8 bonded phase, etc.

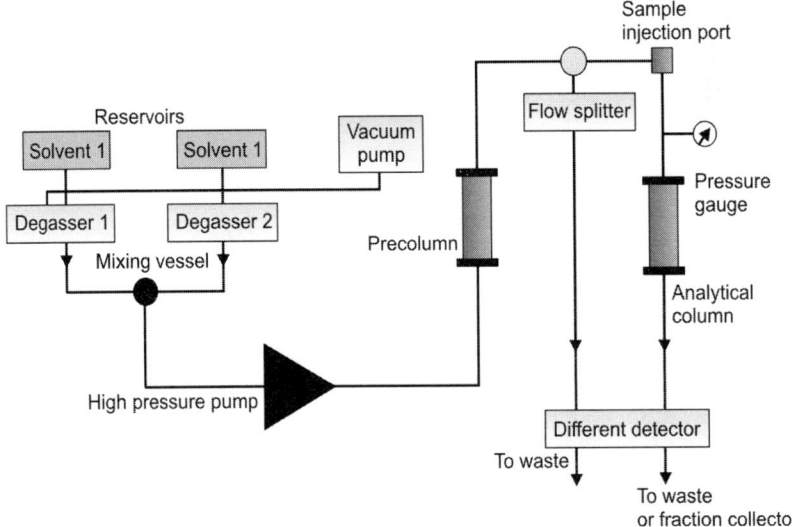

Fig. 1.9: Schematic diagram of binary HPLC system

vi. Specially modified stationary phase like proteins or peptides, cyclodextrins.
2. Pumps: They are required to pump the mobile phase through the column.
3. Detector: UV/visible spectrophotometer are commonly used.
   - The result is expressed in terms of retention time.
   - It is commonly employed for quantitative analysis.
   - HPLC is mainly used for those classes of compounds which are nonvolatile, e.g. high terpenoids, phenolic compounds of all types, alkaloids, lipids and sugars.
   - It works best for compounds which can be detected in UV or visible region.
   - Due to small particle size of stationary phase and its compact arrangement, the column, prone to blocking. Hence, it is necessary to purify and filter plant extract before injecting them.

For example HPLC analysis of *Picrorrhiza*

Standard – Kutkoside and Picroside I

Table: 1.4: Method requirements for HPLC

Drug	Constituents	Solvent	Column
Diterpenoids		Methanol: Water (9:11)	C_{18} column
Sterols	22-Dehydrocampesterol	Methanol: Water (9:11)	RP-18 column
Anthocyanins	Mono, di, tri glycosides	Water: Acetic acid: Methanol (71:10:19)	C_{18}/RP-18 column
Indole alkaloids		Methanol: Water: Formic acid (166:34:1)	RP-8 column

Mobile Phase – Methanol: Water (35:65)
Flow Rate – 1.5 μl/min
Column – C_{18} Bondapak 10 μ
Detection – UV at 270 nm
R_t - Kutkoside-8.5 min, Picroside I -11.4 min

- For the separation of a particular class of plant constituent, a combination of these techniques is used.

d. Gas liquid chromatography

- The separation principal involved is partition.
- The instrument for GLC is complex in nature. It has the following components:
  1. Column: Consist of a long narrow tube in the form of coil which is packed with a thin layer of stationary phase on an inert support.
  2. Oven: It is provided to heat the column.
  3. Carrier gas: e.g. Nitrogen or argon which is inert in nature acts as the mobile phase.
  4. Detector: Flame ionization or electron capture detector are frequently used for detection.
- This is commonly used for the analysis of essential oil (volatile oil) and the fatty acids.
- It is mainly used for volatile compounds and those compounds which are not volatile in nature are connected into their derivatives (specially trimethyl silyl ethers).
- The results are expressed in terms of retention volume R_v or retention time R_t.
- GLC is useful for both qualitative and quantitative analysis.
- In recent years GLC is coupled with mass spectrometer, which can be used for the identification of the components but this method can be used only for pure compounds, e.g. Analysis of volatile oil of *Mentha piperata* using GLC:

Column: Fused silica capillary column with coating of free fatty acid phase.
Oven Temperature: Programmed from 90 to 210°C at 7°C/min.
Injector temperature: 230°C
Detector temperature: 240°C
Carrier gas: Helium
Flow rate: 1.5 ml/min
Injection volume: 0.1 μl
R_t : 16.5 min

e. High performance thin layer chromatography

High Performance thin layer chromatography is a sophisticated and automated form of TLC. This highly efficient method is useful for both qualitative and quantitative analysis, is now referred to as high performance thin layer chromatography

Table 1.5: Method requirements for HPTLC

Drug	Constituents	Solvent	Detection	Stationary Phase
Rheum emodi	Emodin, Chrysophenol	Petroleum ether: Ethyl acetate: Formic acid (7.5:2.5:0.1)	UV – 254 nm	Silica gel G60 F_{254}
Ginseng	Panaxadiol and Panaxatriol	Chloroform: Ether (1:1)	10% Sulphuric acid in mehanol	Silica gel
Liquorice	18 β-Glycyrrhetinic acid	Ethyl acetate: Methanol: Ammonia solution (10:3:1)	UV – 260 nm	Silica gel
Aloe vera	Aloin	Ethyl acetate: Formic acid: Water (17:2:3)	UV – 350 nm	Silica gel

(HPTLC).

High performance thin layer chromatography refers to the layer, which have a smaller particle size (6 µm), which are slightly thinner (100 or 200 µm) and particularly whose particle size distribution is significantly closer than that of conventional TLC sorbets. Because of these specifications, the optimum separation distance of a high performance thin layer chromatography layer is around 50 mm instead of 100–120 mm on a conventional TLC plate.

HPTLC in the analysis of herbal products:

HPTLC is a planer chromatography, where separation of the sample components is achieved on high performance layers with detection and data acquisition using an advanced workstation. These high performance layers are precoated plates, coated with a sorbent of particle size 5–7 microns and a layer thickness of 150–200 microns. The reduction in the thickness of the layer and the particle size results in increasing the plate efficiency as well as nature of the separation. Separations on high performance thin layer plates gives sharper and more compact bands with shorter distances of migration. HPTLC is mainly used to develop analytical profile for tropane alkaloids, flavonoids, anthracene, aglycone, lipids and steroidal compounds.

VI. SPECTROSCOPIC METHODS OF ANALYSIS OF HERBAL DRUGS

Spectroscopy mainly deals with the study of interaction of electromagnetic radiation with the matter. The obtained spectra is divided into a series of regions corresponding to the type of absorption or emission, e.g. electronic transition of atoms and molecules are obtained in UV-visible region while molecular vibration is observed in IR region.

1. **Ultraviolet and Visible Spectroscopy (UV–Visible Spectra)**
   - The absorption spectra of plant constituents are measured in very dilute solution against a solvent, using an automatic recording spectrophotometer.
   - For coloured compounds: Range of measurement is 200 to 400 nm.
     For coloured compounds: Range for measurement is between 200 to 700 nm.
   - The wavelengths of maxima and minima of absorption spectrum so obtained are recorded in nm.
   - The intensity of absorbance at particular maxima and minima is also recorded.
   - Such type of spectral measurements are used in the identification of various plant constituents for monitoring the elutes of chromatographic columns during purification of plant products and for screening crude plant extracts for the presence of polyacetylene compounds.
   - Solvent widely used for UV spectroscopy is 95% ethanol (C_2H_5OH). (commercial absolute alcohol should not be used, as it contains residual benzene which gets absorbed in short UV range). Other solvents used are water, methanol, hexane, petroleum ether.
   - Solvents such as chloroform and pyridine are not used as they absorb strongly in 200–600 nm region. (Hence, they are suitable for making measurements in visible regions of spectrum with plant pigments such as carotenoids.
   - The spectral utility is increased by repeating samples made in neutral solution, e.g.
     - When alkali is added to alcoholic solutions of phenolic compounds, the UV-spectra shifts towards longer wavelengths (i.e. batho-

Table 1.6: Spectral properties of different classes of plant pigments

Class of Pigments	Colour	Ultraviolet range (nm)	Visible spectral range (nm)
Chlorophylls	green	short UV absorption	640–660 and 430–470
Phycobillins	red and blue	short UV absorption	615–650 and 540–570
Cytochromes	yellow	short UV absorption	545–605 and 415–440
Anthocyanins	red	275	475–550
Betacyanins	blue	250–270	530–554
Carotenoids	yellow to orange	–	400–500
Anthraquinones	yellow	3–4 intense peaks between 220 and 290	420–460
Yellow flavonols	yellow	250–270	365–390

chromic shift) with increase in absorbance.
- When alkali is added to neutral solutions of aromatic carboxylic acids, UV spectra shifts in the opposite direction, i.e. towards shorter wavelengths (i.e. hypsochromic shift).
- If a substance shows a single absorption band between 250–260 nm, the compound is a simple phenol, purine/pyrimidine or an aromatic acid.
- If it shows, three distinct peaks in 400–500 nm regions, the compound is carotenoid.

2. **Infrared Spectroscopy (IR Spectra)**
The region which extends about 8000 Å–35000 Å, the wavelength is known as infrared region. Infra red rediations are associated with much lower energy than UV-visible radiation. IR is mainly used to elucidate the functional groups present in the sample.
- IR spectra is measured on plant substances in automatic recording IR spectrophotometers either in solution (in $CHCl_3$ or CCl_4 as 1–5%) or in solid state (mixed with KBr).
- The region in IR spectra above 1200 cm^{-1} shows spectral bands due to the vibrations of individual bonds or functional groups in the molecule under examination.
- The region below 1200 cm^{-1} shows spectral bands due to the vibrations of the whole molecule and because of its complexity it is called as fingerprint region. Thus, in this region multiplicity

Table 1.7: Characteristic infrared frequencies of some natural products

Natural Products	Approximate positions of characteristic bands above 1200 cm^{-1}
Alkanes	2940 (S), 2860 (M), 1455 (S), 1380 (M)
Alkenes	3050 (W M), 1850 (W), 1650 (W-M), 1410 (W)
Aromatics	3050 (W M), 2100–1700 (W), 1600, 1580, 1500 (W-M)
Alcohols and Phenols	3610 (W M), 3600–2400 (Broad), 140 (M)
Aldehydes and ketones	2750 (W), 2680 (W), 1820–1650 (S), 1420 (W-M)
Esters and Lactones	1820 1680 (S)
Carboxylic acids	3520 (W), 3400–2500 (Broad), 1760 (S), 1710 (S)

S = Strong, M = Medium, W = Weak

assures the individual identification of bands, but collectively absorption bands help in identifying the material.
- IR spectroscopy is most frequently used in phytochemical studies as a "finger printing device", for comparing a natural with a synthetic sample.
- IR spectral analysis is extensively used for identifying known essential oil components.

VII. CHEMICAL TESTS FOR VARIOUS CLASSES OF PHYTOCONSTITUENTS

General Tests

1. Alkaloids

Dissolve extracts individually in dilute hydrochloric acid and filter. Test the solution carefully by treating with following alkaloidal reagents:

i. **Dragendorff's test:** To extract, add few a drops of dragendorff's reagent (solution of potassium bismuth iodide). Reddish brown precipitate is formed.

ii. **Mayer's test:** To 2–3 ml of extract, add a few drops of Mayer's reagent (potassium mercuric iodide). It gives cream or buff colored precipitate.

iii. **Hager's test:** To 2–3 ml of extract add Hager's reagent (saturated picric acid solution). It gives yellow colored precipitate.

iv. **Wagner's test:** To 2–3 ml extract, add few drops of Wagner's reagent (iodine in potassium iodide). It gives reddish brown precipitate.

v. **10% Tannic acid solution:** Alkaloids give a buff coloured precipitate.

TLC

Solvent system, Ethyl acetate, Methanol: Water (100:13.5:10)

Spraying reagent: Dragendorff's reagent

Colour: Orange

2. Glycosides

Hydrolyse the extracts with dilute hydrochloric acid and the hydrolysate is subjected to the following glycosides tests:

i. **Modified Borntrager's Test:** Treat the extracts with ferric chloride solution and heat on boiling water bath for about 5 minutes. Cool and shake the mixture with equal volume of benzene. Separate the benzene layer and treat with half of its volume of ammonia solution. Formation of rose pink/cherry red colour in the ammoniacal layer, indicates presence of anthranol type of glycoside.

ii. **Legal's test:** Treat the extract with sodium nitroprusside in pyridine and methanolic alkali. Formation of pink to red colour indicated the presence of cardiac glycosides.

iii. **Baljet test:** Treat extract of drug with sodium picrate. Formation of a yellowish orange colour confirmed the presence of cardiac glycosides.

iv. **Keller–kiliani test:** Take 0.5g of dried extract, dissolved in 2 ml of glacial acetic acid containing one drop of ferric chloride solutions. Add 1 ml of concentrated H_2SO_4. A brown ring shows the presence of a cardenolides.

TLC

Solvent system: Ethyl acetate: Methanol: Water (100:13.5:10)

Spraying reagent: Kedde reagent (cardiac glycoside): Colour-pink/violet

Spraying reagent: KOH reagent (anthraquinone glycoside): Colour-red

3. Steroids and terpenoids

i. **Liebermann Burchard Test:** To the extract, add chloroform and few drops of acetic anhydride, boil and cool. Then, add concentrated sulphuric acid from the side of the test tube, brown ring is formed at the junction of two layers and on shaking upper layer turns green which shows presence of steroids and formation of deep red colour indicates presence of triterpenoides.

ii. **Salkowski Test:** Dissolve the extract in chloroform and few drops of sulphuric acid, red colour at the lower layer indicates the presence of steroids and yellow colour indicates the presence of triterpenoides.

iii. **Liebermann's Reaction:** Mix minimum 3 ml of extract and 3 ml of acetic anhydride, heat and cool. Add few drops of concentrated sulphuric acid then blue colour appears.

TLC

Solvent system: Hexane: Diethyl ether (7:3)

Benzene: Diethyl ether (9:1)

Spraying reagent:

50% H_2SO_4 in ethanol

80% potassium dichromate in H_2SO_4

Colour: Orange

4. **Tannins (Phenolic compounds/Flavonoids)**

   i. **Goldbeater's skin test**

   To a small piece of goldbeater's skin, add 2% of hydrochloric acid, rinse it with distilled water and place in the solution to be tested for five minutes then wash with distilled water and transfer to a 1% ferrous sulphate solution. A brown or black on the skin indicates the presence of tannins.

   ii. **Ferric chloride test:** Treat the extract with 5% neutral ferric chloride solution, a deep blue black colour appears.

   iii. **Lead acetate test:** To the extract add 10% lead acetate solution. White precipitate appears.

   iv. **Gelatin test:** Treat the extract with gelatin solution, a white precipitate is formed.

   v. **Potassium permanganate test:** To the extract add dilute potassium permanganate solution, decolouration of the solution takes place.

   vi. **Alkaline reagent test:** Treat the extract with few drops of sodium hydroxide separately. Formation of intense yellow colour, which turned colourless on addition of few drops of dilute hydrochloric acid, indicates the presence of flavonoids.

   vii. **Shinoda test:** Treat the extract with few fragments of magnesium metal separately, followed by drop wise addition of concentrated hydrochloric acid. The formation of magenta colour indicates the presence of flavonoid.

   viii. **Vanillin hydrochloric test:** Treat the extract with few drops of vanillin hydrochloride reagent. The formation of pinkish red colour indicates the presence of tannins.

   Phenols: Spot a drop of ethanolic extract on a filter paper and add a drop of phosphomolybdic acid reagent on it. Expose the spot to ammonia vapor. Blue coloration of the spot indicates presence of phenols.

5. **Flavonoids**

   i. **Shinoda test:** To the dry powder or extract, add 5 ml of 95% ethanol, few drops of concentrated hydrochloric acid and 0.5 gm of magnesium turnings, a pink colour confirms the presence of flavonoids.

   ii. To a small quantity of residue, add lead acetate solution, a yellow coloured precipitate formed.

   iii. To the above precipitate add increasing amount of sodium hydroxide a yellow colour appears which decolourises after addition of acid.

TLC
Solvent system: Ethyl acetate: Methanol: Water (100:13.5:10)
Ethyl acetate: Formic acid: Glacial Acetic acid: Water (100:11:11:26)
Spraying reagent: NP/PEG reagent
Colour: Orange/yellow/green (UV-365 nm)

6. **Oils and Fats**
   i. **Place a thick section of drug on glass slide.** Add a drop of Sudan red III reagent. After two minutes, wash with 50% alcohol. Mount in glycerin. Observe under microscope. Oil globules appear red.
   ii. **Stain/spot test:** Place a small amount of extract between two filter papers and press them. Oil stain on paper indicates the presence of fixed oil.
   iii. **Saponification test:** Add a few drops of 0.5 ml alcoholic potassium hydroxide to a small quantity of extract along with a drop of phenolphthalein and heat on a water bath for one to two hours. The formation of soap on partial neutralization of alkali indicates the presence of fixed oils and fats.
   iv. **Solubility test:** Oils are soluble in ether, benzene and chloroform, but insoluble in 90% ethanol and water. (Exception: Castor oil is soluble in alcohol).
   v. **Test for complete saponification:** Place 3 ml of the dry acids in a test tube, and add 15 ml of alcohol. Heat the solution to boiling, and add an equal volume of 6N ammonium hydroxide. Clear solution obtained.

7. **Proteins and amino acids**
   a. **Biuret test (general test):** To 3 ml. test solution add 4% NaOH and a few drops of 1% $CuSO_4$ solution. Violet or pink color appears.
   b. *Millons' test*: Mix 3 ml test solution with 5 ml. Millon's reagent. White precipitate forms which turns brick red or the precipitate dissolves giving red colored solution on warming.
   c. **Xanthoprotein test (for protein containing tyrosine or tryptophan):** Mix 3 ml test solution with 1 ml conc. H_2SO_4. White precipitate is formed precipitate turns yellow. Add NH_4OH: precipitate turns orange.
   d. **Test for proteins containing sulpur:** Mix 5 ml test solution with 2 ml 40% NaOH and 2 drops of 10% lead acelate solution. Boil. Solution turns black or brownish due to PbS formation.
   e. **Precipitation test:** The test solution gives white colloidal precipitate with following reagents:
      a. Absolute alcohol
      b. 5% $HgCl_2$ solution
      c. 5% $CuSO_4$ solution
      d. 5% lead acetate
      e. 5% ammonium sulphate
   f. **Ninhydrin test:** Add 0.25% ninhydrin reagent to the extract and boil for few minutes. Formation of blue color indicated presence of amino acid.

8. **Carbohydrates**

   Molisch's test (general test for carbohydrates):
   To 2–3 ml of aqueous extract add few drops of Molisch reagent (alcoholic solution of α-naphthol) shake and add concentrated sulphuric acid from sides of the test tube. Violet ring is formed at the junction of the two liquids.

   Test for Reducing Sugars:
   a. *Fehling's test*: Mix 1 ml Fehling's A and 1 ml Fehling's B solution, boil the mixture for one minute. Add equal volume of test solution. Heat in boiling water bath for 5–10 min. First a yellow, then brick red ppt is observed.
   b. *Benedict's test*: Mix equal volume of Benedict's reagent and test solution in a test tube. Heat in boiling water bath

for 5 min. Solution appears green, yellow or red depending on amount of reducing sugar present in test solution.

Monosaccharides:

Barfoed's test: Mix volume of Barfoed's reagent and test solution. Heat for 1–2 min in boiling water bath and cool. Red ppt is observed.

Test for Pentose Sugars: Pentoses are components of certain gums.

a. **Bial's orcinol test:** To boiling Bial's reagent, add a few drops of test solution. Green or purple coloration appears.

b. **Aniline acetate test:** Boil test solution in test tube. Hold filter paper soaked in aniline acetate in the vapour. Filter paper turns pink.
  i. Mix equal amount of test solution and HCl. Heat and add a crystal of phloroglucinol, red colour appears.

Test for Hexose Sugars:

a. *Selwinoff's test (for ketohexose like fructose)*: Heat 3 ml. Selwinoff's regeant and 1 ml test solution, keep in boiling water bath for 1–2 min. Red colour is formed.

b. **Tollen's phloroglucinol test for galactose:** Mix 2.5 ml conc HCl and 4 ml 0.5% phlorogluncinol. Add 1–2 ml test solution. Heat. Yellow to red colour appears.

c. **Cobalt-chloride test:** Mix 3 ml test solution with 2 ml cobalt chloride. Boil and cool. Add a few drops of NaOH solution. Solution appears greenish blue (glucose) or purplish (fructose) or upper layer greenish blue and lower layers purplish indicates the presence a mixture of glucose and fructose.

Test for Nonreducing Sugars:

a. Test solution does not give response to Fehling's and Benedict's tests.

b. Hydrolyse test solution. Fehling's and Benedict's tests are positive.

Test for Nonreducing Polysaccharides (Starch):

a. *Iodine test:* Mix 3 ml test solution and few drops of dilute iodine solution. Blue color appears. It disappears on boiling, reappears on cooling.

b. *Tannic acid test for starch:* With 20% tannic acid, test solution gives precipitate.

9. **Volatile Oils:**

Take 50 g of powdered material. Subject it to hydrodistillation. Collect the distillate in the graduated tube of assembly in which the aqueous portion is automatically separated from the volatile oil. Separate volatile oil from distillate and perform the following tests:

a. Volatile oils have characteristic odour.

b. Filter paper is not permanently stained with volatile oil.

10. **Amino Acids**

a. **Ninhydrin test (general test):** Heat 3 ml. test solution and 3 drops 5% ninhydrin solution in boiling water bath for 10 min. Purple or bluish color appears.

b. **Test for tyrosine:** Heat 3 ml test solution and 3 drops Million's reagent. Solution shows dark red colour.

c. **Test for tryptophan:** To 3 ml. test solution and add a few drops of glyoxalic acid and conc. H_2SO_4. Reddish violet ring appears at the junction of the two layers.

d. **Test for cysteine:** To 5 ml test solution add a few drops of 40% NaOH and 10% lead acetate solution. Boil. Black precipitate of lead sulphate is formed.

11. **Lipids**

a. **Brown paper test**

Lipids can be tested with a brown paper. If it evaporates after being dropped on the paper, lipids are not present. If transparent spots appear on the paper, lipids are present.

b. **Sudan IV Test**

In the Sudan IV test, dark red Sudan IV (a common dye) is added to a solution. If lipids are present, they will be dyed red.

c. **Test for lipids**

Add ethanol to sample, then shake, add water to the solution, and shake again. If fat is present, the product turns milky white.

Preparation of Specimen for Fats and Fixed Oils

If a specimen of oil shows turbidity owing to separated stearin, warm the container in a water bath at 50°C until the oil is clear, or if the oil does not become clear on warming, pass it through dry filter paper in a funnel contained in a hot-water jacket. Mix thoroughly, and weigh at one time as many portions as are needed for the various determinations, using preferably a bottle having a pipette dropper, or a weighing burette. Keep the specimen melted, if solid at room temperature, until the desired portions of specimen are withdrawn.

1. *Specific gravity*: Unless otherwise stated in the individual monograph, the specific gravity determination is applicable only to liquids and unless otherwise stated, is based on the ratio of the weight of a substance in air at 25°C to that of an equal volume of water at the same temperature. Where a temperature is specified in the individual monograph, the specific gravity is the ratio of the weight of the substance in air at the specified temperature to that of an equal volume of water at the same temperature. When the substance is a solid at 25 °C, determine the specific gravity at the temperature directed in the individual monograph, and refer to water at 25 °C.

   Procedure: Select a clean, dry pycnometer that previously has been calibrated by determining its weight and the weight of recently boiled water contained in it at 25°C. Adjust the temperature of the substance to about 20°C, and fill the pycnometer with it. Adjust the temperature of the filled pycnometer to 25°C, remove any excess of the substance and weigh. Subtract the total weight of the pycnometer from the filled weight of the pycnometer. The specific gravity of the substance is the quotient obtained by dividing the weight of the substance contained in the pycnometer by the weight of water contained, both determined at 25°C unless otherwise directed in the individual monograph.

2. *Melting range or temperature*

   Method I: An example of a suitable melting range apparatus consists of a glass container for a bath of transparent fluid, a suitable stirring device, an accurate thermometer and a controlled source of heat. The bath fluid is selected with a view to the temperature required, but light paraffin is used generally and certain liquid silicones are well adapted to the higher temperature ranges. The fluid is deep enough to permit immersion of the thermometer to its specified immersion depth so that the bulb is still about 2 cm above the bottom of the bath. The heat may be supplied by an open flame or electrically. The capillary tube is about 10 cm long and 0.8 to 1.2 mm in internal diameter with walls 0.2 to 0.3 mm in thickness.

   Heat the bath until the temperature is about 30°C below the expected melting point. Remove the thermometer, and quickly attach the capillary tube to the thermometer by wetting both with a drop of the liquid of the bath and adjust its height so that the material in the capillary is level with the thermometer bulb. Replace the thermometer, and continue the heating, with constant stirring, sufficiently to cause the temperature to rise at a rate of about 30°C per minute. When the temperature is about 3°C below the lower limit of the expected melting range, reduce the heating so that the temperature rises at a rate of about 1 to 2°C per minute. Continue heating until melting is complete. Repeat the determination twice on a freshly melted portion of the test substance. If the variation of three determinations is less than 1°C, take the average of the three as the melting point. If the variation of three determinations is 1 or greater than 1, make two additional determinations and take the average of the five consecutive readings.

The temperature at which the column of the substance under test is observed to collapse definitely against the side of the tube at any point is defined as the beginning of melting, and the temperature at which the test substance becomes liquid throughout is defined as the end of melting or the "melting point". The two temperatures fall within the limits of the melting range.

Method II: An instrument may be used in the procedures. The instrument consists of a block of metal that may be heated at a controlled rate, its temperature being monitored by a sensor. The block accommodates the capillary tube containing the test substance and permits monitoring of the melting process, typically by means of a beam of light and a detector. The detector signal may be processed by a microcomputer to determine and display the melting point or range, or the detector signal may be plotted to allow visual estimation of the melting point or range.

3. *Acid value (free fatty acids)*

The acidity of fats and fixed oils may be expressed as the number of ml of 0.1N alkali required to neutralize the free acids in 10 g of substance. Acidity is frequently expressed as the acid value, which is the number of mg of potassium hydroxide required to neutralize the free acids in 1 g of the substance.

Procedure: Dissolve about 10 g of the, accurately weighed substance in 50 ml of a mixture of equal volumes of alcohol and ether (which has been neutralized to phenolphthalein with 0.1N sodium hydroxide) contained in a flask. If the test specimen does not dissolve in the cold solvent, connect the flask with a suitable condenser and warm slowly, with frequent shaking, until the specimen dissolves. Add 1 ml of phenolphthalein, and titrate with 0.1N sodium hydroxide until the solution remains faintly pink after shaking for 30 seconds. Calculate either the acid value or the volume of 0.1N alkali required to neutralize 10 gm of specimen (free fatty acids), whichever is appropriate.

If the volume of 0.1N sodium hydroxide required for the titration is less than 2 ml, a more dilute titrant may be used, or the sample size may be adjusted accordingly. The results may be expressed in terms of the volume of titrant used or in terms of the equivalent volume of 0.1N sodium hydroxide.

If the oil has been saturated with carbon dioxide for the purpose of preservation, gently reflux the alcohol-ether solution for 10 minutes before titration. The oil may be freed from carbon dioxide also by exposing it in a shallow dish in vacuum desiccators for 24 hours before weighing the test specimens.

4. *Ester value*

The ester value is the number of mg of potassium hydroxide required to saponify the esters in 1 g of the substance. If the saponification value and the acid value have been determined, the difference between these two represents the ester value.

Procedure: Place 1.5 g to 2 g of the substance in a tared, 250 ml flask, weigh accurately, add 20 ml to 30 ml of neutralized alcohol, and shake. Add 1 ml of phenolphthalein and titrate with 0.5N alcoholic potassium hydroxide until the free acid is neutralized. Add 25.0 ml of 0.5N alcoholic potassium hydroxide, and proceed as directed under saponification value, beginning with "Heat the flask" and omitting the further addition of phenolphthalein. The difference between the volumes, in ml, of 0.5N hydrochloric acid consumed in the actual test and in the blank test, multiplied by 28.05 and divided by the weight in grams of the specimen taken, is the ester value.

5. Hydroxyl value

The hydroxyl value is the number of mg of potassium hydroxide equivalent to the hydroxyl content of 1 g of the substance.

Pyridine-acetic anhydride reagent: Mix 3 volumes of freshly opened or freshly distilled pyridine with 1 volume of freshly opened or freshly distilled acetic anhydride just before use.

Procedure: Transfer a quantity of the substance, determined by reference to the accompanying table and accurately weighed, to a glass-stoppered 250 ml conical flask, and add 5 ml of pyridine–acetic anhydride reagent. Transfer 5 ml of pyridine–acetic anhydride reagent to a second glass stoppered, 250 ml conical flask to provide the reagent blank. Fit both flasks with suitable glass-jointed reflux condensers, heat on a steam bath for 1 hour, add 10 ml of water through each condenser, and heat on the steam bath for 10 minutes more. Cool, and to each add 25 ml of butyl alcohol, previously neutralized to phenolphthalein with 0.5N alcoholic potassium hydroxide, by pouring 15 ml through each condenser and after removing the condensers, washing the sides of both flasks with the remaining 10 ml portions. To each flask add 1 ml of phenolphthalein, and titrate with 0.5N alcoholic potassium hydroxide, recording the volume in ml, consumed by the residual acid in the test solution as T and that consumed by the blank as B. In a 125 ml conical flask, mix about 10 g of the substance, accurately weighed, with 10 ml of freshly distilled pyridine, previously neutralized to phenolphthalein, add 1ml of phenolphthalein, and titrate with 0.5N alcoholic potassium hydroxide, recording the volume, in ml, consumed by the free acid in the test specimen as A, or use the acid value to obtain A. Calculate the hydroxyl value taken by the formula:

$$(56.11\ N/W)\ (B + (WA/C) - T)$$

in which W and C are the weights, in g of the substances taken for the acetylation and for the free acid determination, respectively; N is the exact normality of the alcoholic potassium hydroxide; and 56.11 is the molecular weight of potassium hydroxide.

Table 1.8: Hydroxyl value

Sample weights (hydroxyl value range)	Weight of test specimen (g)
0 to 20	10
20 to 50	5
50 to 100	3
100 to 150	2
150 to 200	1.5
200 to 250	1.25
250 to 300	1.0
300 to 350	0.75

6. Iodine value

The iodine value represents the number of g of iodine absorbed, under the prescribed conditions, by 100 g of the substance. Unless otherwise specified in the individual monograph, determine the iodine value by the following method:

Hanu's Method

Procedure: Transfer an accurately weighed quantity of sample, as determined from the accompanying table, into a 250 ml iodine flask, dissolve it in 10 ml of chloroform, add 25 ml of iodobromide solution, insert the stopper in the vessel securely, and allow it to stand for 30 minutes protected from light, with occasional shaking. Then add, in the order named, 30 ml of potassium iodide and 100 ml of water, and titrate the liberated iodine with 0.1 N sodium thiosulfate, shaking thoroughly after each addition of thiosulfate. When the iodine color becomes quite pale, add 3 ml of starch solution, and continue the titration with 0.1N sodium thiosulfate until the blue color is discharged. Perform a blank test at the same time with the same quantities of the same reagents and in the same manner. Calculate the iodine value from the formula:

$$(126.9\ (VB-VS)\ N)/10W$$

in which 126.9 is the atomic weight of iodine; VB and VS are the volumes in ml, of 0.1N sodium thiosulfate consumed by the blank test and the actual test, respectively; N is the exact normality of the sodium thiosulfate; and W is the weight in g of the substance taken for the test.

NOTE: If more than half of the iodobromide is absorbed by the portion of the substance taken, repeat the determination, using a smaller portion of the substance under examination

Table 1.9: Iodine value and sample weight

Iodine value	Expected weight in g
<5	3.000
5–20	1.000
21–50	0.400
51–100	0.200
101–150	0.130
151–200	0.100

7. *Peroxide value*

The peroxide value is the number that expresses, in milliequivalents of active oxygen, the quantity of peroxide contained in 1000 g of the substance (this test must be performed promptly after sampling to avoid oxidation of the test specimen)

Procedure: Place about 5 g of the substance, accurately weighed, in a 250 ml conical flask fitted with a ground-glass stopper. Add 30 ml of a mixture of glacial acetic acid and chloroform (3:2), shake to dissolve, and add 0.5 ml of saturated potassium iodide solution. Shake for exactly 1 minute, and add 30 ml of water. Titrate with 0.01N sodium thiosulfate, adding the titrant slowly with continuous shaking, until the yellow color is almost discharged. Add 5 ml of starch solution, and continue the titration, shaking vigorously, until the blue color is discharged. Perform a blank determination under the same conditions (the volume of titrant used in the blank determination must not exceed 0.1 ml). The difference between the volumes, in ml, of 0.01N sodium thiosulfate consumed in the actual test and in the blank test, multiplied by 10 and divided by the weight, in g, of the specimen taken, is the peroxide value.

8. *Saponification value*

The saponification value is the number of mg of potassium hydroxide required to neutralize the free acids and saponify the esters contained in 1 g of the substance.

Procedure: Place 1.5 g to 2 g of the substance in a tared, 250 ml flask, weigh accurately and add 25 ml of 0.5N alcoholic potassium hydroxide. Heat the flask on a steam bath, under a suitable condenser to maintain reflux for 30 minutes, frequently rotating the contents. Then, add 1 ml of phenolphthalein, and titrate the excess potassium hydroxide with 0.5N hydrochloric acid. Perform a blank determination under the same conditions. The titration also can be carried out potentiometrically. The difference between the volumes in ml, of 0.5N hydrochloric acid consumed in the actual test and in the blank test, multiplied by 56.1 and the exact normality of the 0.5N hydrochloric acid, and divided by the weight in g of specimen taken, is the saponification value. If the oil has been saturated with carbon dioxide for the purpose of preservation, expose it in a shallow dish in vacuum desiccators for 24 hours before weighing the test specimen.

9. *Unsaponifiable matter*

The term *unsaponifiable Matter* in oils or fats, refers to those substances that are not saponifiable by alkali hydroxides but are soluble in the ordinary fat solvents, and products of saponification that are soluble in such solvents.

Procedure: Transfer about 5 g of the oil or fat, accurately weighed, to a 250 ml conical flask, add 50 ml of an alcoholic potassium hydroxide solution prepared by dissolving 12 g of potassium hydroxide in 10 ml of water and diluting this solution with alcohol to 100 ml, and heat the flask on a steam bath under a suitable condenser to maintain reflux for 1 hour, swirling frequently. Cool to a temperature below 25°C and transfer the contents of the flask to a separator having a poly-tetrafluoroethylene stopcock, rinsing the flask twice with 50 ml portions of water that are added to the separator (do not use grease on stopcock). Extract with three 100 ml portions of ether, combining the ether extracts in another separator containing 40 ml of water. Gently rotate or shake the separator for a few minutes. Allow the mixture to separate, and discard the lower aqueous phase. Wash the ether extract with two additional 40 ml portions of water, and discard the lower aqueous phase. Wash the ether extract successively with a 40 ml portion of potassium hydroxide solution (3 in 100) and a 40 ml portion of water. Repeat this potassium hydroxide solution–water wash sequence three times. Wash the ether extract with 40 ml portions of water until the last washing is not reddened by the addition of 2 drops of phenolphthalein. Transfer the ether extract to a tared flask, and rinse the separator with 10 ml of ether, adding the rinsings to the flask. Evaporate the ether on a steam bath, and add 6 ml of acetone to the residue. Remove the acetone in a current of air, and dry the residue at 105 °C until successive weighings differ by not more than 1 mg. Calculate the percentage of unsaponifiable matter in the portion of oil or fat taken by the formula:

$$100(WR/WS)$$

in which *WR* is the weight in g of the residue; and *WS* is the weight in g of the oil or fat taken for the test.

Dissolve the residue in 20 ml of alcohol, previously neutralized to the phenolphthalein endpoint, add phenolphthalein, and titrate with 0.1N alcoholic sodium hydroxide to the first appearance of a faint pink color that persists for not less than 30 seconds. If the volume of 0.1N alcoholic sodium hydroxide required is greater than 0.2 ml, the separation of the layers was incomplete; the residue weighed cannot be considered as "unsaponifiable matter," and the test must be repeated.

10. *Anisidine value*

The anisidine value is defined as 100 times the optical density measured in a 1 cm cell of a solution containing 1 g of the substance to be examined in 100 ml of a mixture of solvents and reagents according to the method described below (carry out the operations as rapidly as possible, avoiding exposure to actinic light).

Test solution A: Dissolve 0.5 g of the substance to be examined in iso-octane, and dilute with the same solvent to 25 ml.

Test solution B: To 5 ml of test solution A, add 1 ml of a 2.5 g per litre solution of p-anisidine in glacial acetic acid, shake, and store protected from light.

Standard solution: To 5 ml of iso-octane add 1 ml of a 2.5 g per litre solution of *p*-anisidine in glacial acetic acid, shake, and store protected from light.

Procedure: Measure the absorbance of test solution A at 350 nm using iso-octane as the blank. Measure the absorbance of test solution B at 350 nm exactly 10 minutes after its preparation, using the standard solution as the compensation liquid. Calculate the anisidine value from the expression:

$$\frac{25(1.2A_s - A_b)}{m}$$

in which A_s is the absorbance of test solution B at 350 nm; A_b is the absorbance of test solution A at 350 nm; and m is the weight, in g, of the substance to be examined in test solution A.

11. *Total oxidation value (totox)*

Total oxidation value is defined by the formula:

$$2PV + AV$$

in which PV is the peroxide value, and AV is the anisidine value.

II. Specific Tests

1. *Alkaloids*

Boil 0.5 gm of powdered or broken drug with 10 ml of 10% sodium carbonate solution, cool and extract with a little chloroform. Evaporate the extract to dryness and apply the particular specific test.

   i. **Vitali Morin test for tropane alkaloids**

   To the residue, add 1–2 drops of fuming nitric acid and evaporate to dryness on a water bath. Cool and moisten it with 2 drops of alcoholic potassium hydroxide (3% potassium hydroxide in ethanol). A transient purple colour is produced.

   ii. **Ehrlich's test for ergot alkaloids**

   To the residue, dissolved in a mixture of 1% sulphuric acid and ethanol, add Ehrlich's reagent, slowly from the side of the tube a blue colour develops.

   iii. **Murexide test for purine alkaloids**

   Mix the residue with a few drops of hydrochloric acid on a watch glass and add a crystal of potassium chlorate. Evaporate carefully to dryness on a water bath, allow to cool and then add 2 drops of dilute ammonia solution, a purple colour appears.

   iv. **Thalleoquin test for cinchona alkaloids**

   To the residue add drop of dilute sulphuric acid and 1 ml water. Add bromine water drop wise until the solution just acquires a permanent yellow tinge and then add 1 ml of dilute ammonia solution. Deep green colour is produced.

   v. **Test for morphine**
   - Heat the residue with concentrated sulphuric acid on a water bath for 15 minutes, cool and add few drops of dilute nitric acid. A violet colour is produced rapidly changing to blood red.
   - To extract add Frohde's reagent (ammonium molybdate in concentrated sulphuric acid) a violet colour.

   vi. **Test for strychnine**

   Mix the residue with concentrate sulphuric acid and add solid potassium dichromate. A purple color appears which changes slowly to red.

   vii. **Test for brucine**

   Mix the residue with concentrate sulphuric acid and add crystal of potassium dichromate. A red color develops immediately. Add concentrate nitric acid a blood red color develops.

2. Glycosides

i. Tests for anthraquinine glycosides

a. *Borntrager's test*

Boil sample drug with dilute H_2SO_4 for 5–6 minute. Filter while hot and then cool the filtrate with an equal volume of organic solvent like benzene or $CHCl_3$, separate organic layer and shake with half of its volume of dilute ammonia. The ammonical layer shows pink to red color.

b. *Modified Borntrager's test*

Boil the sample drug with dilute sulphuric acid and 5% aqueous ferric chloride for 5 min. Filter while hot and then cool the filtrate. Shake the filtrate with an equal volume of organic solvent and perform it in similar way as the Borntrager's test. This test is given by cardiac glycosides. Ferric chloride used causes oxidation to anthraquinones.

ii. Test for cardiac glycosides

a. *Kedde's test*

Extract the drug with chloroform, concentrate the extract to dryness. Add one drop of 90% alcohol and two drops of 2% 3, 5–dinitrobenzoic acid in 90% alcohol. Basify the solution with 20% NaOH, purple colour develops. The colour reaction with 3, 5–dinitrobenzoic acid depends on the presence of a, b-unsaturated lactones in the aglycone.

b. *Baljet test*

To the test solution add picric acid or sodium picrate, orange colour is produced.

c. *Keller kiliani test for deoxy sugars*

Extract the test drug with chloroform and concentrate to dryness. To the residue add glacial acetic acid and one drop of ferric chloride (5%). Carefully add concentrated sulphuric acid through the side of test tube acidic layer shows blue colour.

d. *Legal's test*

To The test solution add pyridine and alkaline nitroprusside solution, blood red colour appear.

e. *Raymond's Test*

Treat the test solution with hot methanolic alkali, violet colour develops.

iii. Test for cyanogenetic glycosides

a. *Grignard reaction or sodium picrate test*

Moistened a filter paper first with picric acid then with 10% sodium carbonate and dry it. Place drug in a conical flask and moisten it with water. Suspend the above filter paper in the neck of the flask by means of the cork, warm gently at about 37°C the filter paper turns reddish purple colour.

Hydrogen cyanide is librated from cyanogenetic glycoside by the enzyme activity and reacts with sodium picrate to form the reddish purple sodium isopurpurate.

iv. Test for saponin glycosides

a. *Foam test*: Shake vigorously drug with water stable foam is formed.

b. *Heamolysis test*: Place a drop of blood on glass slide add a drop of test solution over it. Haemolytic zone appears.

v. Test for coumarin glycosides

Place moistened drug powder in test tube and cover it with a filter paper moistened with dilute sodium hydroxide solution. Heat the covered test tube over water bath for several minutes. Remove the paper and expose to UV light, the paper shows green fluorescence.

TLC

Solvent system: Ethyl acetate: Methanol: Water (100:13.5:10)

Chloroform: Glacial: Methanol: Water (64:32:12:8)

Spraying reagent-AS /VS Reagent
Colour-Blue

3. **Resins**
   i. **Test for Colophony**
      a. Dissolve sample in petroleum spirit, to it add 0.1% solution of cupric acetate. Shake well. Emerald green color slowly develops.
      b. To acetic anhydride add 20 drops of 1% solution of colophony in china dish. Add 2–3 drops of concentrated sulphuric acid. Wine red color is produced which slowly changes to brown.
   ii. **Test for Myrrh**
      a. Triturate the sample with water yellowish brown emulsion is formed.
      b. Ethereal solution of myrrh becomes reddish when treated with bromine vapours and purplish when moistened with nitric acid.
   iii. **Test for Benzoin**
      a. Heat a small amount of powder in a dry test tube. It melts and evolves whitish fumes of cinnamic and benzoic acid. Condense these fumes on a glass slide by placing a slide by to the mouth of the test tubes. Whitish crystalline sublimate is formed on a slide.
      b. Warm gently about 1 gm of powder with 5 ml of potassium permagnate solution in test tube. Due to oxidation of cinnamic acid distinct odour of benzaldehyde is produced which shows the presence of benzoin.
      c. Triturate small amount of benzoin with alcohol, filter and to the filtrate add few drops of alcoholic ferric chloride. Production of bright green colour denotes the presence of tarch benzoin.
      d. Treat 0.2 gm of benzoin with 5 ml of ether for 5 minutes. Pour 1 ml of ethereal solution in a porcelain dish containing 2- 3 drops of concentrated sulphuric acid. Formation of reddish brown colour shows the presence of benzoin.
   iv. **Test for Asafoetida**
      a. *Emulsion test*
         Trituration of sample with water forms yellowish orange emulsion if aloe gum resin present.
      b. Treat the freshly cut surface of sample with 1–2 drops of concentrate sulphuric acid on a glass slide. Red or reddish brown color is obtained which changes to violet when washed with water. Asafoetida is present.
      c. Similarly if sample treated with 50% nitric acid surface turns green in color. Asafoetida is present.
      d. *Combined umbelliferone test*
         Boil 0.5 gm of drug with 3 ml of concentrate hydrochloric acid and 3 ml of water for 5-10 minutes in a test tube. Filter and add the filtrate to test tube containing equal volume of alcohol. Add excess of strong ammonia solution. Blue fluorescence is produced. Asafoetida is confirmed.
   v. **Carbohydrates**
      a. *Tests for gums*
         Heat the test solution with dilute hydrochloric acid to hydrolysis. To it add Fehling's reagent and Benedict's reagent separately. Heat on water bath a brick red precipitate is formed.
      b. *Tests for mucilage*
         - To powdered drug add ruthenium red. Red color is produced.
         - Mucilage containing drug powder swells in water or aqueous potassium hydroxide.

Chapter 2

Powder: Morphological and Microscopical Studies

EXPERIMENT 1

Aim: To study the simple and compound microscopes.

Requirement: Microscope, eyepiece, and objective.

MICROSCOPE

Definition: It is the instrument, which is used to magnify small elements under study, which can not be observed with naked eye. It is an important and delicate scientific instrument, should be handled with care.

Parts of the microscope: It consists of two main parts:

i. Mechanical parts:
1. The base or foot, a heavy piece used to support the other parts
2. The pillar, used to handle the part of the microscope under study

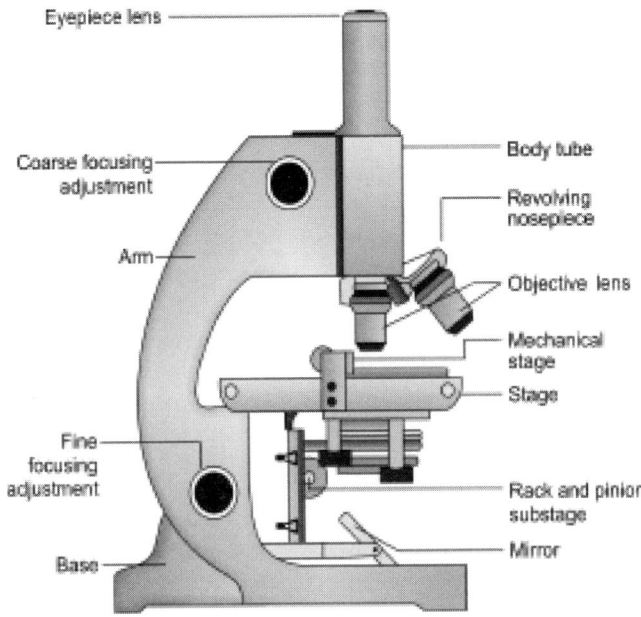

Fig. 2.1: Labelled diagram of a compound microscope

3. The stage, a platform with two clips to hold the slide while being studied
4. The arm, a cured handle used for carrying the microscope
5. The body tube, which bears the magnifying lenses
6. The nosepiece, a rotating structure carrying the lower lenses or objectives
7. The coarse adjustment, for raising and lowering the stage to obtain a sharp image of the examined object, the course use to move the stage for long distances.
8. The fine adjustment, for more accurate focusing especially at high magnifications; and used to move the stage for very short distances.
9. The draw tube, found on top of the body tube. It may be pulled upwards to give a greater magnification.

ii. **Optical parts:**
   1. **The light source:** Found below the stage and used to give light over the examined object. It may electrical or sun light.
   2. **The condenser:** Found between the light source and the stage. It increases illumination when high power objectives are in use.
   3. **The iris diaphragm:** Fitted at the base of the condenser. It controls the amount of light reaching to the object.
   4. **The objectives or object lenses:** Serve to form a real image of the object within the body tube. The objectives usually used in ordinary microscope are:
      a. Low–power objective (4X): It is used to have a view by the coarse adjustment.
      b. Mid–power objective (10X): It used to search the slide to find the objects.
      c. High–power objective (40X): It used to draw the objects.
      d. Oil immersion lens: (100X) this lens is used in bacteriological, cytological and other studies require the highest magnifications.
   5. The oculars or eyepieces: are other lenses, which fit on the top of the drawtube.

The magnification power of each of these lenses is marked on it, thus 5X, 10X, and 15X, these lenses serve for further magnification of the images produced by the objectives (Fig. 2.1).

EXPERIMENT 2

Aim: To study the section cutting technique of stem, root and leaf and staining and mounting of a section.

Theory
Section cutting of the stem, root and stolon

Different sections are obtained from the Stem, Root and Stolon depending upon the plane of cutting each section reveling detail from a different angle.

A. **Transverse section (TS)**

TS is obtained by cutting along the radial plane of cylindrical portion of stem, root, stolon and perpendicular to long axis.

B. **Longitudinal section (LS)**
   a. **Tangential longitudinal section:**
      A section cut along the long axis parallel to the tangent.
   b. **Radial longitudinal section:**
      A section cut along the long axis and the cutting plant passing through the long axis and radial.

Section of leaf

Leaf is an important aspects to study. Section through the midrib is taken perpendicularly and in case of bilateral leaves, observation of the surface preparation, i.e. either surface may be observed.

Section of bark

In case of bark TS is important as it reveals the horizontal arrangement of cell.

Section of fruit and seed

In case of fruits and seed, generally TS of various parts is observed under microscope.

Staining: Staining is a process in which chemical dyes are used to impart colour to various tissue. A section of drug sample, enable to distinguish the arrangement of various tissues in the sample.

Staining process: Take a clean watch glass and a staining solution in it. With the help of brush, transfer the section from water to stain solution and keep it for 2–3 min. Then transfer it in watch glass containing plain water, so that excess stain is washed away.

Mounting process: Take a clean slide. Transfer the section for study on it. Add 2–3 drops of water. If any air bubbles are seen, slightly lift the cover slip and add a drop of water and replace the cover slip. With a help of blotting paper, wipe excess of water present outside and observe under microscope.

EXPERIMENT 3

Aim: To measure the length and breadth of fibers in the given sample.

Requirement: Compound microscope, stage micrometer, eyepiece micrometer, chloral hydrate solution, phloroglucinol, hydrochloric acid and glycerin.

Theory

Fibers are made up of sclerenchymatous tissues. They are narrow with conspicuously pointed ends and lack intercellular spaces.

Fibers are of two types:

1. **Libriform fibers** are very long with simple and mostly oblique pits, e.g. fibers of cortex, pericycle and phloem.
2. **Tracheidal fibers** are short as compared to libriform and have bordered pits, e.g. fibers of xylem.

Fibers give mechanical support to plant. They also help in the identification of crude drugs.

Procedure

Calibrate the eyepiece micrometer under both low and high power using stage micrometer and calculate the factor. Boil a little quantity of powdered drug with chloral hydrate solution and stain with phloroglucinol and hydrochloric acid (1:1). Mount the stained sample in glycerin. Focus the fibers under high power and measure the breadth with help of the calibrated eyepiece micrometer by noting the number of divisions being covered by the fibers. Similarly focus the fibers in low power, measure the length using calibrated eyepieces micrometer. Multiply the number of divisions by the factor so as to get the actual dimensions of fibers in micrometer. Calculate the average value and report the maximum and minimum values.

Observation Table

Table 2.1: Calibrations of eyepiece micrometer at 10X

Sl. No.	Number of divisions of eyepiece micrometer	Number of divisions of stage micrometer	Calibrated value (µm)	Average value

Table 2.2: Calibrations of eyepiece micrometer at 40X

Sl. No.	Number of divisions of eyepiece micrometer	Number of divisions of stage micrometer	Calibrated value (µm)	Average value

Table 2.3: Length and breadth of fibres

Sl. No.	Length		Breadth	
	Number of division covered by fiber	Size (Number of divisions × calibrated value)	Number of divisions covered by fiber	Size (Number of divisions × calibrated value)

EXEPERIMENT 4

Aim: To measure the size of calcium oxalate crystals in the given powdered sample.

Requirement: Compound microscope, chloral hydrate solution, glycerin, stage micrometer, eye piece micrometer.

Theory

Calcium oxalate crystals are the by-products of diverse metabolic reactions occurring in plant cells. It is an excretory product of plants and is therefore deposited in various tissues. Crystals of calcium oxalate occurs in various tissues in different shapes.

1. Raphides: Needle shaped crystal
   Example: Colacasia, Boerhavia.
2. Sphaeroraphides or conglomerate crystals– groups of numerous prisms
   Example: Rhubarb, Senna leaf.
3. Prismatic: Prism shaped occur singly or in groups
   Example: Liquorice, Quassia wood
4. Rosette: Star shaped
   Example: arjuna bark
5. Microcrystals/microphenoid/fine sandy crystals: Amorphous mass.
   Example: Cinchona, Belladona leaf
   - Calcium oxalate crystals are very useful in identification of plant drugs, as different plant species differ in the form and arrangement of crystals which helps in identification and evaluation.
   - Chloral hydrate solution is a clearing agent and it aids in the clear visualization of calcium oxalate crystals.

Pizzoloto method for observation of calcium oxalate crystals:

Place uniformly a thin section of the drug in 2N acetic acid for 15 minutes. Remove and treat with 1% solution of silver nitrate in 15% hydrogen peroxide. After 15 minutes remove the sections and wash with distilled water. Stain the sections with 2% safranin solution. Mount the section on a slide and observe under the microscope. Black crystals of calcium oxalate are seen against the red background.

Procedure

Calibrate the eyepiece micrometer using stage micrometer under high powder and calculate the factor. Heat the powdered sample with chloral hydrate solution. Mount the cleared powdered sample in glycerin. Focus the calcium oxalate crystals under high power and measures the size with the help of eyepiece micrometer by counting the numbers of divisions being covered by the crystals. Multiply the number of divisions by the factor so as to get the actual dimensions of calcium oxalate crystals in micrometer. Calculate the average value and note the minimum and maximum value.

Observation Table

Table 2.4: Calibrations of eyepiece micrometer at 40X

Sl.No.	Number of divisions of eyepiece micrometer	Number of divisions of stage micrometer	Calibrated value (μm)	Average value
1				
2				
3				
4				

Table 2.5: Size of calcium oxalate crystals

Sl. No.	Number of divisions covered by the crystal	Size in micrometer (number of divisions × average calibrated value)
1.		
2.		
3.		
4.		
5.		
6.		
7.		
8.		
9.		
10.		
11.		
12.		
13.		
14.		
15.		

EXPERIMENT 5

Aim: To measure the diameter of starch grains in the given powdered sample.

Requirement: Compound microscope, stage micrometer, eyepiece micrometer, lactophenol.

Theory

Starch, a polysaccharide is a food product and occurs in the form of grains in all green plants. The principle source of starch are maize (Zeamays; Graminae), Rice (*Oryza sativa*; Graminae), potato (*Solanum tuberosum*; Solanaceae), wheat (*Triticum aestivum*: Graminae) starch grains are of particular shape and size and differ in different plants. Each starch grain has a dark rounded spot known as hilum which is surrounded by layers of starch. Starch grains depending upon the position of hilum can be divided in to two categories:

1. *Eccentric:* Hilum situated towards one side.
2. *Concentric:* Hilum is situated at the center.

Starch grains are of two types depending upon the number of hilum.

1. *Simple:* one hilum
2. *Compound:* more than one hilum

Example: potato starch

Type: Simple and compound

Shape: Subspherical or ovoid

Size: 20–100 μm

Hilum and striations: Eccentric hilum is surrounded by well marked concentric striations.

Table 2.6: Calibrations of eyepiece micrometer at 40X

Sl. No.	Number of divisions of eyepiece micrometer	Number of divisions of stage micrometer	Calibrated value (μm)	Average value
1.				
2.				
3.				
4.				

Table 2.7: Size of calcium oxalate crystals

Sl. No.	Number of divisions covered by the particles	Size in micrometer (number of divisions × average calibrated value)
1.		
2.		
3.		
4.		
5.		
6.		
7.		
8.		
9.		
10.		
11.		
12.		
13.		
14.		
15.		

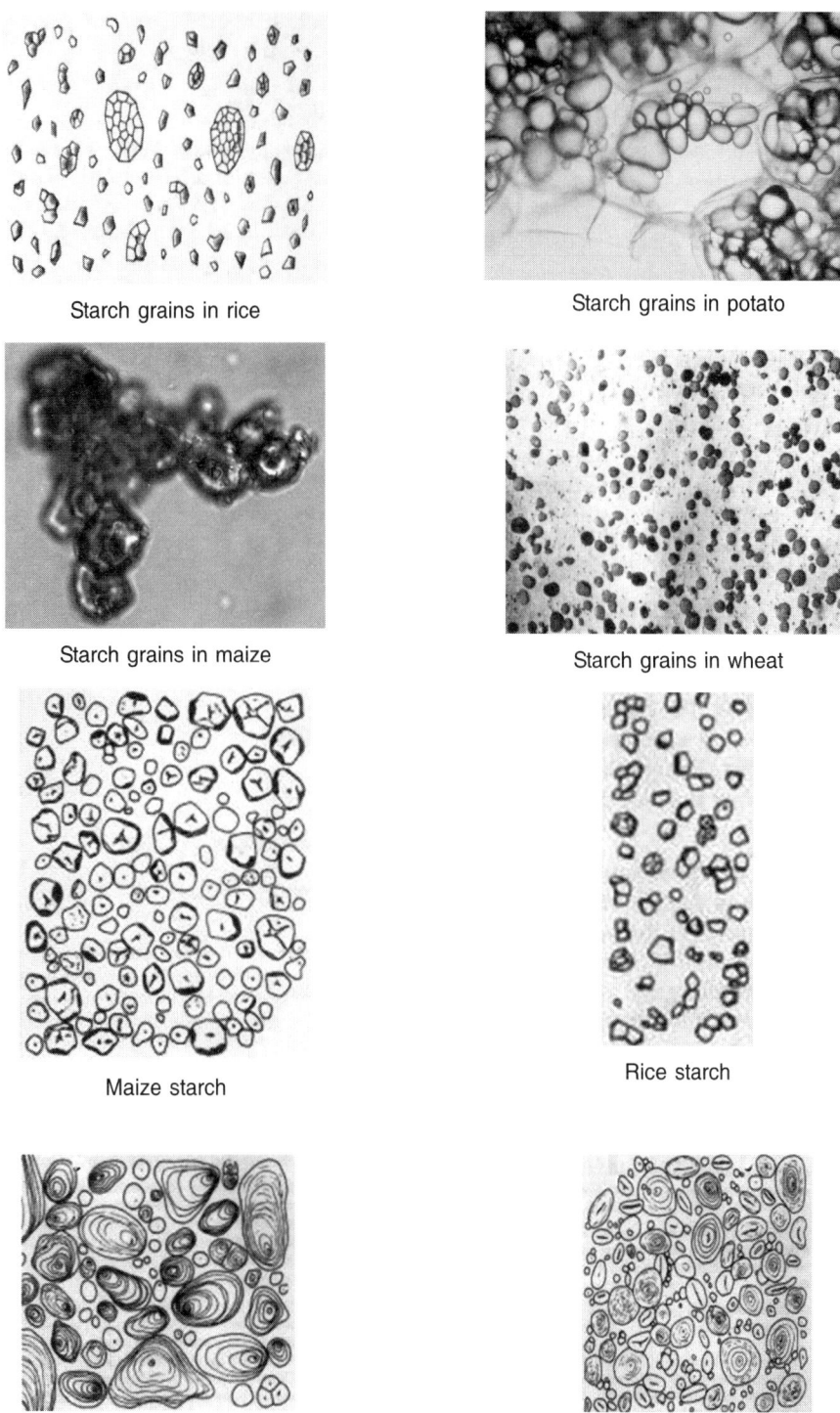

Fig. 2.2: Microscopy of different types of starch grains

Procedure

Calibrate the eyepiece micrometer using stage micrometer under high power and calculate the factor. Suspend the drug powder in lactophenol water mixture (1:1) stain with dilute iodine solution (2%). Place a drop of this suspension on a clean glass slide and place the cover slip over it. Focus the starch grain under high power and measure the size with the help of eyepiece micrometer by counting the number of divisions being covered by the starch grains. Multiply the number of divisions by the factor so as to get the actual dimension of starch grains in micrometer. Calculate the average value and repeat the minimum and maximum values.

EXPERIMENT 6

Aim: To determine the palisade ratio in the leaf sample.

Requirement: Compound microscope, stage micrometer, camera lucida, chloral hydrate solution, glycerol.

Theory

Palisade ratio is defined as the average number of palisade cells beneath each epidermal cell. It can be determined with powdered drugs. Palisade ratio is constant for a given species of the plant and is used as characteristic for the identification of the allied species. For example senna varieties are distinguished by the palisade ratio.

Procedure

Cut a piece of leaf from the lamina region. Clear the leaf piece by boiling in chloral hydrate solution and mount the cleared leaf piece in glycerol. Fix the camera lucida to the microscope and at low power trace off the outlines of four cells of epidermis. Focus over the palisade layer and trace off the cells to cover the tracings of the epidermal walls. Count the palisade cells under the four epidermal cells while counting the palisade cells; a cell is being counted if at least half of its area lies within the area of epidermal cell. Calculate the average number of cells beneath a single epidermal cell.

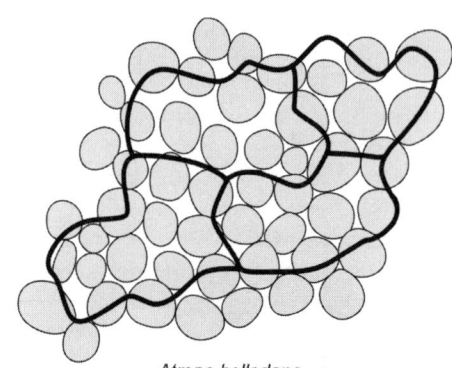
Atropa belladona

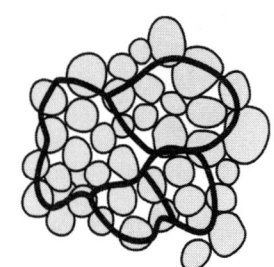
Datura stramonium

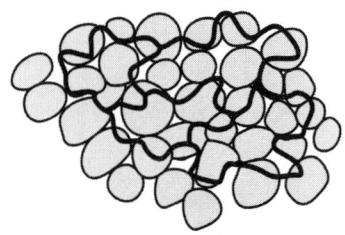
Scopolia carniolica

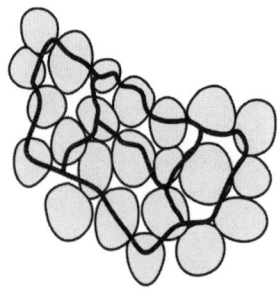
Solanum nigrum

Fig. 2.3: Cell count

Observation Table

Table 2.8: Objective lensing power

Sl. No.	Optical combination	Number of palisade cells beneath four epidermal cells	Average number of palisade cells
1.	5X × 10X		
2.	5X × 10X		
3.	5X × 10X		
4.	5X × 10X		

EXPERIMENT 7

Aim: To determine the stomata number and stomata index of leaf.

Requirement: Compound microscope, stage micrometer, camera lucida, chloral hydrate solution, glycerol.

Theory

Stomata number is the average number of stomata per square mm of the epidermis of the leaf. Stomatal index is the percentage by which the number of stomata forms to the total number of epidermal cells; each stomata being counted as one cell. It is determined by the using the formula

$SI = S/(S + E) \times 100$

S = No. of stomata per unit area

E = No. of epidermal cells in the same unit area

The actual number of stomata/mm^2, may vary for the leaves of the same plant grown in different environmental conditions. But the stomata index is constant for any age of the plant and plants grown under different climatic conditions.

Procedure

Peel off the epidermis and clear it by heating with chloral hydrate solution. Mount in glycerin. Fix up the camera lucida to microscope and draw a square on a black paper under high power using stage micrometer. Remove the stage micrometer and place the prepared slide. Trace the epidermal cells and stomata in the squares already prepared. Count the number of stomata and epidermal cells in the square. While counting the epidermal cells, a cell is being counted if at least half of its area lies within the square provided two adjacent sides are considered for the purpose of counting.

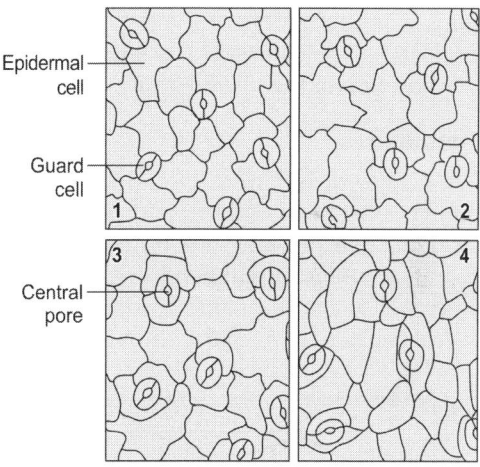

Fig. 2.4: Stomata number

Observation Table

Table 2.9: Calculation of stomatal index

Square number	Number of epidermal cells in 1 mm^2 area	Number of stomata in 1 mm^2 area	Stomata number	Stomatal index

EXPERIMENT 8

Aim: To determine the *vein islet number* and *vein termination number* of leaf.

Requirement: Compound microscope, stage micrometer, camera lucida, chloral hydrate solution, glycerin.

Theory

Vein islet is a small area of the green tissue encircled by the veins (vein islets).

Vein islet number is the number of vein islets present per square mm of the leaf surface midway between midrib and margin.

Veinlet termination number is number of veinlet terminations per square mm of the leaf surface midway between midrib and margin. An ultimate free end or termination of a vein islet is called as *veinlet termination*.

Vein islet number and *veinlet termination number* are constant for a given species of the plant and are used as a characteristic for the identification of the allied species.

Procedure

Cut a piece of leaf from the middle region lamina between the midrib and the margin. Clear the leaf piece by boiling with chloral hydrate solution. Mount the cleared leaf piece in glycerin. Fit the camera lucida to the microscopes and prepare square of using

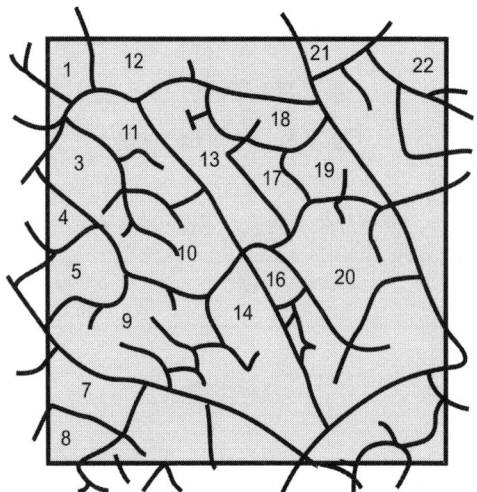

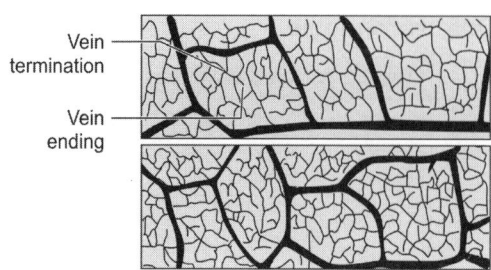

Fig. 2.5: Veinlet termination and vein islets number

stage micrometer in low power on a white paper. Replace the stage micrometer with the prepared slide and trace the vein islets in the drown squares in low power using 5X eyepiece. Count the number of vein islets and veinlet terminations present within the square and also taking into consideration incomplete vein islets on any two adjacent sides of the square. Calculate the average number of *vein islets* and *veinlet termination number* from the four adjoining squares.

Observation Table

Table 2.10: Calculation of vein termination and vein islets no

Square	Optical combination	Vein islet number	Veinlet termination number
1.	5X × 10X		
2.	5X × 10X		
3.	5X × 10X		
4.	5X × 10X		

EXPERIMENT 9

Aim: To determine the swelling index of the given sample drug.

Requirement: Stoppered measuring cylinder.

Theory

Swelling index is the volume in ml taken up by one gram of plant material under specified conditions. Many medicinal plant materials are of specific therapeutic or pharmaceutical utility for their swelling properties, especially gums and those containing an appreciable amount of mucilage, pectin and starch. Drug such as ispaghula and linseed containing mucilage are used for their demulcent and laxatives properties. The determination is based on addition of water or a swelling agent as given in the list procedures for an individual plant material. The volume occupied by the one gram of the plant material is majored including the sticky mucilage.

Procedure

Accurately weigh the specified quantity of sample powder (isapgol seeds: *Plantago ovata*) and place in a 25 ml of stoppered cylinder. Add 25 ml of water to it. Agitate gently and occasionally during 24 hr and allow to stand for one hour. The volume occupied by the seeds including the sticky mucilage is measured. The difference in the final and initial volumes indicates the swelling index. Perform in triplicate.

Calculation

Swelling index = Final volume – initial volume

EXPERIMENT 10

Aim: To determine the total ash, acid insoluble ash and water soluble ash of the given crude drug.

Requirement: Silica crucibles, ashless filter paper, funnels, dilute hydrochloric acid, muffle furnace and distilled water.

Theory

The residue remaining after the incineration is the ash content of the drug which consists of inorganic material (metallic salts and silica). A high ash value is indicative of contamination, substitution, adulteration or carelessness in preparation of crude drug. Different types of ash values are used such as total ash, acid insoluble ash and water soluble ash.

1. *Total ash:* It is the measure of the amount of material remaining after ignition. This includes "physiological ash" which is derived from the tissue itself and "non physiological ash" which is residue of the extraneous matter (e.g. sand and soil) adhering to the plant surface. Total ash consists of carbonates, phosphates, silicates and silica.

2. *Acid insoluble ash:* It is the part of total ash which is insoluble in dilute hydrochloric acid. This measures the amount of silica present as sand and siliceous earth.

3. *Water soluble ash:* It is the part of total ash which is soluble in water. It is used to detect the presence of exhausted drug.

Procedure

1. Total ash
- Weigh accurately 2–3 gm of the air dried crude drug in tared platinum or silica dish and incinerate at a temperature not exceeding 450°C until free from carbon, cool and weigh.
- If a carbon free ash cannot be obtained in this way, exhaust the charred mass with hot water, collect the residue on an ashless filter paper, incinerate the residue and filter paper until the ash turns white or nearly so, add the filtrate, evaporate to dryness and ignite at a temperature not exceeding 450°C,
- Calculate the percentage of ash with the reference to the air dried drug.

2. Acid insoluble ash
- Boil the total ash with 25 ml of 2N HCl for 5 min, collect the insoluble matter on an ashless filter paper, wash with hot water, ignite, cool in dessicator and weigh.
- Calculate the percentage of acid insoluble ash with reference to the air dried drug.

3. Water soluble ash
- Boil the ash for 5 min with 25 ml of water, collect the insoluble matter on

an ashless filter paper. Wash with hot water and ignite for 15 min at a temperature not exceeding 450°C. Subtract the weight of the insoluble matter from the weight of the ash, the difference in weight represents the water soluble ash.
- Calculate the percentage of water soluble ash with reference to the air dried drug.

Calculation

i. **Total ash value:**

Weight of empty dish = A

Weight of the drug taken = B

Weight of the dish + ash (after complete incineration) = C

Weight of the ash = $(C - A)$ gm

X gm of the crude drug gives $(C - A)$ gm of the ash

Therefore, 100 gm of drug gives = $(C - A)/X \times 100$ gm of ash

II. **Acid insoluble ash:**

Weight of the ash = Y gm

X gm of drug gives = Y gm of acid insoluble ash

Therefore, 100 gm of drug gives = $Y/X \times 100$ gm acid insoluble ash

iii. **Water Soluble ash:**

Weight of water insoluble ash = Z gm

Therefore, water soluble ash = Total ash $(C - A)$ – Water insoluble ash (Z) = W gm

X gm of drug gives W gm of ash

100 gm of drug gives = $W/X \times 100$ gm of ash

EXPERIMENT 11

Aim: To determine the extractive value of the given crude drug.

Requirement: Stoppered flask, alcohol, ether, water, funnel, filter paper.

Theory

Extractive value gives an idea about the amount of active principles present in the plant drug when extracted with solvents. Different solvents like ethyl alcohol, chloroform, water and diethyl ether are used to determine the extractive value but the amount of phytoconstituents in the particular solvent depends upon the chemical nature of drug and solvent. This method is employed for those materials for which no chemical or biological assay method exists. It is used for the evaluation of crude drug.

Procedure

To a 5 gm of air dried coarsely powdered drug add 100 ml of solvent (90% alcohol in case of alcohol soluble extractive value, similarly ether and chloroform water for ether and water soluble extractive values respectively) in stoppered flask for 24 hr, shaking frequently for first 6 hours and allowing to stand for 18 hours. After 24 hours, filter rapidly. Take 25 ml of filtrate and evaporate to dryness in a tared flat bottomed shallow dish at 100°C and weigh. Calculate the percentage of extractive value with reference to the air dried drug.

Calculation

Weight of empty china dish = a gm

Weight of empty china dish + residue = b gm

Weight of residue = $b - a = c$ gm

25 ml of extract gives = c gm of the residue

Therefore 100 ml of extract will give = $c/25 \times 100$ gm of residue

= $4c$ gm of residue

5 gm of air dried drug give = $4c$ gm of residue

Therefore, 100 gm of air dried drug will give = $4c/5 \times 100$ gm of residue

= $80c$ gm of soluble residue.

EXPERIMENT 12

Aim: To determine the moisture content of given crude drug by loss on drying method.

Requirement: Crude drug sample, petriplate, desiccators.

Theory
Moisture content of crude drug determine its chemical and microbial stability, as presence of high water content in crude drugs favours microbial growth and enzymatic destruction of active principles. Therefore, it becomes necessary to set limits for water content of crude drug especially for those materials which absorb moisture easily or deteriorate quickly in the presence of water.

Procedure
Place 2 gm of sample drug in a tared petriplate. Dry in oven at 105°C for one hour, cool in a desiccators and weigh. Repeat the procedure till the two consecutive readings are same. The moisture content is expressed in percentage with reference to the air dried drug.

Calculation
Weight of empty petriplate (*a*) = ?
Weight of sample + petriplate (*b*) = ?
Weight of sample *I* = ?
After heating for 1 hour
Weight of petriplate + drug (*d*) = ?
Therefore, loss on drying = *d* − *b* = *e*
% moisture content of the given crude drug sample =
(loss on drying/weight of sample) × 100

EXPERIMENT 13

Aim: To study the morphological, microscopical and powder characteristics of leaf of *Digitalis lanata*.

Theory
Synonym Fox glove leaf, Austrian digitalis
Biological source It consist of dried leaves of *Digitalis lanata*; family Scrophulariaceae

Morphology
a. *Type* simple
b. *Shape* linear lanceolate to oblong lanceolate
c. *Margin* entire
d. *Apex* acuminate
e. *Petiole* absent (sessile)
f. *Size* long up to 30 cm and broad up to 4 cm
g. *Colour* green
h. *Odour* faint
i. *Taste:* bitter

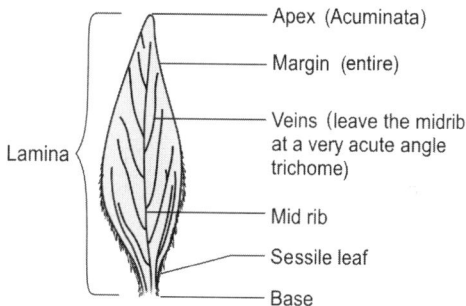

Fig. 2.6: Microscopy of *Digitalis lanata*

Microscopy
The leaf is dorsiventral type. In the lamina and mid rib region following tissue are present:
A. Lamina:
   a. **Upper epidermis:** It is single layered, covered with thick cuticle, very less number of glandular trichomes (when compare to *D purpurea*) with unicellular stalk and unicellular or bicellular head are seen. Stomata are also occasionally present.
   b. **Mesophyll:** Differentiated into:
      i. **Palisade:** bilayered, loosely arranged and absent above vascular bundles of lamina region.
      ii. **Spongy parenchyma:** multilayered, transversely cut vascular bundles are present, same as in midrib.
   c. **Lower epidermis:** Same as upper epidermis but has numerous stomata.

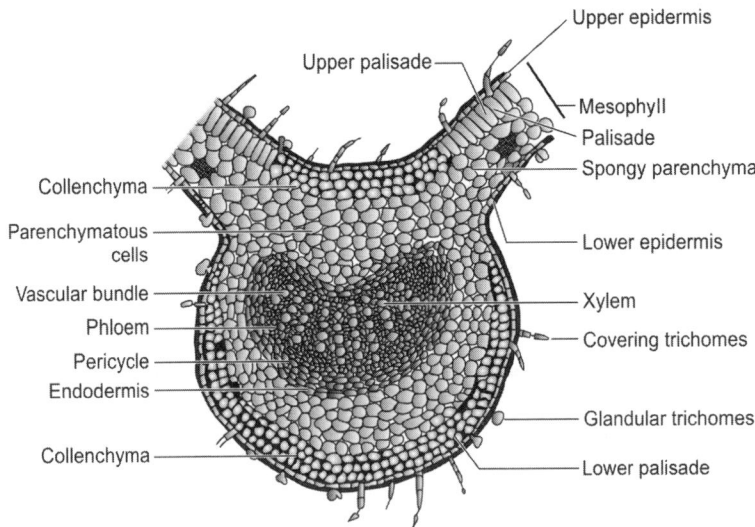

Fig. 2.7: Microscopy of *Digitalis lanata*

B. Midrib: Almost triangular in outline with pronounced pointed projection on dorsal side. Cells of epidermal layer are smaller in midrib region when compared to that of lamina region. Remaining tissues are identical to the *D purpurea*.

In the centre of the midrib an arc shaped vascular bundle is present which is surrounded by one or two layer of endodermis containing starch. Xylem is seen towards the ventral (upper) surface while phloem is present below it towards the dorsal (lower) surface. Inside endodermis, pericycle is present which is parenchymatous below the phloem.

Surface preparation reveals straight or slightly heavy walls of upper epidermis and more heavy walls of lower epidermis as well as presence of anomocytic type of stomata and trichomes.

Chemical Constituents

It contains five primary glycosides and in all about 70 cardiac glycosides. The primary glycosides identified as lantoside A, B, C, D and E. It also includes digoxigenin and diginatigenin.

Diginatigenin

Powder microscopy: It shows the following identifying characters

i. **Trichomes:**

a. **Covering trichomes:** numerous, multicellular with acute apex, finely warty cuticle and collapsed cells.

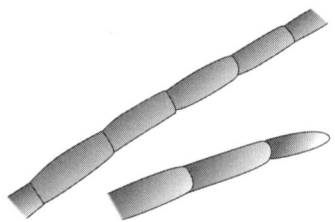

Fig. 2.8: Covering trichomes in *Digitalis lanata*

b. **Glandular trichomes:** less in number, with unicellular stalk and a unicellular or bicellular head.

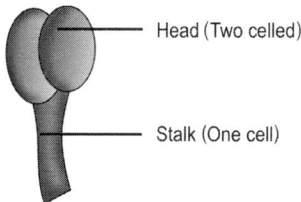

Fig. 2.9: Glandular trichomes *in Digitalis*

ii. **Stomata:** anomocytic or ranunculaceous type.

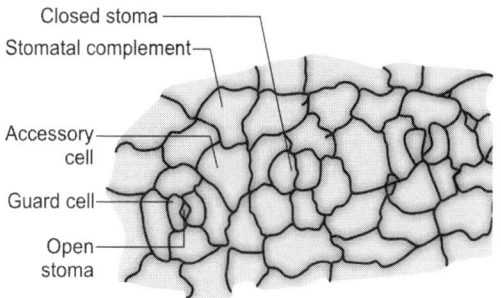

Fig. 2.10: Stomata in *Digitalis*

iii. **Calcium oxalate crystals and sclerenchymatous fibre** are absent.

iv. **Chemical tests:**
   a. *Legal's test (for glycosides and aglycones)*: Add sodium nitroprusside solution to the leaf extract in pyridine. Make the solution alkaline with sodium hydroxide solution. Pink or red colour appears.
   b. *Killer–Kiliani test (for digitoxose)*: Boil the powdered drug with 70% alcohol and then filter. To the filtrate add a few ml of distilled water and a few drops of strong solution of lead acetate. Shake well and filter. Treat the clear filtrate with equal volume of chloroform. Separate the chloroform layer and evaporate the chloroform. Dissolve the residue in glacial acetic acid and add ferric chloride solution drop by drop. Add concentrated sulpphuric acid from the side of the test tube. A reddish brown ring is developed between the two rings which turned bluish green on standing (due to presence of digitoxose).
   c. *Baljet test (for aglycones and glycosides)*: Yellow to orange colour is observed when leaf section is treated with sodium picrate reagent.

Substituents

1. *Digitalis lutea* (Straw foxglove)
2. *Digitalis thapsi* (Spanis foxglove)
3. *Digitalis purpurea*
4. *Digitalis dubia*

Uses: It is used in the treatment of congestive heart failure, supraventricular arrhythmia, atrial fibrillation, atrial flutter and paroxysomal atrial tachycardia (cardiotonic).

EXPERIMENT 14

Aim: To study the morphological, microscopical and powder Characteristics of leaf of *Digitalis purpurea*.

Theory

Synonym: Purple foxglove leaves

Biological source: *Digitalis* consists of the dried leaves of *Digitalis purpurea*; family Scrophulariaceae

Morphology

a. *Type* simple
b. *Venation* pinnate, veins curving towards apex and near the margin.
c. *Shape* ovate lanceolate to broadly ovate
d. *Margin* crenate or dentate
e. *Apex* subacute

f. *Surface* both are hair; upper surface – pubescent and lower surface – strongly pubescent
g. *Petiole* petiolate
h. *Colour* dark grayish green (dried leaves)
i. *Size* 10–30 cm (L); 4–10 cm (W)
j. *Odour* no marked odour
k. *Taste* bitter

A. **Lamina:**

a. **Upper epidermis:**

It is single layered consists of rectangular cells with a distinct cuticle. Covering and glandular trichomes emerges from this layer. Few stomata (anomocytic type revealed in surface preparation) are also seen.

b. **Mesophyll:**

It lies between upper and lower epidermis. It is divided into:

i. **Palisade:** single layered made up of compactly arranged radially elongated cells.

ii. **Spongy parenchyma:** 4–6 layered and mainly obliquely cut veinlets are seen.

c. **Lower epidermis:**

Similar to upper epidermis but has more anomocytic stomata and glandular trichomes as compared to upper epidermis.

B. **Midrib:**

The epidermal layers continue over the midrib region. Below and above epidermal

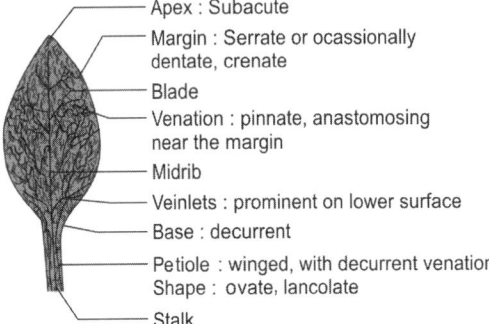

Fig. 2.11: Digitalis leaf

Microscopy

Leaf of *Digitalis purpurea* is dorsiventral (bifacial) in nature. Different tissues in the lamina and midrib region as follows –

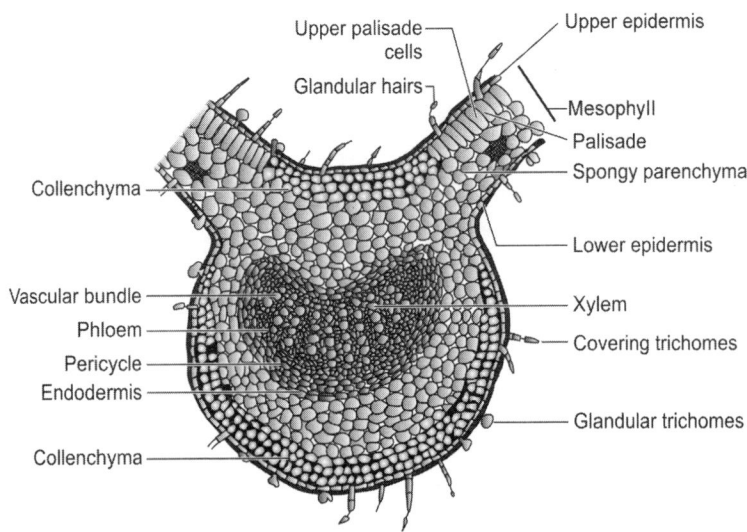

Fig. 2.12: Microscopy of *Digitalis purpurea*

layers, few layers of mesophyll are present. Remaining tissue of the midrib are cortical parenchyma.

Surface preparation: revealed irregularly beaded anticlinal walls of the epidermal cells (diagnostic feature), anomocytic stomata.

Chemical Constituents

Digitalis contains glycoside A and B and glucogitaloxin and primary glycosides possessing at C 3 of the aglycone, a linear chain of 3 digitoxose moieties terminated by glucose. Digitalis also contains several other glycosides such as odoroside H, gitaloxin, verodoxin and glucoverodoxin. The products of hydrolysis of purpurea glycoside A and purpurea glycoside B, the chief active constituents of the drug are digitoxigenin and gitoxigenin. Additionally it contains 2 saponin glycosides such as digitonin and gitonin.

Powder Microscopy

A. Epidermal Cells: Irregularly beaded cells.

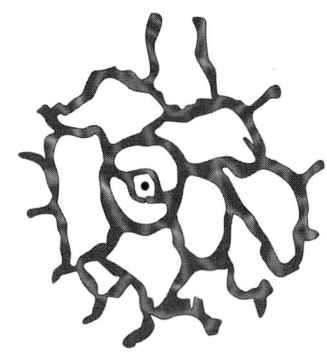

Fig. 2.13: Epidermal cells

B. Stomata: Anomocytic type and the subsidiary cells are not differentiated from the other epidermal cells.

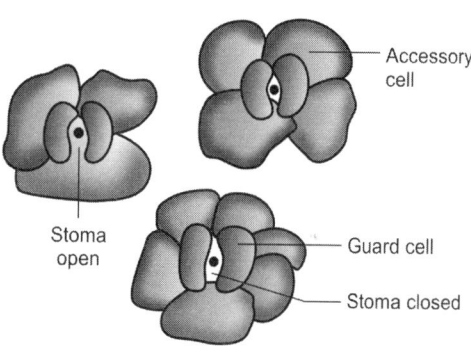

Fig. 2.14: Types of stomata

C. Trichomes: Very rare; two types:

a. **Covering trichomes:** 10 – 14 celled

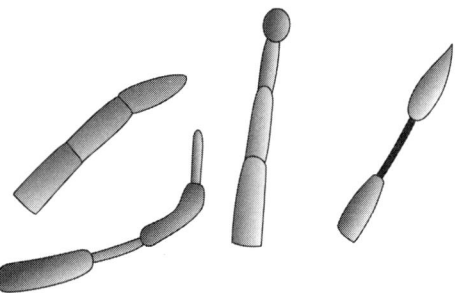

Fig. 2.15: Types of covering trichomes

b. **Glandular trichomes:** Unicellular stalk and bicellular head or with unicellular head and 2–8 celled uniseriate stalk.

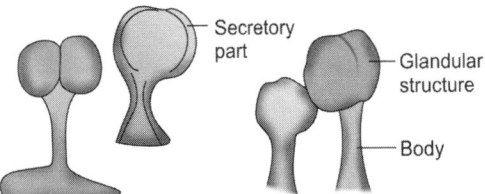

Fig. 2.16: Types of glandular trichomes

Note – Pericyclic fibres and crystal of calcium oxalate are absent.

Chemical Tests

Legal's test (for glycosides and aglycones): Add sodium nitropruside solution to the leaf extract in pyridine. Make the solution alkaline with sodium hydroxide solution. Pink or red colour is produced.

Keller–Kiliani test (for digitoxose): Boil the powdered drug with 70% alcohol and then filter. To the filtrate, add a few ml of distilled water and a few drops of strong solution of lead acetate. Shake well and filter. Treat the clear filtrate with equal volume of chloroform. Separate the chloroform layer and evaporate the chloroform. Dissolve the residue in glacial acetic acid and add ferric chloride solution drop by drop. Add concentrated sulphuric acid from the side of the test tube. A reddish brown ring is developed between the two rings which turned bluish green on standing (due to presence of digitoxose).

Baljet test (for aglycones and glycosides): Yellow to orange colour is observed when leaf section is treated with sodium picrate reagent.

Adulterants

1. *Verbascum thapsus*; family Scrophulariaceae
2. *Primula vulgaris*; family Primulaceae
3. *Symphytum officinale*; family Boraginaceae

Uses: It is used in the treatment of congestive heart failure, supraventricular arrhythmia, atrial fibrillation, atrial flutter and paroxysomal atrial tachycardia.

EXPERIMENT 15

Aim: To study microscopical powder, characteristics of Digitalis leaf.

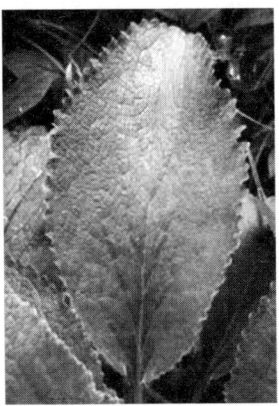

Fig. 2.17: Digitalis leaf

Synonym: *Digitalis purpurea* L, Digitalis leaf, Foxglove Leaf.

Biological Source: Digitalis consists of dried leaves of *Digitalis purpurea*.

Family: Scrophulariaceae.

A pale green powder with a slight odour and a bitter taste.

The diagnostic characters are:

a. The fragment of the *lamina in surface view*. The *upper epidermis* is composed of rather irregularly shaped cells with slightly thickened walls which may show slight beading and pitting; stomata are absent or very infrequent; the underlying palisade cells are fairly large and loosely packed. The *lower epidermis* is composed of smaller cells with thinner, conspicuously sinuous walls; circular *anomocytic stomata* are very abundant. Both upper and lower epidermis show occasional *cicatrices* where trichomes were attached; those formed by the glandular trichomes occur in the center of a smaller cell in the epidermis, while those formed by the covering trichomes occur either in the center of a single cell or over the junction of two or more epidermal cells.

b. The *trichomes*, both *covering* the *glandular* types; they are found scattered and attached to fragments of the epidermis. The covering trichomes are very numerous; they are uniseriate, usually three to five cells long, conical and bluntly pointed with thin, faintly warty walls; frequently one or more of the cells may be collapsed. The glandular trichomes are of two types; those which are more numerous are composed of a single-celled stalk and a bicellular (or rarely unicellular) head; others, less numerous, have a uniseriate multicellular stalk and a unicellular head.

c. The occasional fragments of thin-walled *parenchyma* from the cortex of the midrib and the larger veins composed of longitudinally elongated cells.

d. Fragments of the *epidermis* and *underlying tissues* occasionally occur in *sectional view* but complete sections through the lamina are rare; the epidermal cells may show slight pitting on the side walls. The leaf is dorsiventral but sometimes the palisade is not well differentiated.

EXPERIMENT 16

Aim: To study the morphological, microscopical and powder Characteristics of Senna leaf.

Procedure

Synonym: Sonamukhi, Indian Senna, Tinnevelley Senna, Swarn patti

Biological Source: It consists of dried leaflets of *Cassia angustifolia*, contains not less than 2.0% of glycosides calculated as Sennoside B.

Family: Leguminosae

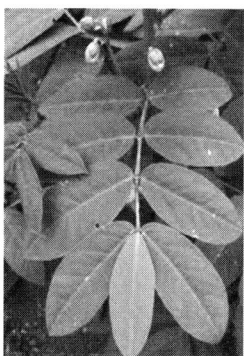

Fig. 2.18: Senna leaf

Morphology

- *General appearance:* Entire and less broken
- *Size:* 2.5 to 6 cm long; 7 to 8 mm wide
- *Shape:* Lanceolate
- *Margin:* Entire
- *Venation:* Pinnate, veins anastomosing towards margin
- *Apex:* Less acute with sharp spine at the apex
- *Base:* Less asymmetrical
- *Surface:* Less pubescent with press makings
- *Texture:* Firm, flexible
- *Colour:* Pale green
- *Odour:* Faint
- *Taste:* Mucilaginous and slightly bitter

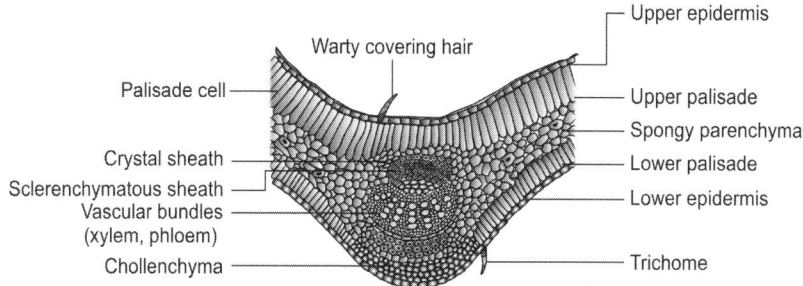

Fig. 2.19: TS of Senna leaf

Surface Preparation

Paracytic stomata: Rubiaceous or parallel celled stomata with two subsidiary cells around the guard cells.

Epidermal cells: Polygonal, thin and straight walled, parenchymatous.

Trichome: Covering unicellular, conical, bulbous base, thick walled, pitted, lie appressed to epidermis.

Transverse Section

Lamina: Isobilateral

Upper epidermis: Single layered, polygonal, straight, anticlinal walls, few cells contain mucilage, epidermis is covered with cuticle.

Lower epidermis: Similar to upper epidermis.

Trichomes: Conical, unicellular, thick walled, covering trichome, distinctly warty.

Stomata: Paracytic type (Rubiaceous)

Mesophyll

Upper Palisade: Single layered, elongated, compactly arranged, narrow, thin walled parenchyma, continued over midrib region.

Spongy Parenchyma: Thin walled, loosely arranged, large intracellular spaces, spheroaphides present.

Lower Palisade: Only in lamina, loosely arranged, large wavy walls, cells smaller than upper palisade

Midrib

Palisade parenchyma: Single layer.

Crystal sheath: Parenchymatous layer containing calcium oxalate prism. Present at dorsal and ventral side.

Sclerenchymatous sheath: Lignified, thick walled cells, covering the vascular bundle.

Vascular bundle:

Xylem: Lignified cells, present at ventral surface.

Phloem: Nonlignified cells present at dorsal surface.

Collenchyma: Multilayered, thick walled parenchyma containing cellulose. Present only at ventral side

Microscopical Characteristics of Powdered Drugs

Epidermal cells–stomata and trichome–xylem vessels–Calcium–oxalate crystals

Epidermal cells: Polygonal, straight walled, epidermal cells with paracytic stomata.

Paracytic stomata: Rubiaceous or parallel celled stomata with two subsidiary cells around the guard cells.

Covering trichomes: Unicellular, thick warty walls, acute apex, bulbous base, narrow lumen, conical shape.

Length = 70–260 µm

Width = 12–18–25 µm

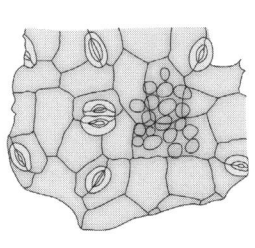 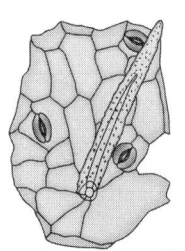 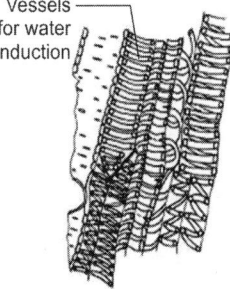 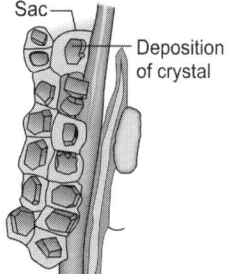

Epidermal cells　　Stomata and trichome　　Xylem vessels　　Calcium oxalate

Fig. 2.20: Microscopic characterstic of powdered drug

Xylem vessels: Angular thickening, lignified

Calcium oxalate: Crystal isolated or in parenchymatous cells. Very abundant, occur as prism and also as cluster crystals.

Staining and Microchemical Tests:

1. Add conc. HCl (1:1) to phloroglucinol: Red coloured lignified tissue: Xylem sclerenchyma observed.
2. Rhuthenium Red: Red/pink mucilagenous cells of epidermis observed.
3. With Sudan Red III: Red cutical observed.
4. With acetic acid: insoluble calcium oxalate crystals observed.
5. With 60% sulphuric acid: Crystal soluble calcium sulphate needle observed.

Chemical Constitutents

Mainly anthraquinone glycosides: Sennosides A, B, C and D

Chemical Tests

Anthraquinone (Borntrager test): Hydrolyse the leaf powder by boiling with sulfuric acid and the filter. Add carbon tetrachloride/benzene to the filtrate and shake the tube. Add strong ammonia solution to the organic layer, shake and set aside for some time. Red/pink colour of the aqueous layer shows presence of anthraquinone.

Uses: Irritant purgative.

Preparation

Ingredient of compound Liquorice powder IP

Allied Drugs and Substitutes

1. Arabian, Bombay and Mecca senna.(*Cassia angustifolia*)
   i. Leaflets more elongated and darken in colour.
   ii. Veinislet number is different.
2. **Dog senna (*Cassia obvota*):**
   i. Leaves are broadly obovate with abruptly tapering apexes, the venation is pinnate.
   ii. Lower epidermis shows papillose cells.
      a. Argel leaves (*Solenostemma argel*)
         Family –Asclepiadaceae
         i. Texture is thick and rigid.
         ii. Surface is finely wrinkled.
         iii. Base is equal.
         iv. Leaves are curved or twisted.
         iv. Two or three celled hairs.

B. To study the morphology of Senna pods

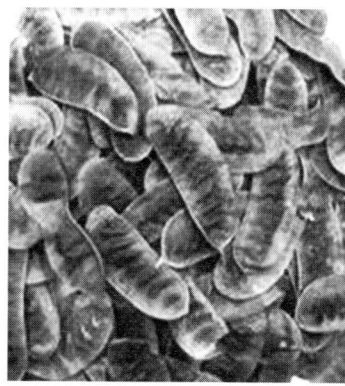

Fig. 2.21: Senna pods

Biological Source

Senna pods are the dried ripe fruits of *Cassia senna* L. (*Cassia acutifolia Delile*) known as Alexandrian senna pods and of *Cassia angustifolia* Vahl known as Tinnevelly Senna pods.

Family: Leguminosae

Morphology

- *General appearance:* Superior, unilocular laterally flattened, dehiscing by both sutures
- *Size:* About 5 cm long and 1.5 to 2 cm broad
- *Shape:* Oblong and sutures slightly curved
- *Surface:* Brownish-green, veins less prominent and less regular
- *Apex:* Rounded, on the ventral surface, remains of the style distinct.
- *Seeds:* 5–8 attached to the ventral surface by funicle.

- *Colour:* Dark chocolate brown
- *Odour:* Sickly
- *Taste:* Sweet

EXPERIMENT 17

Aim: To study the morphological, microscopical and powder Characteristics of Vinca leaf.

Theory

Synonym: Catharanthus, Sada phuli, Periwinkle, Barmasi, Sadabahar

Biological Source: It is dried whole plant of *Catharanthus roseus*, G. Don.

Family: Apocyanaceae.

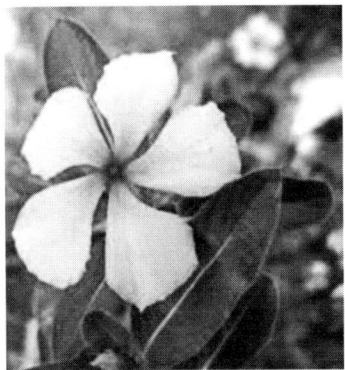

Fig. 2.22: Vinca leaf and flower

Morphology

- *General appearance:* Erect, pubescent herb with branched tap-root
- *Size:* 2–3 cm in length, 1.0–1.2 cm in width
- *Shape:* Ovate or oblong
- *Apex:* Acute
- *Base:* Petiolate
- *Margin:* Entire
- *Surface:* Pubescent

Organoleptic Characters

Colour: Green.

Odour: Faint.

Taste: Bitter.

Microscopy

Surface Preparation

Epidermal cell: Rectangular cells. Thin and straight walled.

Covering trichomes: Unicellular with bulbous base, warty.

Stomata: Anisocytic or unequal celled stomata. Three subsidiary cells, one is smaller than other two.

Transverse Section

- *Lamina:* Dorsiventral nature.

  Upper Epidermis: Single layered, rectangular cells, the outer wall of which is cuticularized. Covering trichomes and anisocytic stomata are also present.

  Lower Epidermis: Similar to upper epidermis but number of stomata are more.

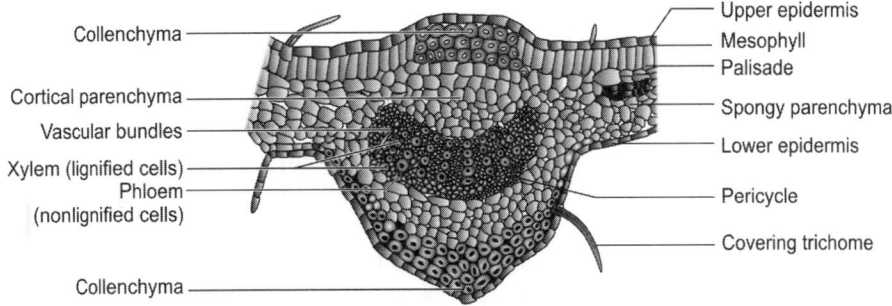

Fig. 2.23: TS of Vinca leaf

Covering trichome: From epidermal layer, which are unicellular, long, dagger shaped, warty with bulbous base.
- *Mesophyll: Palisade:* Single layered cells, elongated and compact.
  Spongy parenchyma: Five to eight layered cells, loosely arranged with intercellular spaces. Vascular strands are seen, but calcium oxalate crystals are absent.
- *Midrib:*
  Collenchyma: Strips of spongy parenchyma appear below the upper epidermis, and above lower epidermis.
  Vascular bundle: Xylem: Lignified.
  Phloem: Nonlignified.

Microscopical Characteristics of Powdered Drugs

Stomata: Anisocytic or unequal celled stomata. Three subsidiary cells, one is smaller than other two.

Trichomes: Covering, unicellular, dagger shaped, warty with bulbous base.

Epidermal cells: Cells are slight rectangular in shape with thin and straight wall.

Mesophyll: Palisade and spongy parenchyma with epidermis.

Vessels: Lignified vessels (from veins)

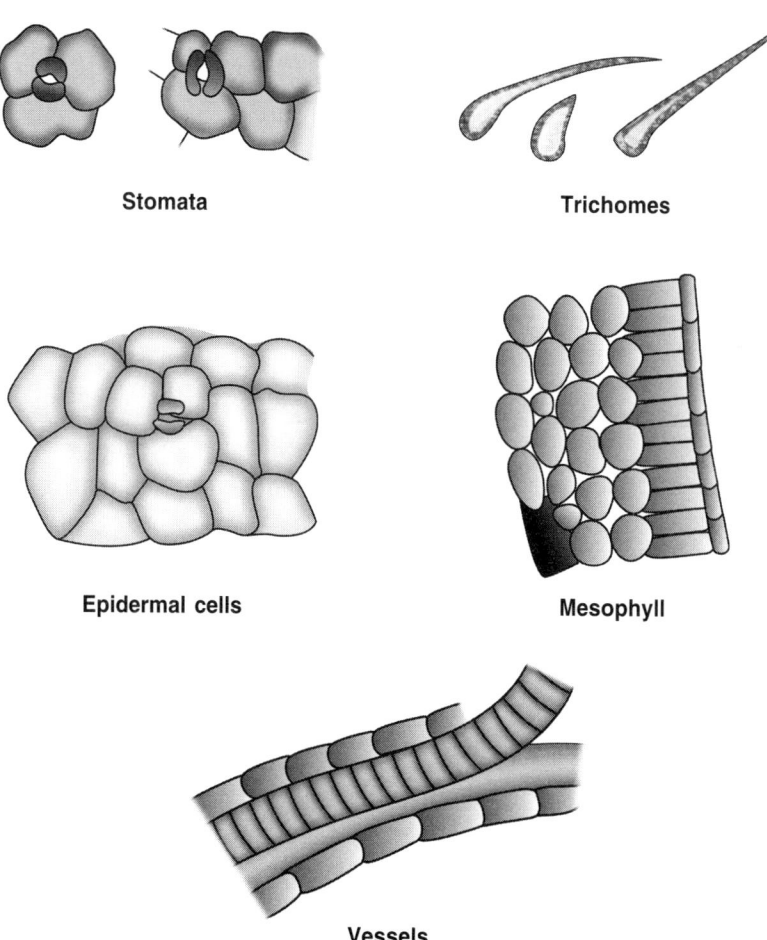

Fig. 2.24: Microscopic characterstics of powdered *Vinca*

Staining and Microchemical Tests

1. Add conc.HCl (1:1) to phloroglucinol: Red coloured xylem (vascular bundle) observed.

2. With Sudan Red III: Red cutical observed.

Chemical Constituents

A large number of indole alkaloids are present in Vinca. Out of them, about 20 dimeric indoledyhydroindole alkaloids possess oncolytic activity and among them, vinblastine and vincristine are most significant. Vinblastine contains indole part called catharanthine and dihydroindole moiety vindoline. The other alkaloids are ajmalicine, serpentine, lochnerine and tetrahydroalstonine.

Chemical Tests

It gives general tests for alkaloids as follows:

Dragendroff's Test

To extract add few drops of dragendroff's reagent. Reddish brown precipitate is formed.

Mayer's Test

To 2–3 ml of extracta, add a few drops of Mayer's reagent. It gives cream or buff coloured precipitate.

Hager's Test

To 2–3 ml of extract add a few drops Hager's reagent. It gives yellow colored precipitate.

Wagner's Test

To 2–3 ml extract add a few drops of Wagner's reagent. It gives reddish brown precipitate.

10% Tannic Acid Solution

Alkaloids give a buff coloured precipitate.

Uses

Vincristine sulphate is an antineoplastic agent. It is given in the treatment of acute leukemia in children. In adults, it is used in the treatment of Hodgkin's disease, lymphosarcoma, etc.

EXPERIMENT 18

Aim: To study the morphological, microscopical and powder Characteristics of Vasaka leaf.

Theory

Synonym: Ardushi, Vrisha, Vishnu, Adulsa

Biological Source: Vasaka consists of the fresh or dried leaves of *Adhatoda vasica* Nees.

Family: Acanthaceae.

Morphology

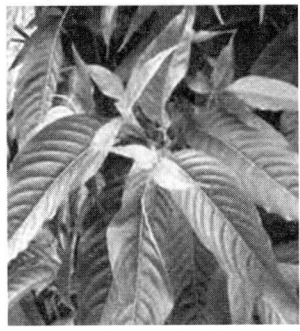

Fig. 2.25: Vasaka leaf

- *General Appearance:* Fresh leaves, dried crumpled and in broken fragments.
- *Size:* 12 to 20 cm long, 2.5 to 6 cm broad
- *Shape:* Ovate-lanceolate
- *Margin:* Entire or slightly crenate
- *Venation:* Pinnate, prominent midrib and 8 to 12 pairs of lateral veins
- *Apex:* Acuminate
- *Base:* Tapering
- *Surface:* Glabrous, slightly pubescent
- *Texture:* Thin and leathery
- *Petiole:* 2 to 8 cm long, grooved

Organoleptic Characters

- *Colour:* Light green
- *Odour:* Characteristic
- *Taste:* Bitter

Microscopy

Surface Preparation

Epidermal cell: Polygonal thin walled parenchymatous cells with wavy and anticlinial walls.

Glandular trichome: Sessile, with quadricellular heads.

Caryophyllaceous Stomata (Cross celled stomata).

Covering trichome: 2–4 cell blunt, thick walled, pointed.

Transverse Section

Lamina

Upper Epidermis

Single layered, rectangular cells, wavy anticlinal walls, cuticularized covering and glandular trichomes (sessile without stalk) and stomata are present.

Lower Epidermis: Resembles upper epidermis, but number of trichomes and stomatal pores are more.

Covering Trichome: 2– 4 celled, blunt, thick walled, pointed.

Glandular Trichome: Sessile, with quadricellular heads.

Caryophyllaceous (Diacytic) stomata.

Mesophyll: Dorsiventral.

Palisade: Two layered compact and radially elongated cells.

Spongy parenchyma: 4 to 6 layered, loosely arranged with intercellular spaces. Presence of calcium oxalate crystals in acicular and prismatic form.

Collenchyma: 2 to 4 layers, below upper epidermis. Also present above lower epidermis.

Cytoliths: Few cystoliths can be seen in cortical parenchyma.

Mid Rib

Vascular bundle: There are arc shaped, Collateral.
Xylem: With annular to spiral thickening and lignified
Phloem: Nonlignified
Collenchyma: Thick walled cellulosic cells.

Microscopical Characteristics of Powdered Drugs

Epidermal cells: Polygonal thin walled parenchymatous cells with wavy and anticlinal walls.

Stomata: Two subsidiary cells at right angle to stoma (cross celled stomata).

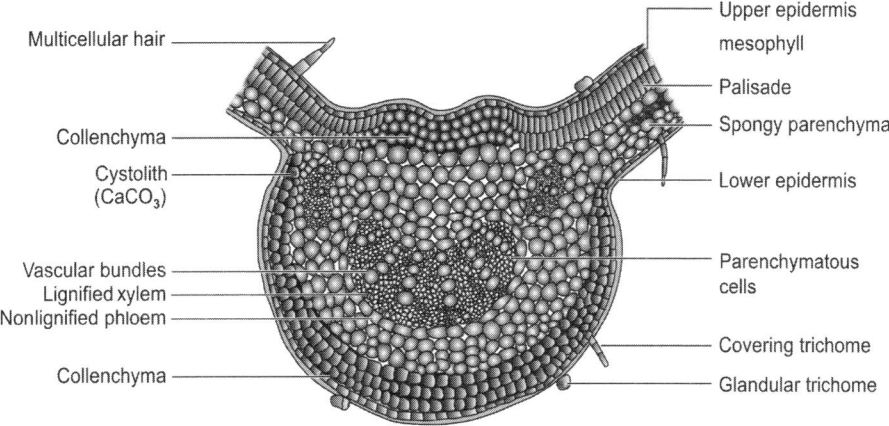

Fig. 2.26: TS of Vasaka leaf

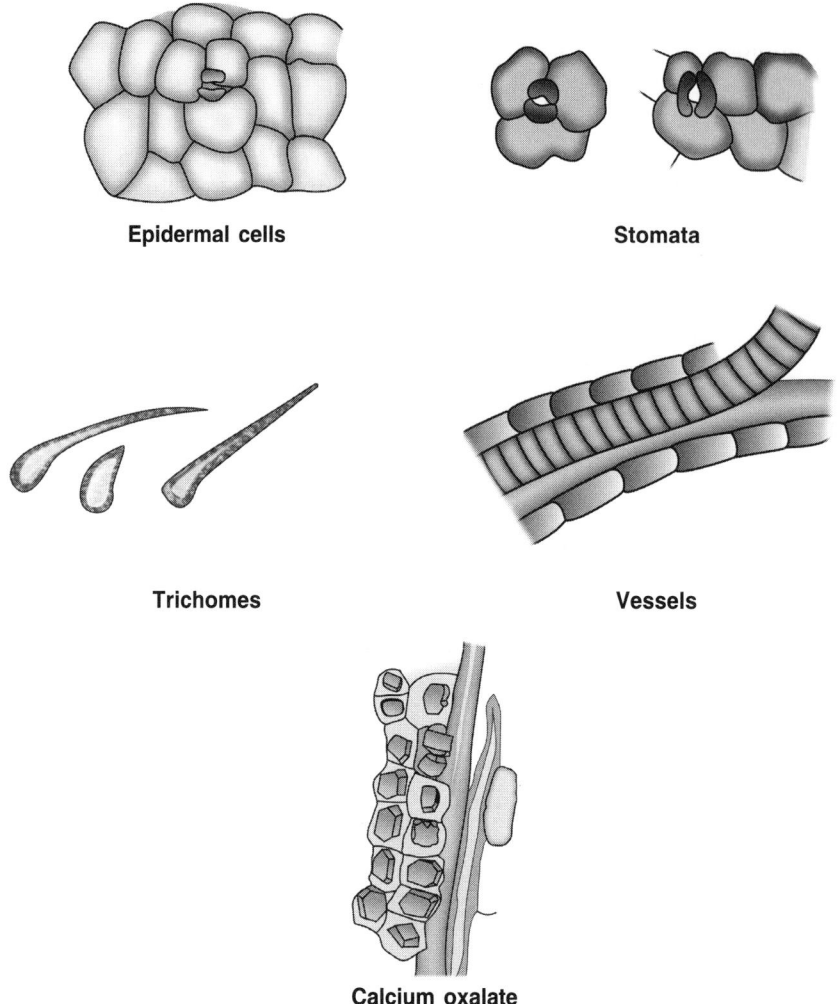

Fig. 2.27: Microscopical characterstics of powdered Vasaka

Covering trichomes: Two to four celled, bent, thick walled, pointed, uniseriate.

Glandular trichome: Sessile with Quadri cellular heads

Xylem vessels: With annular to spiral thickening and lignified.

Cystoliths: Calcium carbonate crystals, dissolves in hydrochloric acids with effervescences.

Calcium oxalate: Crystals in acicular and prismatic form.

Microchemical Tests

1. Phloroglucinol + Conc HCl (1:1): Red coloured lignified xylem (vascular bundle)
2. Insoluble in acetic acid: Calcium oxalate crystals
3. Needle shaped crystals of calcium sulphate are formed with sulphuric acid (60% w/v): Calcium oxalate crystals
4. Soluble with effervescence in hydrochloric acid: Cystolith

Chemical Constituents

Leaves contain quinazoline derivatives such as vasicine, vasicinone, vincristine, vinblastin, vasicine and vindoline. The drug also contains volatile oil, betain and vasakin. It also contains adhatodic acid.

Chemical Tests

It gives general tests for alkaloids as follows:

Dragendroff's Test

To extract, add a few drops of dragendroff's reagent. Reddish brown precipitate is formed.

Mayer's Test

To 2–3 ml of extract, add few drops of Mayer's reagent. It gives creamy or buff coloured precipitate.

Hager's Test

To 2–3 ml of extract, add Hager's reagent. It gives yellow colored precipitate.

Wagner's Test

To 2–3 ml extract, add a few drops of Wagner's reagent. It gives reddish brown precipitate.

10% Tannic Acid Solution

Alkaloids give a buff coloured precipitate.

Uses

Expectorent and bronchodilator, vasicine also shows oxytocic property similar to oxytocin.
Preparations: Vasaka syrup, Vasaka liquid extract, vasavaleha,

EXPERIMENT 19

Aim: To study the morphological, microscopical and powder Characteristics of Datura leaf.

Theory

Synonym: Devil's Apple

Biological Source: Datura herb consists of the dried leaves and flowering tops of *Datura metel* Linn. and *Datura metel* var *fastuosa*

Family: Solanaceae.

Plant Habit: *Datura metal* known as white Datura is dichotomously branched and spreading. Usually this plant is herbaceous but sometimes becomes like a shrub. Lower branches and base of the plant are woody. In *Datura metal* var.*fastuosa*, stem, flowers and main veins of leaves are purple coloured. Corolla is bilobed. Other characters of *D. metel*, var *fastuosa* are similar to *D. metel*.

Morphology

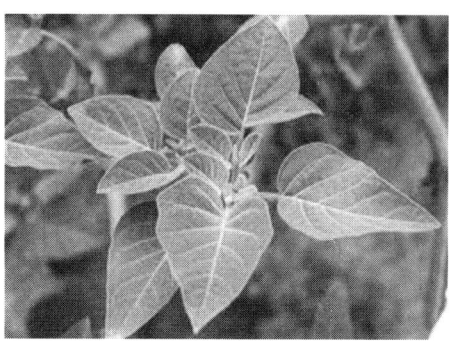

Fig. 2.28: Datura leaf

- *Appearance:* Nearly glabrous and has three to four coarse teeth on each side and there are 4 to 6 secondary veins on each side of the midrib.
- *Size:* 8–13 cm long, 7 cm broad
- *Shape:* Ovate.
- *Apex:* acute.
- *Base:* asymmetrical
- *Margin:* Angular but sometimes entire.
- *Colour:* dark grayish green
- *Odour:* Disagreable and Characteristic
- *Taste:* Unpleasantly bitter
- *Flowers*: Large, white and funnel–shaped. Calyx is tubular and has five triangles, acuminate margin teeth. Corolla is thin, acuminate and circular to triangular.
- *Fruit*: Muricate or tubercled on short, thick curved pedicel.

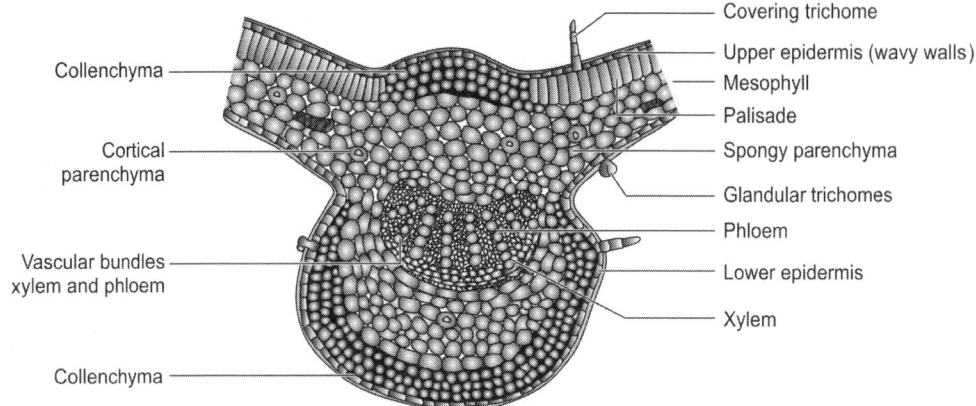

Fig. 2.29: TS of Datura leaf

D. metel var *fastuosa:* It is known in commerce as black datura. The stem, branches main veins of leaves and flowers are purple-coloured. Corolla is double or triple. Outer corolla has five teeth and inner corolla has six to ten teeths. Other characters of this plant are similar to *D. metel*.

Microscopy

Surface Preparation

Covering trichomes: Uniseriate, multicellular, warty, blunt at apex approximately 115 to 220 μ long.

Glandular trichomes: Unicellular stalk, 2 to 4 celled head. 23 to 35 μ in diameter and 50 μ in length.

Epidermal cells: Wavy wall, rectangularly arranged.

Cruciferous stomata: Stomata surrounded by three cells, where one is smaller than other two, i.e. anisocytic stomata (unequal celled stomata).

Transverse Section

Lamina

Dorsiventral nature.

Epidermis: Epidermal layers are continuous.

Upper epidermis: Straight walls, 600 to 1100 cells/mm^2, single layered, rectangular.

Lower epidermis: Similar to upper epidermis, stomata and numerous trichomes are seen; wavy walls and cuticle. 700 to 1250 cells/sq. mm.

Covering trichomes: Uniseriate, multicellular, waxy, blunt tip.

Glandular trichomes: Stalk unicellular, head 2–4 celled.

Stomata: Cruciferous or unequal celled.

Collenchyma: Below upper and above lower epidermis.

Cortical parenchyma containing prisms of calcium oxalate and microphenoidal crystals.

Mesophyll

Palisade: Single layered, compact cells, radially elongated, covering $2/5$ th of lamina.

Spongy parenchyma: 6–8 layers, loosely arranged, intercellular spaces, cluster crystals (sphaeraphides), Microspheroidal crystals and vascular strands are found in upper layers.

Vascular Bundles

Xylem: Spiral to annular, lignified.

Phloem: Nonlignified

Microscopical Characteristics of Powdered Drugs

Cruciferrous stomata (anisocytic): Stomata surrounded by three cells, where one is

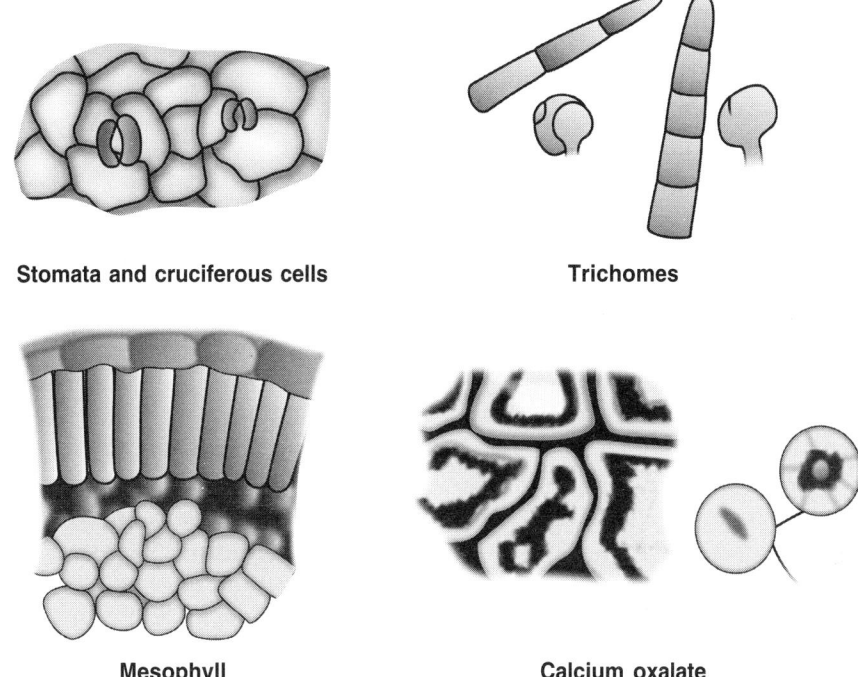

Fig. 2.30: Microscopical characterstic of powdered Datura

smaller than other two, i.e. Anisocytic stomata (unequal celled stomata).

Epidermal cells: Slightly straight in upper epidermis, wavy walled in lower epidermis.

Trichomes

Covering trichome: Uniseriate, multicellular, wavy covering trichomes with blunt apex.

Length: approximately 115 to 200 cm

Glandular trichome: One celled stalk and 2-4 celled head.

23 to 35 m in diameter and 50 m in length.

Lamina/Mesophyll: Palisade parenchyma, elongated, compactly arranged.

Calcium oxalate crystals (spherophides), vascular element, spongy parenchyma.

Calcium oxalate crystals: Spheroraphide crystals: Occur in spongy parenchymatous cells and scattered in the powder.

Microchemical Tests

1. **Phloroglucinol and conc HCl (1:1):** Pink coloured xylem (vascular bundle)
2. **Insoluble in dil acetic acid:** Calcium oxalate crystals
3. Soluble in sulphuric acid (60% w/w), on standing forms needles of calcium sulphate: Calcium oxalate crystals

Chemical Tests

1. Vitali–Morin reaction: The tropane alkaloid is treated with fuming nitric acid, followed by evaporation to dryness. Addition of methanolic acid, potassium hydroxide solution to an acetone solution of nitrated residue violet colour is developed.
2. On addition of silver nitrate solution to solution of hyoscine hydrobromide, yellowish white precipitate is formed, which is insoluble in nitric acid, but soluble in dilute ammonia solution.
3. General chemical tests for alkaloids.

Chemical Constituents

Scopolamine (hyoscine up to 0.5 %) is the main alkaloid. Hyoscyamine and atropine are present in tracer amounts.

Uses: Parasympatholytic with anticholinergic and CNS depressant effect. Also used as mydriatic, antispasmodic and cerebral sedative. Hyoscine hydrobromide is used in motion sickness, gastric or duodenal ulcers.

Preparations

- Datura liquid extract IP
- Tincture datura IP

Allied Drugs

i. *Datura innoxia:*
   a. Leaves are oval with entire margin (few teeth may be present).
   b. Numerous glandular trichomes occur, composed of 2 to 4 celled uniseriate stalk and an unicellular spherical head.
   c. The basal cell of the covering trichomes measures less than 50 mm in diameter.

ii. *Datura tatula:*
   a. Leaves are smaller.
   b. Covering trichomes are generally longer.
   c. Petiole gives a pink colour with hydrochloric acid.

EXPERIMENT 20

Aim: To study microscopical powder characteristics of Hyoscyamus leaf.

Theory

Synonym: *Hyoscyamus niger* L, Henbane leaf, Hyoscyamus herb, Hyoscyamus leaf

Biological Source: Hyosyamus consists of the dried leaves and flowering tops of *Hyocyamus niger* Linn.

Family: Solanaceae.

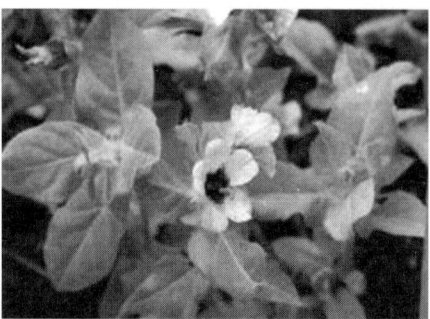

Fig. 2.31: Hyoscyamus leaf

A yellowish–green powder with a characteristic, unpleasant odour and a bitter, slightly acrid taste. The diagnostic characters are:

a. Fragments of the lamina in *surface view*. The *upper epidermis* is composed of large cells with thin, slightly sinuous walls; fairly numerous *anisocytic stomata* are present; the underlying palisade cells are moderately large and loosely packed. The cells of the *lower epidermis* are also large and have thin, markedly sinuous walls; numerous anisocytic stomata are present. Fragments of the epidermis from over the veins also occur, composed of elongated cells with straight, slightly thickened walls; these fragments usually have attached trichomes or show the *cicatrices* left by them.

b. The *glandular trichomes*, which are very abundant; they are found scattered or attached to fragments of the epidermis and they are frequently broken. They are very characteristic, with a uniseriate stalk composed of two to six cells with thin, smooth walls and an ovoid, multicellular head containing two to twelve or more cells; occasional trichomes have a unicellular stalk and a multicellular head. *Covering trichomes* also occur but they are not very numerous; they are uniseriate and conical, composed of two to four thin walled cells.

c. The abundant *calcium oxalate crystals*, which occur in a layer of cells in the spongy mesophyll immediately below the palisade. They show great variation in form and may be *prisms, cluster crystals* with a few components or, occasionally, *microsphenoids*; a number of the prisms have dense cylindrical outgrowths, which appear to penetrate the crystal forming a plug. The crystals are found scattered in the powder as well as in the cells of the crystal layer.

d. The fragments of the *lamina in sectional view* showing the epidermis with a smooth cutical, a single layer of palisade cells, the crystal layer and the irregular parenchymatous cells forming the remainder of the mesophyll.

e. The occasional fragments of the *corolla in surface view*; the *epidermal cells* have thin, wavy anticlinal walls with well marked infoldings which are very characteristic; occasional glandular trichomes may be attached to the fragments.

f. The *fibrous layer of the anthers*; these fragments are reddish-purple and in surface view the thickening on the walls of the cells appears as rods with beaded ends; they are usually lignified or partially lignified.

g. The occasional subspherical *pollen grains* with three pores and three furrows; the exine is covered with numerous small pits in an irregular arrangement.

EXPERIMENT 21

Aim: To study the morphological, microscopical and powder Characteristics of clove.

Theory
It consists of dried flower buds of *Eugenia caryophyllus (Syzygium aromaticum)*; family Myrtaceae.

Morphology
A. *Color:* dark brown
B. *Odour:* aromatic, strong
C. *Taste:* pungent, aromatic
D. *Size:* length 10–17mm
E. *Flower:* The flower bud has a dome shaped head and a subcylindrical hypanthium. Head consists of calyx, corolla, stamens and styles.
  a. *Calyx:* 4, thick and hard sepals with oil glands.
  b. *Corolla:* 4 petals imbricate, enclose the stamens and form the head of the bud.

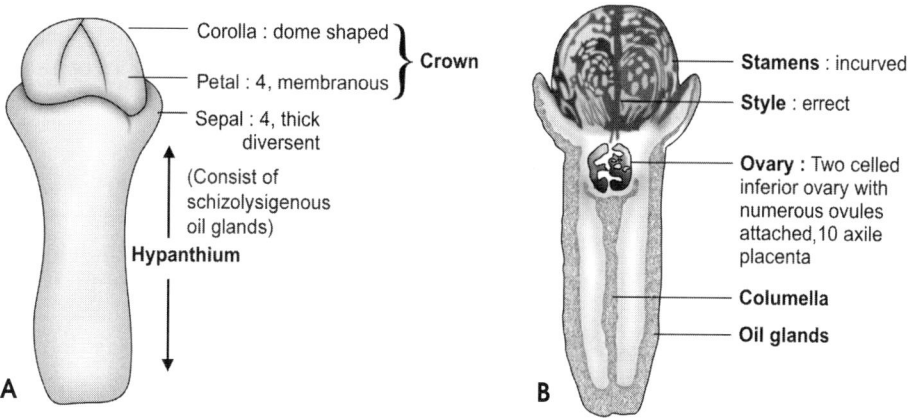

Shape: Subcylindrical slightly flattened.

Fig. 2.32: (A) Morphological diagram and (B) LS of clove bud

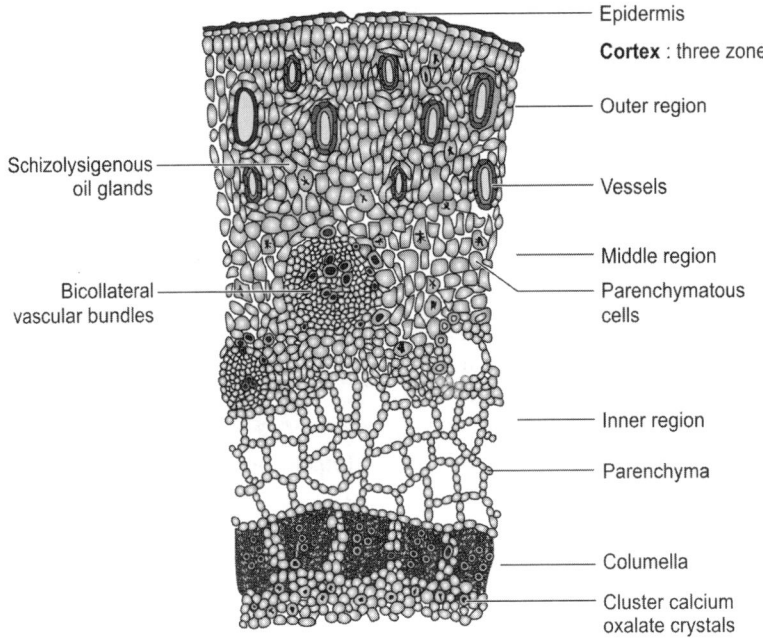

Fig. 2.33: TS of Clove bud

c. *Androcieum:* Numerous stamens, free and introse.
d. *Gynocieum:* Bilocular, inferior ovary, numerous ovules with axils placentation. Style single and erect. The oil glands are present throughout the flower bud.

Microscopy

In transverse section through hypanthium following tissues are seen from periphery to the centre.

A. **Epidermis:** single layered thick cuticle, in between the cells anomocytic (ranunculaceous) stomata are present.

B. **Cortex:** is divided into three distinct regions:

The **outer region** contains 2–3 layers of big ellipsoidal schizolysigenous oil glands in between the radially elongated parenchymatous cells.

The **middle region** is made up of parenchymatous cells containing bicollateral vascular bundles arranged in one or two rings, associated with a few pericyclic fibers.

The **inner region** is made up of aerenchyma.

C. **Columella:** Made up of parenchymatous cells with a ring of bicollateral vascular bundles present towards the periphery. Calcium oxalate crystals in clusters (sphaerophides) are present throughout the columella and a few in middle cortical region.

Chemical Constituents

Clove contains about 15 to 20% of volatile oil; 10 to 13% of tannin (gallotannic acid), resin, chromone and eugenin. The volatile oil of the drug contains eugenol (about 70 to 90%), eugenol acetate, caryophyllenes and small quantities of esters, ketones and alcohols.

Powder Microscopy

A. Oil glands: Fragments of parenchyma containing entire or a portion of oil glands.

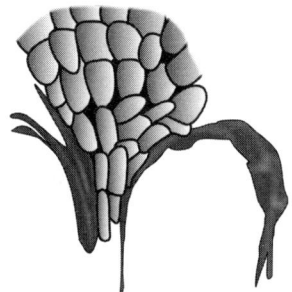

Fig. 2.34: Oil glands in Clove

B. Parenchyma: Parenchymatous cells and large intercellular spaces.

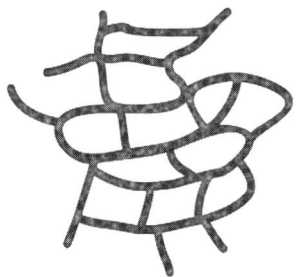

Fig. 2.35: Parenchyma cells

C. Fibres: Sclerenchymatous fibers attached with parenchymatous cells.

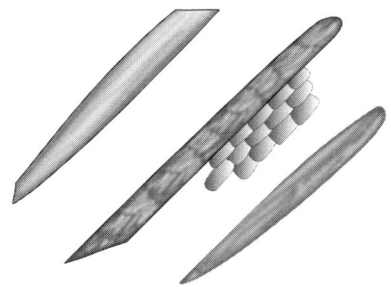

Fig. 2.36: Fibres

D. Pollen grains: Small, biconvex with rounded or triangular in shape.

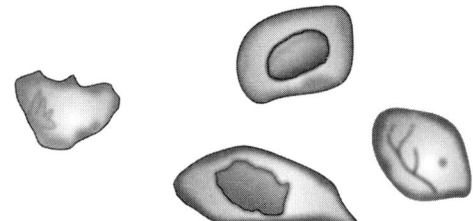

Fig. 2.37: Pollen grains

E. Anther: Fibrous layer of anther.

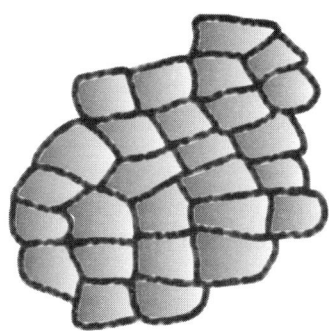

Fig. 2.38: Anther

F. Calcium oxalate: In the form of clusters.

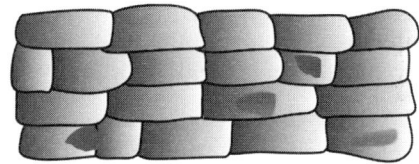

Fig. 2.39: Calcium oxalate crystals

G. Starch grains: Absent (present in mother clove)

Chemical Tests

Tannins

i. To the aqueous extract, add lead acetate solution. White precipitate is formed.

ii. To the aqueous extract, add 5% ferric chloride solution. Dark colour is formed.

Eugenol

To the alcoholic solution of clove oil, add 5% ferric chloride solution. Blue colour is formed.

Eugenolate

i. To the chloroform extract, add 3% sodium hydroxide solution. Crystals of sodium eugenolate are formed.

ii. To the thick section of hypanthium, add 5% potassium hydroxide solution. Needle shaped crystals of potassium eugenolate are observed under the microscope.

Substituents

1. Mother cloves
2. Blown cloves
3. Clove stalks
4. Exhausted cloves

Uses

Dental analgesic, carminative, stimulant, flavouring agent and antiseptic.

EXPERIMENT 22

Aim: To study the morphological, microscopical and powder Characteristics of Ginger.

Theory

It consists of the rhizome of *Zingiber officinalis* family Zingiberaceae, scrapped to remove the dark outer skin and dried in the sun.

Morphology

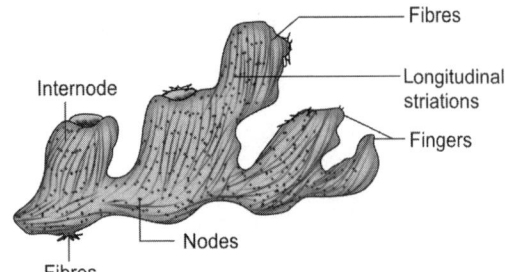

Shape: Laterally flattened

Fig. 2.40: Morphological structure of Ginger

A. *Color:* Buff colored
B. *Odour:* Agreeable and aromatic
C. *Taste:* Pungent
D. *Size:* Length: 5–15 cm,
   width: 3–6 cm
E. *Extra features:* Irregularly branched (sympodial), branches known as fingers arise obliquely from the rhizome. Nodes, internodes and scales are not clearly seen on the dried ones. Longitudinal striations are present on the surface. Fractures are short and fibrous.

Microscopy: In a cross section of an unpeeled rhizome, following tissues are seen from the periphery to the centre.

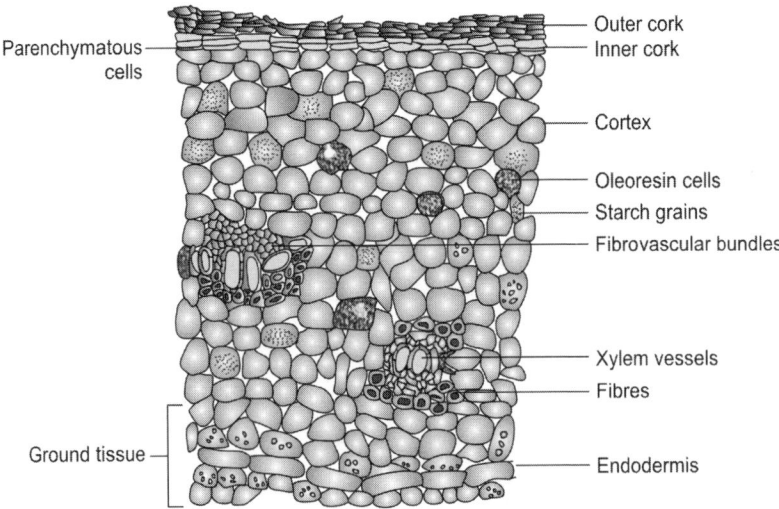

Fig. 2.41: Microscopy of Ginger

A. **Cork:**
- *Outer cork:* Few layered, irregularly made up of parenchymatous cells, dark brown coloured.
- *Inner cork:* Few layered, radially arranged in regular rows, made up of colourless parenchymatous cells.

B. **Cortex:** Consists of thin walled loosely arranged parenchymatous cells. Starch grains are abundant in this region. Inter spread within cortex are found, numerous yellow oleoresin cells and fibro vascular bundles (sclerenchymatous fibers covers the vascular bundle hence called fibrovascular bundle)

C. **Endodermis:** Single layered with radial walls thickened, starch grains are absent.

D. **Ground tissues:** Similar to that of cortex, made up of parenchymatous cells containing in large amounts starch grains, oleoresin cells and vascular bundles. Vascular bundles present below the endodermis are not covered by the sclerenchymatous fibers while that present in the center of the ground tissues are covered by the same. Vascular bundles are conjoint, collateral and closed.

Chemical constituents

Ginger consists 1 to 4% volatile oil (terpenes, cineol, citral, borneol), starch (40 to 60%), fibres (5%), inorganic material (6%), residual moisture (10%) and acrid resinous matter (5 to 8%). Ginger oil is constituted of monoterpene hydrocarbons, sesquiterpene hydrocarbons, oxygenated mono and sesquiterpenes, and phenyl propanoids. Sesquiterpenes hydrocarbons includes α-zingiberene, β-bisabolene, β-sesquiphellandrene and α-curcumin.

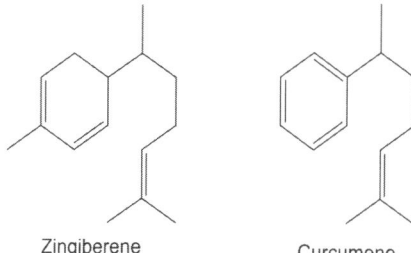

Zingiberene Curcumene

Powder Microscopy

A. **Parenchyma:** Parenchyma cells containing yellow brown oleoresinous bodies and or starch grains.

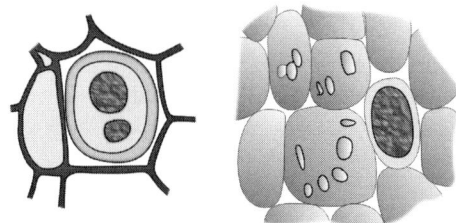

Fig. 2.42: Parenchyma

B. **Fibres:** Occurs in groups associated with vessels. Fibres are septate and pitted and mostly nonlignified.

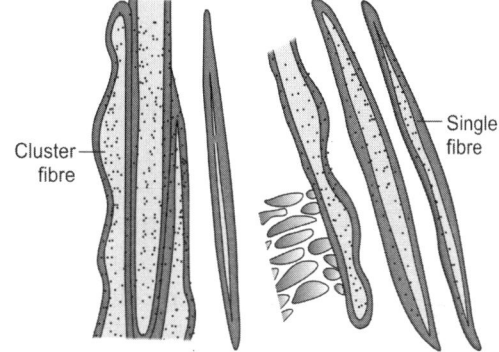

Fig. 2.43: Fibres

C. **Vessels:** occurs in groups with reticulatily thickened and pitted.

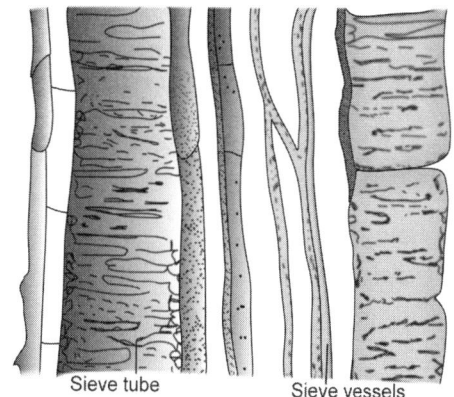

Sieve tube   Sieve vessels
Fig. 2.44: Vessels

D. **Starch grains:** Abundant sack shaped with terminal beak like projection, hilum is eccentric 5–60 μ in length.

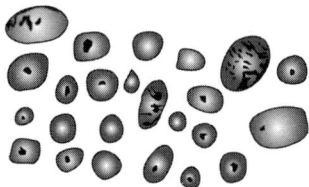

Fig. 2.45: Strach grains in Ginger

E. **Calcium oxalate crystals:** Calcium oxalate crystals are absent.

Chemical Tests

Pungency (due to gingerol) of the ginger powder is destroyed when boiled with 5% potassium hydroxide solution.

Substituents

1. Japanese ginger obtained from *Zingiber mioga*
2. Greater galangal obtained from *Alpinia galanga*
3. Galangal rhizome obtain from *Alpinia officinarum*

Uses: Ginger is used as stomachic, an aromatic, a carminative, stimulant and flavouring agent. Ginger oil is used in mouth washes, ginger beverages and liquors. Ginger powder is effective in motion sickness.

EXPERIMENT 23

Aim: To study the morphological, microscopical and powder Characteristics of coriander.

Theory: It consists of the dried ripe fruits of *Coriandrum sativum*, family Umbelliferae.

Morphology

a. *Type of fruit:* Cremocarp
b. *Shape:* Subspherical or subglobular or globular or oval with 5 calyx teeth and a short stylopod at the apex.
c. *Size:* 2.3 – 4.3 mm
d. *Color:* Straw yellow or brownish yellow
e. *Odour:* Aromatic
f. *Taste:* Spicy and agreeable
g. *Surface:* Each mericarp has 5 primary ridges (wavy and in conspicuous) and 4 secondary ridges (straight and more prominent)

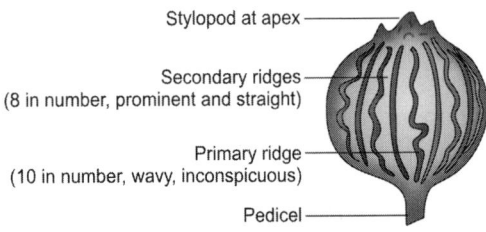

Fig. 2.46: Morphology of Coriander

Microscopy: TS of mericarp show 3 regions from periphery to centre

A. **Pericarp:**
  i. *Epicarp:* Single layer with thick walled cells
  ii. *Mesocarp:* differentiated into 3 regions
    a. *Outer layer:* Comprises loosely arranged tangentially elongated parenchymatous cells
    b. *Middle layer:* Made up of sclerencymatous cells. In the outer region of this layer and below the primary ridges longitudinally elongated sclerenchymatous cells are present while the inner region corresponding to secondary ridges comprised of tangentially elongated sclerenchymatous cells. Vascular bundles are present over the sclerenchymatous band below the primary ridge.
    c. *Inner layer:* Made up of irregular, polygonal and lignified parenchymatouas cells.
  iii. *Endocarp:* Show typical parquetry arrangement of cells.

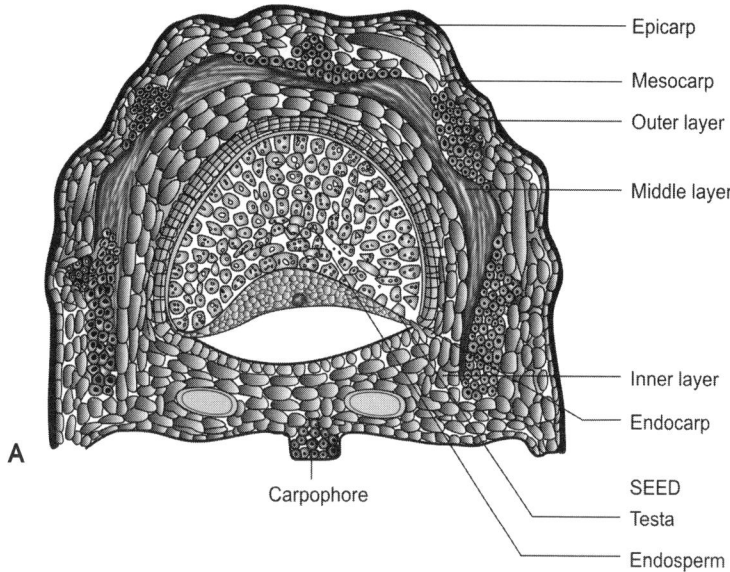

Fig. 2.47A: TS of Coriander

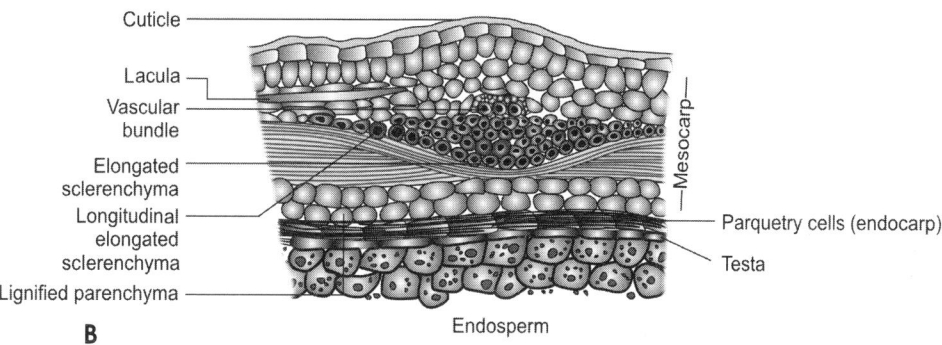

Fig. 2.47B: LS of endosperm (Coriander)

B. Testa: Single layered, yellow colored

C. Endosperm: Thick walled, polygonal, colorless parenchymatous cells containing fixed oils and aleurone grains

Chemical Constituents

Coriander yields 0.3–1% of volatile oil. Volatile of drug contains 60–70% of D-linalool (coriandrol) and coriandryl acetate and a small quantity of L- borneol, geraniol and pinene.

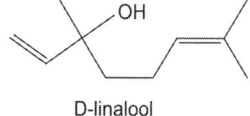

D-linalool

Powder Microscopy

- **Sclerenchymatous layer:** Groups of fusiform fibers running wavy, crossing each other or with thin walled lignified cells of mesocarp.

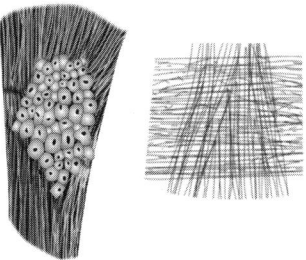

Fig. 2.48: Sclerenchymatous cells

- **Endocarp:** Fragments of parquetry arrangement of thin walled lignified cells with polygonal cells of mesocarp.

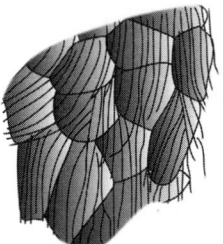

Fig. 2.49: Endocarp

- **Vittae:** Few yellowish brown fragments of vittae.

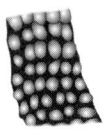 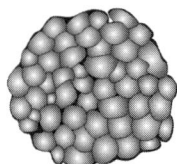 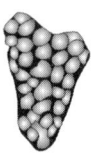

Fig. 2.50: Vittae

- **Endosperm:** Fragments of endosperm with aleurone grains and oil globules.

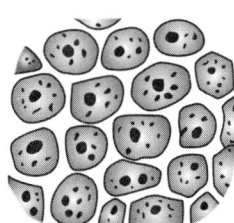

Fig. 2.51: Endosperm

Substitutent: Bombay coriander fruits (contain less volatile oil).

Uses: Fruits as well as volatile oil are used as an aromatic, carminative, stimulant and flavouring agent. Coriander oil is used along with purgatives to prevent gripping.

EXPERIMENT 24

Aim: To study the morphological, microscopical and powder Characteristics of Rauwolfia.

Theory

Synonym: Sarpagandha, Chhotachand, Indian snake root, Rauwolfia roots

Biological Source: Rauwolfia consists of dried roots and rhizomes of 3 to 4 years old plants of *Rauwolfia serpentina*. Percentage of active constituent, i.e. Reserpine (0.15%).

Family: Apocynaceae.

Geographical Source: India, Pakistan, Burma, Thailand and Java

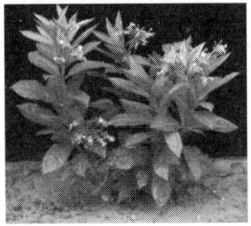 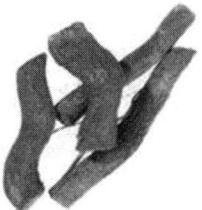

Fig. 2.52: Rauwolfia plant and roots

Morphology

External characters of roots and rhizomes are nearly similar but rhizomes can be distinguished by the presence of small central pith. In pieces of some rhizomes small pieces of aerial stems are attached. Drug consists of pieces which are 2 to 15 cm long and of 3 to 22 mm diameter. Pieces are cylindrical, slightly tapering tortuous and rarely branched. Rootlets are rarely present and when present their diameter is 0.5 to 1 mm. Outer surface is grayish-yellow, pale brown or brown. In young pieces wrinkles and in old pieces longitudinal ridges and sometimes scars of rootlets are seen. In pieces of especially old roots, exfoliation of bark takes place at some places and patches of pale yellow to white wood are exposed. Roots break easily compared to roots of other species of *Rauwolfia* because of absence of sclerenchyma and fracture is short. Smoothed transverse surface shows narrow yellow to brown bark and dense pale yellow radiate wood, with 2 to 8 growth rings occupying nearly three quarters of the diameter. Starch is abundant in bark and wood. Drug is odourless and taste is bitter.

Microscopy

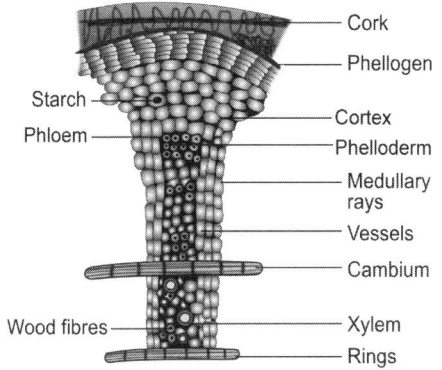

Fig. 2.53: Microscopy of Rauwolifa roots

Periderm

Cork: One to seven layers of small cells, one to three layers of larger cells. Stratified cells in alternating bands of unlignified cells (broder cells upto 90 µ in redial length) and lignified cells (narrow upto 75 µ in tangential width).

Phellogen: Indistinct

Phelloderm

Ten to twelve rows of tangentially elongated to isodiametric parenchyma cells. Few cells contains starch grains and calcium oxalate crystals.

Starch grains: Simple or compound, spherical to sub-spherical, star shaped hilum. Calcium oxalate crystals: Angular crystals, 3–20 µ in length.

Secondary Phloem: (Unlignified)

Sieve tubes, companion cells and phloem parenchyma with starch grains and calcium oxalate crystals.

Secondary xylem: (Lignified)

Xylem vessels: Few lignified, upto 350 µ in length and 50 µ or more in width, simple or bordered pits.

Xylem fibres: Highly thickened with pointed or bifurcated ends, 200–250 µ in length, in tangential bands and radial rows.

Xylem parenchyma: Moderately thick, lignified, pitted walls, containing starch.

Medullary rays: Run radially from the centre to the cortex through the phloem, one to five cells in width.

The tissues of the rhizomes have characters similar to those of the root; with a cortex, a paricycle with unlignified pericycle fibres and a small pith.

Stone cells are absent from both rhizome and root.

Microscopical Characteristics of Powdered Drugs

Cork cells: Stratified isodiametric cells, sometimes lignified.

Parenchyma: Lignified, pitted, xylem parenchymatous cells. Filled with starch grains

Xylem vessels: Few with oblique end walls, lignified.

Calcium oxalate crystals: Few number prismatic.

Starch grains: Mostly simple, spherical, star-shaped hilum.

Staining and Microchemical Tests

1. Pink colour is obtained with Phloroglucinol and conc. HCl (1:1 mixture) which shows lignified cork, xylem region and lower part of medullary rays
2. Blue colour is obtained with iodine solution shows presence of starch
3. Insoluble in acetic acid, shows presence of calcium oxalate
4. Soluble in hydrochloric acid, shows presence of calcium oxalate

Chemical Constituents

Alkaloids: 0.8–1.3% indole alkaloids, reserpine, rescinnamine, ajmaline, serpentine.

Uses: Antihypertensive and tranquillizing agent.

Preparations

Rauwolfia dry extract, Rauwolfia liquid extrat, Rauwolfia tablets.

Allied Drugs/Substitutes

i. *Rauwolfia vomitoria* (African Rauwolfia):
   a. Five discontinued bands of schlerenchyma.
   b. Large vessels.

ii. *Rauwolfia densiflora:* Contains sclerenchyma.

iii. *Rauwolfia tetraphylla*:
   a. Uniform cork
   b. Abundant sclerides and fibres
   c. Absence of rescinnamine.

EXPERIMENT 25

Aim: To study the morphological, microscopical and powder Characteristics of Cinchona bark.

Theory

Synonym: Jesuit's bark, Peruvian bark, Cinchona bark.

Biological Source: Cinchona is the dried bark of the stem or the root *Cinchona calisaya*, *Cinchona ledgeriana*, *Cinchona officinalis* and *Cinchona succirubra* or hybrids of the first two species with any of the last two species.

Family: Rubiaceae.

Geographical Source: Indonesia, Zaire, India, Guatemala and Bolivia.

Morphology

1. *General characters of stem bark:* Shape of bark is curved, quill or double quill. Outer surface is rough mainly due to longitudinal and transverse cracks, fissures, ridges and protuberances
2. *Root bark:* It occurs in channeled pieces. Outer surface is sometimes scaly and inner-striated.

Histology

Cork: Cork consists of several rows of radially arranged thin-walled cells with reddish-brown contents. Phelloderm is narrow zone of regular cells.

Cortex: Cortex consists of thin-walled parenchymatous cells. Cells contain amorphous reddish brown matter, small rounded starch grains and occasionally microcrystals of calcium oxalate. Few idoblasts or secretory cells appearing oval in the transaction are present on the inner side.

Phloem: It is wide. It consists of sieve tubes, phloem parenchyma and phloem fibres. Phloem fibres are isolated or in small radial groups. They are spindle-shaped and lignified with striated walls. Medullary rays are 2 to 3 celled wide and radially elongated.

Microscopy
Periderm

Cork: Several layers of thin walled, flat, polygonal cells with reddish brown content, impregnated with suberin.

Phellogen: 2 to 3 layers of thin walled cells without any cellular content.

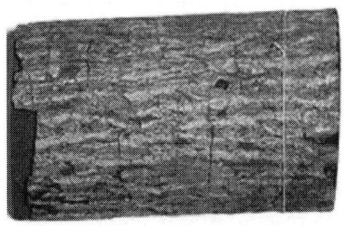 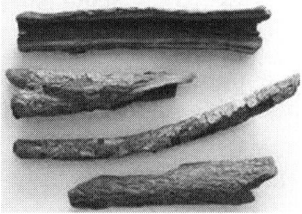

A   B

Fig. 2.54: Cinchona (A) stem bark (B) Root barks

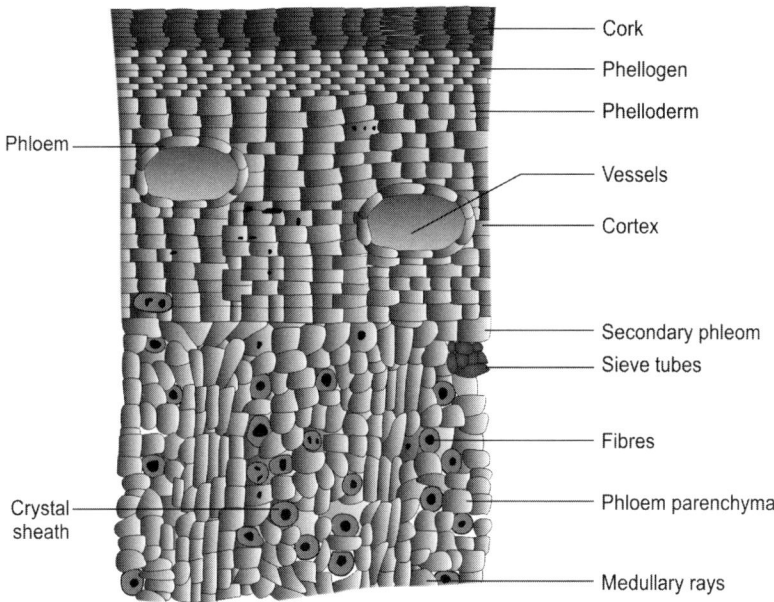

Fig. 2.55: Microscopy of Cinchona bark

Phelloderm

6 to 8 layers of thin walled rectangular cells without any cellular content.

Cortex

Several layers of thin walled tangentially elongated cells containing reddish brown matter.

Calcium oxalate crystals: 2 to 6 µm long, microsphenoidal crystals.

Starch grain: Rounded, 6 to 10 µm in diameter. Sclereides are absent. Cavities (secretion canals) are present.

Secondary Phloem

Sieve tubes: The compact cells are about 200 µ long and 15 to 20 µ wide and having narrow companion cells; most of the sieve tubes are compressed and collapsed.

Fibres: Numerous large, fusiform, lignified phloem fibres, having striated walls and conspicuous tubular or funnel-shaped pits, mostly isolated, some times in groups of 2 to 3 fibres.

Phloem parenchyma: Thin, dark-reddish brown wall, some with microprisms of calcium oxalate.

Medullary Rays: One to three seriate extended upto cortex cells, radially elongated and contains starch grains.

Microscopical Characteristics of Powdered Drugs

Cork: Thin walled, flat, polygonal cells with reddish brown matter.

Phloem fibres: Numerous large, fusiform, lignified phloem fibres, striated walls having simple pores or branched pores. 30 to 60 µ in width and 500 to 800 µ in length.

Calcium oxalate crystals: Microprisms of calcium oxalate crystals, about 2 to 6 µ long, in dark coloured parenchyma.

Starch grains: Minute, simple or compound (2 to 5) individual grain, about 2 to 5 µ in diameter.

Stone cells and sphaerophides are absent.

Staining and Microchemical Tests

1. Pink colour is obtained with Phloroglucinol and conc HCl (1:1 mixture): shows presence of Lignified phloem fibres.
2. Blue colour is obtained with Iodine solution shows presence of starch.
3. Insoluble in Acetic acid and soluble in dilute Hydrochloric acid shows presence of calcium oxalate crystals.
4. Calcium sulphate crystals formed on addition of dilute Sulphuric acid. Shows presence of calcium oxalate crystals.

Chemical Constituents

Alkaloids: Quinine, Quinidine, Cinchonine, Cinchonidine.

Chemical Tests

1. Heat 1 gm bark powder in a test tube. Purple vapours evolved.
2. Treat with dilute sulphuric acid and observe under UV light. Blue fluorescence observed.
3. Thalloquin test: Heat bark powder, add bromine water and ammonia. Emerald green colour is obtained.

Uses: Antimalarial and antipyretic.

Preparations

Cinchona extract, compound cinchona tincture.

Allied Drugs

i. *Cupea bark:* Coppery-red, dense, very hard, with a granular and splintery fracture. Sclereides are present and the fibres are partly associated in small groups.
ii. *Colombian bark (Cinchona lancifolia):* Occurs in flat pieces or single, quill reddish brown in colour and spongy in texture. Outer surface bears patches of silvery cork. Abundant sclereids are present.

EXPERIMENT 26

Aim: To study the morphological, microscopical and powder characteristics of Cassia bark.

Theory

Synonym: Chinese Cinnamon, Dalchini (Hindi)

Biological source: It consists of the dried bark of *Cinnamomum cassia*; family Lauraceae

Morphology

a. *Shape:* Channeled to single quill
b. *Size:* Length: up to 40 cm
   Thickness: 1–5 mm
   Width: 1–2 cm
c. *Color:* Outer surface is dark reddish brown with rough patches of grey cork, inner surfaces is finally striated and brownish.
d. *Odour:* less aromatic
e. *Taste:* aromatic, astringent and mucilaginous

Microscopy: TS of Cassia bark shows following tissues from outside to centre.

Periderm

i. *Cork:* Few layered, outer layer of cells are thin walled while the inner ones are lignified and thick walled.
ii. *Phellogen and Phelloderm:* Cannot be distinguished

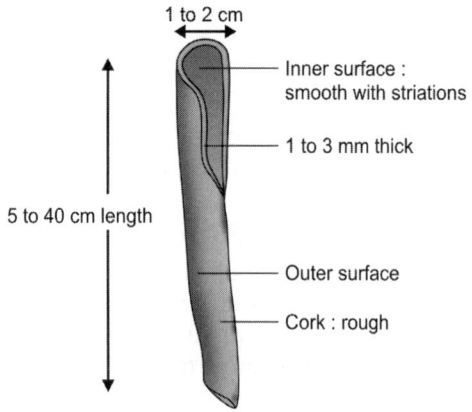

Fig. 2.56: Morphology of Cassia bark

Cortex

10–15 layered parenchymatous contain acicular raphides and abundant starch as well as sclereids scattered, either isolated or in groups.

Stone Cell Layer

Sclereids are lignified and pitted (typically characteristic of cassia bark). The inner and radial walls of the sclereids are thicker than the outer wall giving the appearance of letter 'U'.

On the outside of the sclerenchymatous band a few groups of small pericyclic fibres are found.

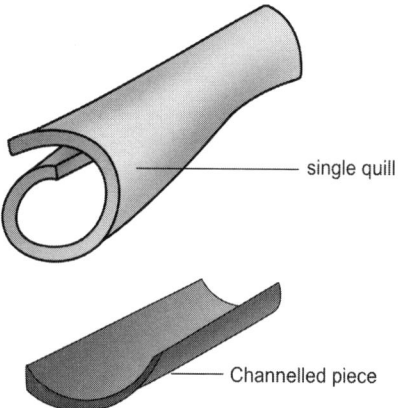

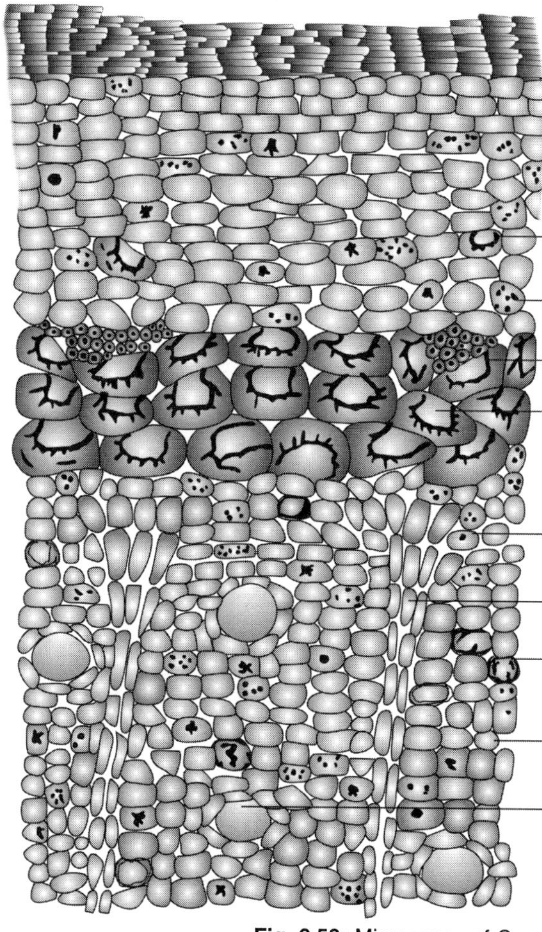

Fig. 2.57: Types of Cassia bark

Fig. 2.58: Microscopy of Cassia bark

Secondary Phloem

Comprises phloem parenchyma, phloem fibres and medullary rays.

i. Phloem parenchyma cells contain starch grains (10μ–20μ) with little acicular calcium oxalate crystals. The most characteristic feature of cassia bark is the presence of big isolated oil cells in the phloem parenchyma.

ii. Phloem fibres occur singly and are isolated. The fibres are almost circular and lignified with starch.

iii. Medullary rays are narrow at inner side and broader towards the stone cell layer, contains starch and acicular raphides.

Chemical Constituents

Cassia bark contains 1–2% of volatile oil known as cassia oil. It also contains mucilage, starch, calcium oxalate and tannins. Cassia oil contains not less than 85% of cinnamaldehyde and very small amount of eugenol. It also contains cinnamyl acetate.

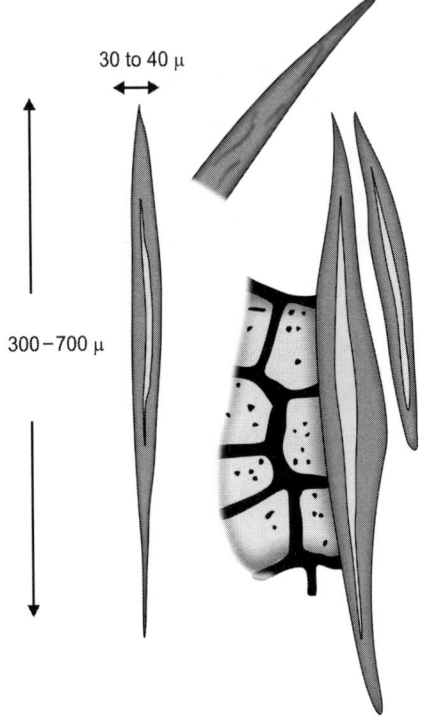

Fig. 2.59: Fibres in Cassia

Eugenol

Cinnamyl acetate

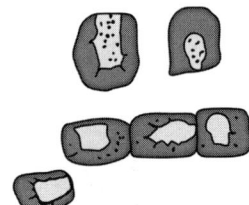

Fig. 2.60: Stone cells in Cassia

- **Oil cells:** Entire or fragments of big oil cells associated with parenchyma cell.

Powder Microscopy

- **Fibres:** 250–700 μ long and 15–40 μ wide, thin, narrow, lignified fibres with pointed ends.
- **Stone cells:** Appear as 'U' shaped as one wall is not thickened and pitted.

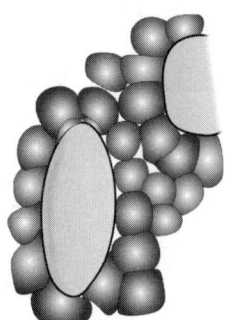

Fig. 2.61: Oil cells in Cassia

- **Cork:** Reddish brown fragments

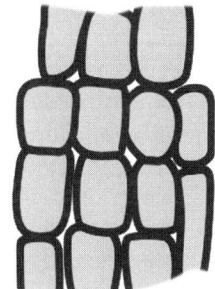

Fig. 2.62: Cork in Cassia

- **Starch:** 5–20 µ, abundant

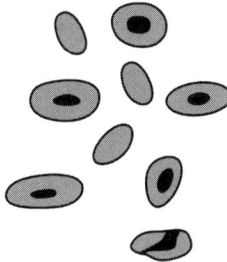

Fig. 2.63: Starch cells in Cassia

- **Calcium oxalate crystals:** In the form of acicular raphides.

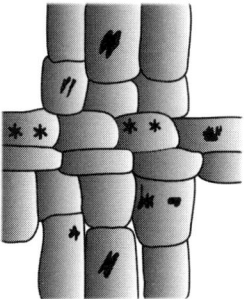

Fig. 2.64: Calcium oxalate crystals in Cassia

Chemical Tests

1. 5% ferric chloride solution is added to the aqueous extract. Dark colour shows presence of tannins.
2. Lead acetate solution is added to the aqueous extract. White precipitate shows presence of tannins.
3. 5 ml alcohol and added 5% ferric chloride solution is to the volatile oil. Brown colour shows presence of Cinnamaldehyde.
4. One drop volatile oil is taken on a slide one drop of 10% aqueous phenyl hydrazine HCl solution is added. Rod shaped crystals shows presence of Cinnamaldehyde.

Substituents

1. Jungle cinnamon
2. Cinnamon chips
3. Java cinnamon
4. Saigon cinnamon

Uses: Carminative, stimulant, flavouring agent and spices.

EXPERIMENT 27

Aim: To study the morphological, microscopical and powder characteristics of root of Liquorice.

Theory

Synonyms: Mulethi, Glycyrrhiza, Glycyrrhiza Radix, Jethimath.

Biological Source: It consists of dried, peeled or unpeeled, roots and stolon of *Glycyrrhiza glabra* Linn. and other Glycyrrhiza species, yielding a drug having a sweet taste and almost free from bitterness.

Family: Leguminosae.

Morphology

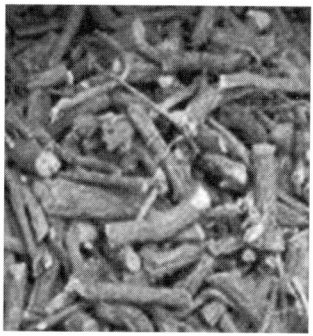

Fig. 2.65: Liquorice root

General Appearance: Spanish liquorice consists of peeled or unpeeled stolons and roots.

Organoleptic Characters

a. *Shape:* Peeled pieces – angular, unpeeled pieces–straight, unbranched and cylindrical.
b. *Size:* Up to 20 cm in length and 1 to 2 cm in diameter.
c. Surface:
   - *Unpeeled:* Yellowish brown with longitudinal wrinkles.
   - *Peeled:* Yellow colored with fine longitudinal ridges.
   - *Stolons:* Bear scars of buds.
d. Fracture:
   - *Peeled*: Fibrous
   - *Unpeeled*: Very fibrous
     Fractured surface shows long fibers projecting outwards.
e. *Colour:* Peeled: pale yellow, unpeeled: yellowish brown to dark brown.
f. *Odour:* Faint and characteristic.
g. *Taste:* Sweet, free from bitterness.

Microscopy: TS of stolon shows the following tissues

A. Periderm:
- **Phellem (cork):** Multilayered, composed of tubular cells; outer layers reddish brown colored while inner layers are colorless.
- **Phellogen:** Indistinct
- **Phelloderm:** 3–5 layered, composed of parenchymatous cells, some of which becomes collenchymatous. Cells contain prisms of calcium oxalate and starch grains.

B. Secondary Phloem: Bundles of phloem fibres (yellowish and slightly lignified) are arranged concentrically and each bundle is covered by a parenchymatous sheath which contains prisms of calcium oxalate crystals.

C. Secondary Xylem: Consists of xylem fibres (highly liginified), vessels of various sizes and xylem parenchyma in small amount. The vessels show sclariform and bordered pitted thickenings. Xylem fibres are also surrounded by parenchymatous cells containing prismatic calcium oxalate crystals. Starch is also present.

D. Medullary Rays: Distinct, bi- to multi-seriate parenchymatous. In the xylem region the rays are narrower and become wider in phloem region.

E. Pith: Parenchymatous with intercellular spaces and also contains a few starch grains.

Note: The histology of root is similar to that of stolon except the absence of pith and arrangement of protoxylem towards outer layer.

Chemical Constituents

The main constituent of liquorice is a triterpenoid saponin known as glycyrrhizin

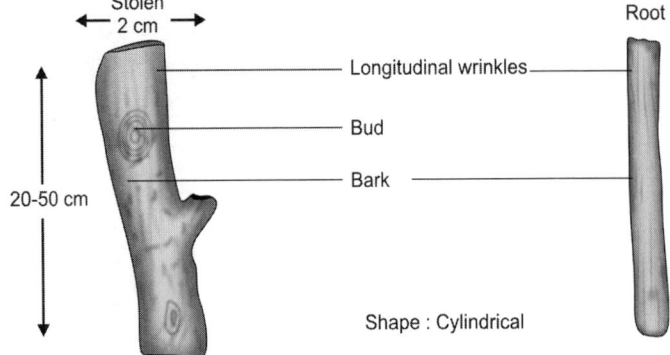

Fig. 2.66: Morphology of liquorice root

(glycyrrhizic acid 3–9%), which is potassium and calcium salt of glycyrrhizic acid. Glycyrrhizic acid is a glycoside and on hydrolysis yields glycyrrhentinic acid (glycyrrhitic acid), which has a triterpenoid structure.

It also contains flavonoid glycosides (isoliqueritin and liqueritin) and coumarin derivatives (herniarin and umbelliferone).

Powder Microscopy

A. Fibres: Yellow colored fibres in bundles of about 10–15 associated with crystal

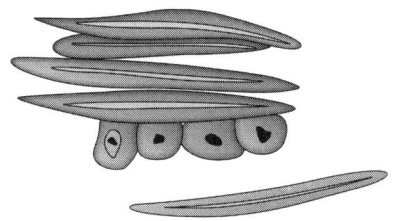
Glycyrrhentinic acid

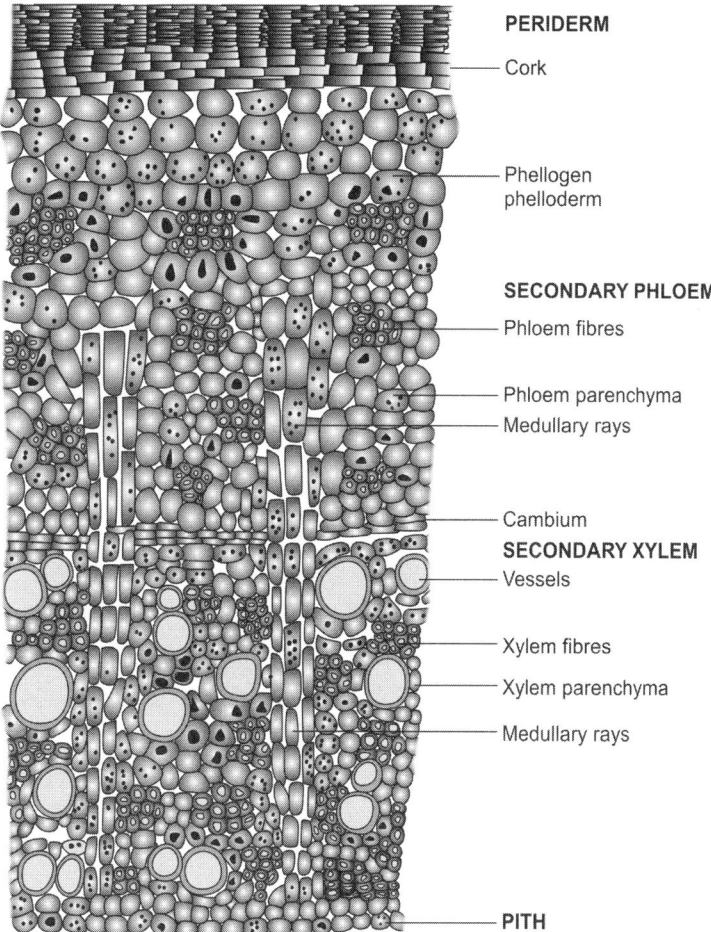

Fig. 2.67: Fibres and calcium oxalate crystals

Fig. 2.68: Microscopy of Liquorice root

sheath of parenchymatous cells each containing single prism of calcium oxalate.

B. **Calcium oxalate crystals:** Prismatic Calcium oxalate crystals occur in parenchymatous cells as well as many are scattered in the powder.

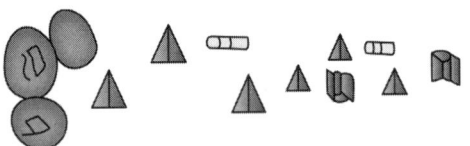

Fig. 2.69: Prismatic calcium oxalate crystals

C. **Vessels:** Large with numerous bordered pits.

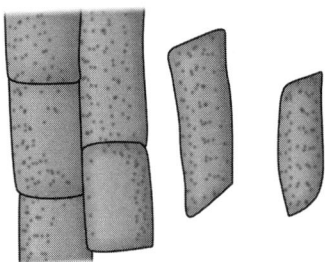

Fig. 2.70: Vessels

D. **Starch grains:** Minute, both simple (oval to elongated) and compound (less in number) showing no striations.

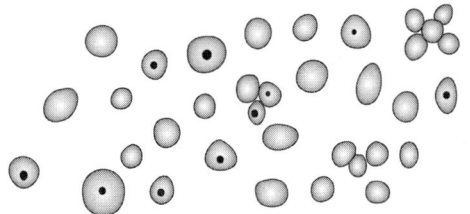

Fig. 2.71: Starch grains

Staining and Microchemical Tests

1. Add concentrated HCl in Phloroglucinol: Pink Lignified xylem fibres, phloem fibres seen.
2. With Iodine solution: Blue coloured solution shows presence of Starch.
3. With Acetic acid: Insoluble Calcium oxalate crystals observed.
4. With 60% Sulphuric acid Crystal soluble Calcium sulphate needles observed.

Chemical Tests

Flavonoids

To the aqueous extract, add sulfuric acid or hydrochloric acid. Reddish orange colour is produced which decolorize on addition of alkali and reappears on addition of acid.

Phenolic Compounds

- To the aqueous extract add 5% ferric chloride solution. Dark colour is produced.
- To the aqueous extract add lead acetate solution. White precipitate is produced.

Reducing Compounds

To the aqueous extract add 5% potassium permanganate solution. Decolourization of potassium permanganate solution is observed.

Saponins

Shake a pinch of powder drug with distilled water in a test tube. Stable foam shows presence of saponins.

Substituents

1. Manchurian liquorice obtained from *Glycyrrhiza uralensis*
2. Russian liquorice obtained from *Glycyrrhiza glabra* variety *glandulifera*

Preparation

Liquorice compound powder, liquid extract, ammoniated glycyrrhizin, Liquorice lozenges, stick liquorice.

Varieties and Allied Drugs

1. Russian Liquorice root (*Glycyrrhiza glabra* var.*glandulifera*) Regal and Herder.
   i. Larger than *Glycyrrhiza glabra* var. typical, pieces are often longitudinally split

ii. Texture is coarser and more fibrous.

iii. Occurs mainly in the peeled state, exhibiting a smooth yellow exterior with loose fibre. Unpeeled resembles Spanish Liquorice but mainly consists mainly of roots with no stolons. It is purplish in colour and the cork may be scanty. Taste is sweet with slight bitterness.

2. Persian liquorice root (*Glycyrrhiza glabra* var. *violacea*, Boiss)

   i. Usually unpeeled and occurs in large, coarse pieces resembling unpeeled Russian root.

3. Manchurian Liquorice root (*Glycyrrhiza uralensis*)

   i. Bears a chocolate-brown exfoliating cork

   ii. Medullary rays are curved or wavy and the wood exhibits Lacunae

Uses: Expectorant, demulcent, flavouring agent, anti spasmodic, used in the treatment of rheumatoid arthritis, inflammations and addison's disease.

EXPERIMENT 28

Aim: To study the morphological, microscopical and powder Characteristics of Kurchi bark.

Theory

Synonym: Holarrhena (Eng.), Kura Kurchi (Hindi), Kidvo indrajav (Marathi), Kutaja (Sans), Kada Chhal (Guj.)

Biological Source: Kurchi consists of dried stem bark of *Holarrhena antidysenterica*, collected from 8 to 12 years old trees and freed from attached wood.
Family: Apocynaceae.

Morphology

- *Size and Shape:* Small recurved pieces of varying sizes and thickness.
- *Outer Surface:* Buff to brownish, longitudinally wrinkled and bearing horizontal lenticels.
- *Inner Surface:* Brownish, rough, wood sometimes attached to inner bark.
- *Fracture:* Short and granular.
- *Taste:* Bitter.
- *Odour:* None.
- *Smoothed Transverse Surface:* Shows outer cork wide phelloderm containing stone cells and wide phloem with medullary rays and tangentially arranged stone cells.

Transverse Section

Periderm

Cork: Four to twelve rows of tangentially elongated cells. Few with yellowish brown matter.

Phellogen: Two layers of colorless thin walled tangentially elongated cells.

Phelloderm: Six to ten rows, thin walled rectangular cells, rhomboidal crystals and starch grains.

Cortex: Wide, parenchymatous, interspersed with groups of stone cells.

Stone cells: Lignified, pitted, rectangular and oval, contain calcium oxalate prisms. Continuous band of stone cells with rhomboidal calcium oxalate crystals.

Few nonlignified pericyclic fibres.

Secondary Phloem

Contain phloem parenchyma, sieve tubes and campanion cells.

Stone cells: Tangentional rows, separated by medullary rays and encircled by a sheath of parenchyma containing rhomboidal crystals of calcium oxalate.

Medullary rays: Two to three celled wide towards the outer part, consists of thin walled redially elongated parenchymatous cells, contains starch grains.

Phloem fibres absent.

Microscopical Characteristics of Powdered Drugs

Cork Cells: Thin walled, few colourless and few are with yellowish brown matter.

Stone cells: Rectangular to oval in shape, walls striated, pitted and lignified. Surrounded by sheath of parenchymatous cells containing calcium oxalate prisms. Show green colour with conc. Sulphuric acid.

Medullary rays: Parenchymatous cells at right angle.

Starch: Few, simple grains.

Calcium oxalate crystals.

Phloem fibres are absent.

Table 2.11: Staining and Microchemical Tests

S.No	Reagent	Observation	Characteristic
1.	Phloroglucinol +conc HCl (1:1 Mixture)	Pink	Lignified stone cells
2.	Iodine solution	Blue	Starch
3.	Conc. Sulphuric acid	Green	Stone cells
4.	Acetic acid	Insoluble crystals	Calcium oxalate
5.	Dil. Hydrochloric acid	Soluble crystals	Calcium oxalate
6.	Sulphuric acid 60% w/w	Soluble, needle shaped crystals of sulphate on standing	Calcium oxalate

Microscopy

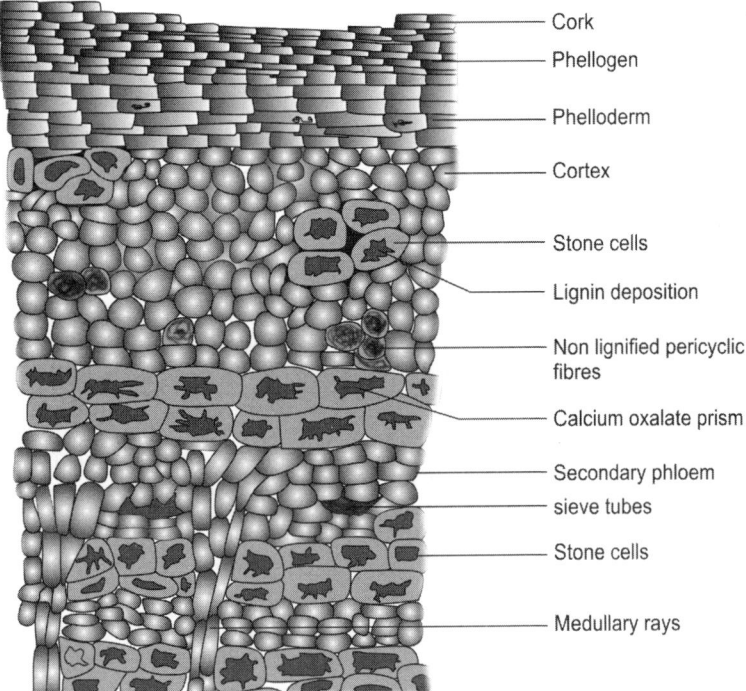

Fig. 2.72: Microscopy of Kurchi bark

Chemical Tests
Green stained stone cells are obtained on addition of conc H_2SO_4 in the solution of bark.

Chemical Constituents
Alkaloids: Steroidal alkaloids 2 to 4%, Conessine 30% of the total alkaloids, Nor-conessine, Isoconessine and kurchicine.

Uses: Antiprotozoal, externally as in case of skin troubles, dysentery; astringent, anemia, epilepsy, stomach pain, etc.

EXPERIMENT 29

Aim: To study the morphological, microscopical and powder Characteristics of Ephedra (Ma-Huang) leaf.

Theory
Biological Source: Dried young stem of *Ephedra gerardiana* (Wall) Stapf and also of *Enebrudensis* (Tineo) stapf collected in autumn. It contains not less than 1.0% of total alkaloids calculated as ephedrine.
Family: Gnetaceae (Ephedraceae).

Morphology
Enebrodensis
Size: Length	: 15 – 35 cm
Thickness	: 1 – 2 mm
Shape	: Cylindrical
Number of ridges	: 21 – 27 – 32
Surface	: Rough because of longitudinal ridges
Fracture	: Fibrous in the cortex. Pitch contains brownish powdery mass
Leaves	: Brownish to whitish brown, scaly, connate, opposite and dicussate
Apex	: Acute
Colour	: Greenish yellow
Odour	: Aggreable and slightly aromatic
Taste	: Astringent and bitter

Egeradiana
Size: Length	: 12 – 33 cm
Thickness	: 0.8 – 1.5 mm
Shape	: Cylindrical
Number of ridges	: 24 – 28 – 36
Surface	: Rough because of longitudinal ridges
Fracture	: Fibrous in the cortex. Pitch contains brownish powdery mass
Leaves	: Brownish to whitish brown, scaly, connate, opposite and dicussate
Apex	: Obtuse
Colour	: Greenish yellow
Odour	: Aggreable and slightly aromatic
Taste	: Astringent and bitter

Esinica
Size: Length	: Up to 30 cm
Thickness	: 1 – 2 mm
Shape	: Cylindrical
Number of ridges	: 9 – 20
Surface	: Rough because of longitudinal ridges
Fracture	: Fibrous in the cortex. Pitch contains brownish powdery mass
Leaves	: A pair of leaves at the nodes, fused at the base
Apex	: Acute and recurred
Colour	: Brownish
Odour	: Aggreable and slightly aromatic
Taste	: Astringent and bitter

Eequisetina
Size: Length	: Above 25 cm
Thickness	: 1.5 – 2 mm
Shape	: Cylindrical
Surface	: Smooth

Fracture : Fibrous in the cortex. Pitch contains brownish powdery mass

Leaves : Fused leaf encircling the node

Apex : Short but not recurred

Colour : Grey to pale green

Odour : Aggreable and slightly aromatic

Taste : Astringent and bitter

Microscopy

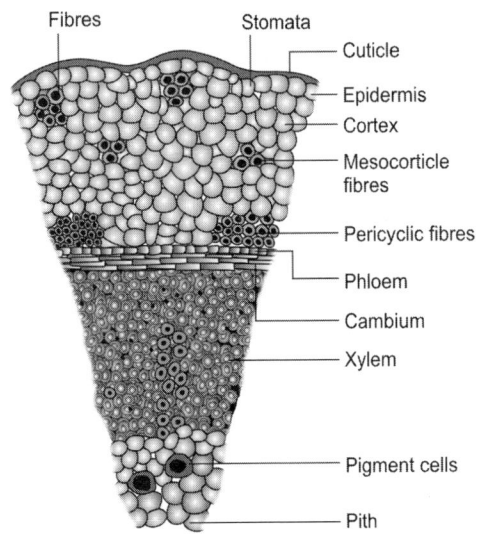

Fig. 2.73: TS of Ephedra leaf

Transverse Section

Epidermis: Single layered, quadrangular cells, with thick and smooth cutical. Verticle rows of sunken stomata present between many vertical ridges on the stem.

Cortex: Many layers of thin walled cellulosic parenchyma, below epidermis, two to three layers of loosely arranged palisade like cells are present (containing chloroplast).

Unlignified fibres: Like bunch of grapes, occur below the ridges where no palisade cells are present.

Fibres: Scattered, isolated or in groups of two to four cells, lignified.

Pericyclic Fibres: Lignified, crown the phloem on its outer side (strengthening cells).

Vascular Bundle: Around 10, collateral, conjoint, open and arranged in ring.

Phloem: Containing sieve tubes and companion cell.

Xylem: Well developed, consists of vessels, tracheides, fibrotracheids and parenchyma.

Pith: Large, thin walled, lignified big polygonal parenchyma with intercellular space. Some cells contain dark brownish mucilaginous substance.

Microchemical Tests

Phloroglucinol and conc HCl (1:1): Lignified fibres, vascular bundles, pericyclic fibres shows pink colour.

Chemical Test

Test for ephedrine: Dissolve 10 mg in 1 ml of water, add 0.2 ml of dilute hydrochloric acid and add 0.1 ml of copper sulphate solution followed by 1 ml of sodium hydroxide solution. The liquid becomes violate. Add 1 ml of solvent ether and shake, the etherical layer is purple and the aqueous layer is blue.

Chemical Constituents

It contains 0.5 to 2% Alkaloids, Alkaloidal amines and Ephedrine.

Uses: Sympathomimetic; in asthamatic condition, causes mydriasis.

Substitutes: *Ephedra sinica.*

Allied Species

Ephedra equisetina, Ephedra sinica, Ephedra intermedia, Ephedra major, Ephedra alata.

EXPERIMENT 30

Aim: To study the morphological, microscopical and powder Characteristics of Ipecacuanha root.

Synonym: Ipecac, Brazilian Ipecac

Biological Source: Ipecacuanha consists of dried root or rhizome of *Caphealis ipecacuanha* (Brot.) A. Rich. (Rio or Brazilian ipecac) or of *Cephealis aluminata* Karsten (Cartagena, Nicaragua or Panama Ipecac).

Family: Rubiaceae.

Morphology

- *Size:* Length 5 to 15 cm; diameter 3 to 5 mm (usually 4 mm).
- *Shape:* Cylindrical, slightly tortuous.
- *Surface:* Annulated or annulated ring encircles the root from the half to three quarters; annulations are broad and round; sometimes attached rhizome or its free pieces and lateral roots or their scars are seen.
- *Colour:* Brick red to brown.
- *Odour:* Slight, powder irritant and sternutatory.

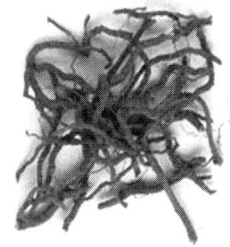

Fig. 2.74: Ipecac root

- *Taste:* Bitter and acrid.
- *Fracture:* Short and starchy in the bark, splintery in the xylem.
- *Fractured surface:* Wide grayish bark occupying two-third diameter and central yellowish-white wood occupying one-third diameter.
- *Extra feature:* Absence of annulations and presence of transverse ridges at an interval of 1–3 mm. They partially encircle the roots.

Microscopy

Transverse Section

Cork: Narrow, tangentially elongated isodiametric cells, with dark brown granular matter, shape is not regular.

Phelloderm: Two or three rows of tangentially elongated thin walled cells. Few cells contain starch grains.

Cortex: Many layers of thin walled cellulosic parenchyma, with very small intercellular spaces. Cells are packed with starch grains. Scattered idioblasts contain bundle of acicular raphides of calcium oxalate.

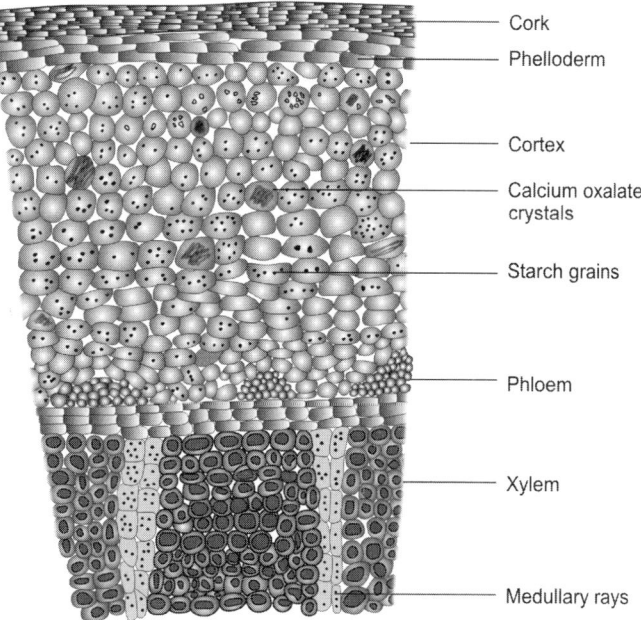

Fig. 2.75: Microscopy of Ipecac root

Starch grain: Rarely single, mostly compound with 2–4 grains. Few cells show more than 4 grains too. Individual diameter about 4 to10 µ (not more than 15 µ in diameter).

Calcium oxalate crystals: 30 to 80 µ in length.

In powdered drug, these raphides are generally broken and crystals are scattered singly throughout the powder.

Phloem: Many patches of small group of sieve tissues embedded in parenchymatous cells, above the cambium.

Xylem: Entirely lignified, consists of tracheids, tracheidal vessels, xylem parenchyma and medullary rays. Tracheids have pitted wall. Vessels are not easily distinguished from the tracheids. Xylem parenchymatous cells are packed with starch grains like those of cortex.

Medullary Rays: Consists of lignified, radially elongated cells arranged in radial rows. Cells are usually filled with starch grains.

There are no vessels or normal fibres.

Microscopical Characteristics of Powdered Drugs

Cork: Polygonal, isodiametric cells with granular brown matter.

Parenchyma: Thin walled polyhedral cells with interacellular space and starch grains.

Calcium Oxalate Crystals: Idioblast of acicular raphides of calcium oxalate crystals either in bundles or scattered all over singly.

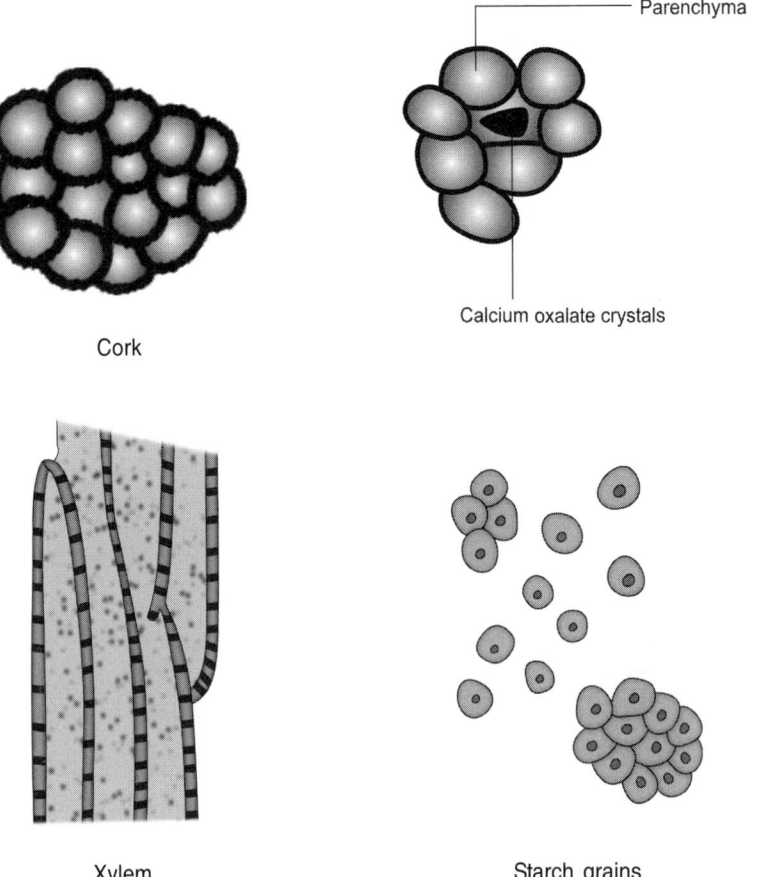

Fig. 2.76: Microscopical characterstics of powedered Ipecac

Xylem: Tracheids with pitted wall. Mostly pointed and frequently perforated at the ends.

Starch Grains: Single and compound. Individual grain diameter is up to 4 to 10 μ. Few grains show prominent pointed hilum.

Vessels, sclerenchymatous cells and fibres are absent.

Staining and Microchemical Tests

1. Pink colour is obtained with Phloroglucinol and concentrated HCl (1:1 mixture): Shows presence of lignified xylem and medullary rays.
2. Blue colour is obtained with iodine solution shows presence of starch.
3. Insoluble in Acetic acid and soluble in dilute hydrochloric acid shows presence of calcium oxalate crystals.

Chemical Tests

Heat 1 gm powder and 5 ml dilute HCl for few minutes and filter. Add 10 mg potassium chlorate to the filtrate. Colour of filtrate changes from yellow to red, shows presence of Emetin.

Chemical Constituents

Mainly it contains following Alkaloids:

Isoquinoline alkaloids: 1.4–1.7% Emetin, 0.5–1.2% Cephaeline, 0.05% Psychotrine, Psychotrine methylether and emetamine.

Uses: Expectorant, emetic, antiamoebic.

Preparations

Ipecacuanha liquid extract, Ipecacuanha tincture, prepared Ipecacuanha.

Adultrants

Limit of adulterations should not be more than 5%.

i. *Carthagena Ipecacuanha*:
   a. Larger in diameter (about 4 to 9 cm).
   b. Greenish-brown in colour.
   c. Root is annulated; showing raised narrow, distinct ridges which do not extend entirely around the root.
   iv. Starch grains are larger.
i. Ipecacuanha stems:
   a. Slender and longitudinally striated.
   b. The transverse section shows a bark, a ring of wood and distinct pith.
iii. East Indian Root (*Cryptocoryne spiralis*, fam: Araceac):

   TS shows monocotyledonous structure.
iv. White Ipecacuanha (*Ionidium ipecacuanha*, fam: Violaceac)
   a. White or yellowish in colour.
   b. Wood is large, porous and yellowish.
   c. Stems are slender and ash-coloured, knotted with radicles.

EXPERIMENT 31

Aim: To study the morphological, microscopical and powder Characteristics of Nux vomica seed.

Theory

Synonym: Zer Kacholu

Biological Source: Nux vomica consists of dried ripe seeds of *Strychnos nux-vomica* containing not less than 1.2% strychnine.

Family: Loganiaceae.

Morphology

- *Size:* 10 to 30 mm in diameter; 3 to 5 mm thick.
- *Shape:* Disc-shaped, flat, some concavo-convex, few seeds irregularly bent, margin rounded or acute.
- *Outer surface:* Grey to greenish-grey covered with numerous, closely appressed silky hairs, radiating from the center, hairs impart characteristics sheen. Hilum is present in the center of the flat surface of the seed. From the hilum a ridge which is not raphe, connects the position of the micropyle at the circumference.

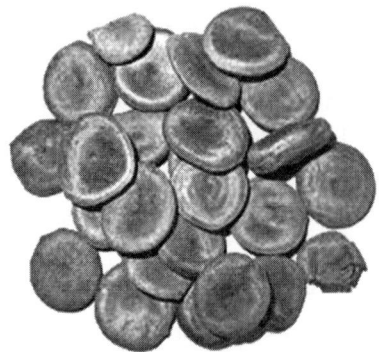

Fig. 2.77: Nux vomica seeds

- *Endosperm:* It is present below the testa and is grey and horny. Below the endosperm in the center a narrow slit like cavity is present.
- *Embryo:* It is seen at the micropylar end with a cylindrical radical and two cordate cotyledons.
- *Odour:* None.
- *Taste:* Very bitter.

Chemical Tests: It gives general tests for alkaloids as follows:

Dragendroff's test
To the extract, add few drops of dragendroff's reagent. Reddish brown precipitate is formed.

Mayer's test
To 2–3 ml of extract, add a few drops of Mayer's reagent. It gives cream or buff colored precipitate.

Hager's test
To 2–3 ml of extract, add Hager's reagent. It gives yellow colored precipitate.

Wagner's test
To 2–3 ml of extract, add few drops of Wagner's reagent. It gives reddish brown precipitate.

10% Tannic acid solution
Alkaloids give a buff coloured precipitate.

Microscopy

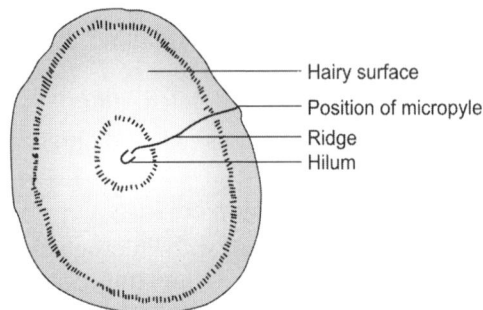

(A) Whole drug

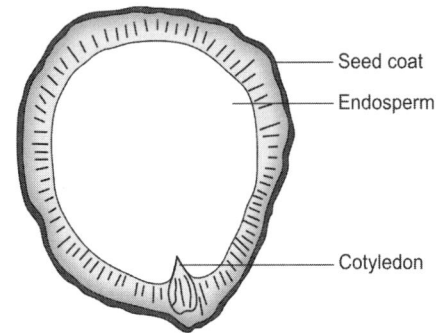

(B) Longitudinal surface of seed

Fig. 2.78: Nux vomica

Transverse section

Testa: Lignified trichomes: Thick walled, bent and twisted lignified trichomes, immerged from epidermis, parallel in one direction.

Length: 600–1000 µ, diameter about 25 µ

Epidermal cell: Single layer, forms lignified trichomes, large thick walled with oblique linear pits (base of trichomes)

Collapsed parenchyma: 2 layers, flattened parenchyma.

Endosperm: Thick walled cellulosic parenchymatous cells. Cell shows following characteristics:

Plasmodesma: Fine protoplasmic strands between the walls of endospermic cells.

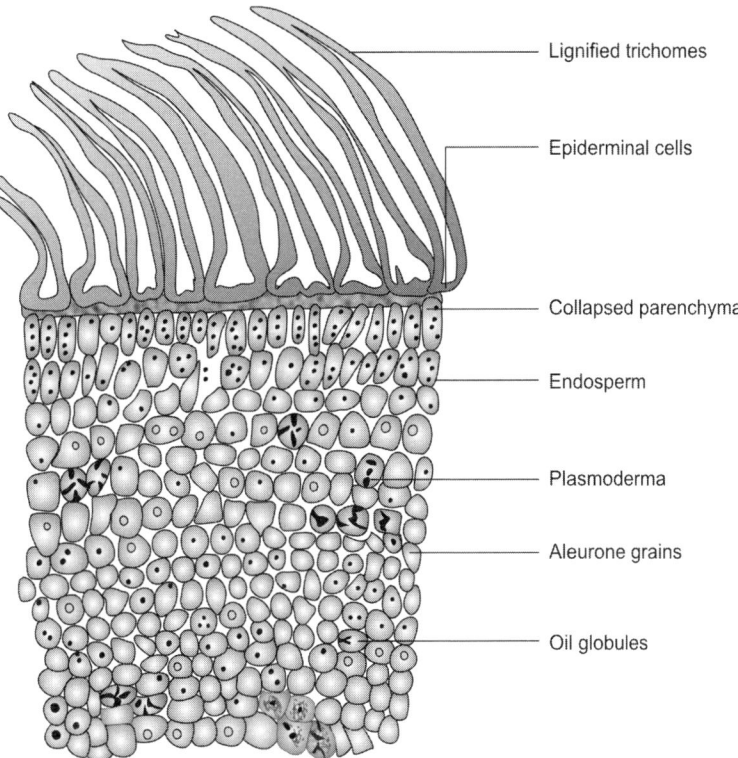

Fig. 2.79: TS of Nux vomica seed

Aleurone grains: About 30 μ in diameter. Only globoids are present.
Oil globules: Fixed oil as small oil droplets in the cells.

Microscopical Characteristics of Powdered Drugs

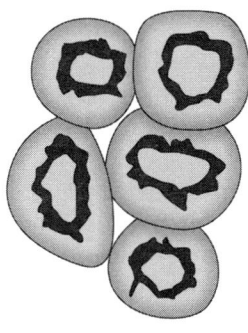

Fig. 2.80: Trichome

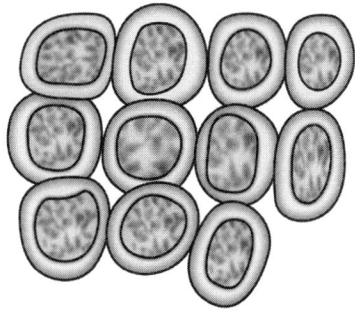

Fig. 2.81: Endosperm

Trichomes: Entire or fragments of trichomes, lignified. Base is pitted and broad. Apex is rounded. Ridges are present on the surface.

Length: 60–1000 μ.

Diameter: about 25 μ

Endosperm: Polygonal cellulosic cells, with oil globules and aleurone grains.

Staining and Microchemical Tests

1. Phloroglucinol and concentrated HCl (1:1 mixture): Pink coloured lignified cells-epidermal trichomes.
2. Dilute iodine solution + conc. sulphuric acid; blue coloured hemicellulose-Endospermic walls (plasmodesma).
3. Alcoholic picric acid: Yellow coloured Aleurone grains present in the cells of endosperm.
4. Sudan red III: Red coloured oil globules present in the cells of endosperm.

Microchemical Tests

1. To the defatted thick section, add Ammonium vanadate and concentrated H_2SO_4: Violet colour to the cells in central region of endosperm: Strychnine present.
2. To the defatted thick section add concentrated HNO_3: Orange yellow colour to the cells of peripheral region of endosperm: Brucine present.

Chemical Constituents

Alkaloids (2.5–5%): Strychnine, strychnicine, brucine, etc.

Glycoside: Loganin fixed oil (2–4%) and proteins

Uses: Bitter stomachic, spinal cord stimulant, nerve tonic.

Preparations

Nux vomica liquid extract, prepared Nux vomica and Tincture Nux vomica.

Adultrants

i. *Strychnos potatorum* seeds:
   a. Smaller and thicker than *Strychnos nuxvomica*.
   b. Free from alkaloids and do not have a bitter taste.
   c. Strychnine is absent, hence a section does not show purple colour when treated with Ammonium Vanadate and conc. Sulphuric acid.

ii. *Strychnus Nux-blanda*
   a. Appearanes are like *Strychnos nuxvomica*, but more yellowish in colour (ii) and (iii) same as above.
   b. Pale in colour with a distinct ridge on the edge of the seed.

Allied Drugs

i. Ignatius Bean (*Strychnos ignati* Berg.)
   a. Larger that the seeds of *Strychnos nuxvomica*
   b. Irregularly ovate shape and dark green colour
   c. Seed coat can be easily removed.
   d. Trichomes are unlignified.

EXPERIMENT 32

Aim: To study powder Characteristics of Rhubarb.

Theory

Biological Source: Rhubarb consists of the dried rhizome of *Rheum emodi* Wall *Rheum Webianum* Royle and other species of *Rheum*.

Family: Polygonaceae

Morphology

- *General appearance:* Compact, firm
- *Shape:* Subcylindrical, conical or barrel shaped, plano-convex pieces.
- *Size:* 2 to 20 cm in length, 1.5 to 8 cm in diameter.
- *Surface:* Outer surface is yellowish to purplish brown. It is longitudinally wrinkled, furrowed or ridged. Star spots or abnormal vascular bundles are absent and xylem vessels are lignified.
- *Colour:* Yellowish-brown to dark brown
- *Odour:* Faint and characteristic
- *Taste:* Bitter and astringent

Chemical Tests
1. Pink colour is obtained when powder is treated with ammonia solution.
2. Red colour is obtained when powder is treated with potassium hydroxide solution.

Microscopical Characteristics of Powdered Drugs

Cluster crystals of calcium oxalate: The fairly abundant cluster crystals of calcium oxalate which are found scattered and in some of the parenchymatous cells. They are very large and frequently fragmented.

Xylem vessels: Occur singly or in small groups and are frequently found in fragments. They are large, reticulately thickened and do not give reaction for lignin.

Starch grain: Which are simple and spherical, or sometimes compound with two to five granules.

Parenchyma of medullary rays: The abundant parenchyma of medullary rays are filled with starch grains and associated with vessels.

Chemical Constituents

Indian Rhubarb contains free anthraquiones 1.12% while combined anthraquiones as O-glycosides are 4.5%. The anthraquinones both free and in glycosidal combination are chrysophenol, aloe emodin, emodin and rhein, Sennosides A and B have been isolated. The hydrolysable tannins are present. Rhapontic is absent in Indian rhubarb. The greater purgative activity of rhubarb may be attributed to a greater percentage of both free and combined anthraquiones.

Uses

In small doses, it is used as a bitter stomachic especially of children and in larger doses as a purgative because of anthracene derivatives and in the treatment of diarrhoea.

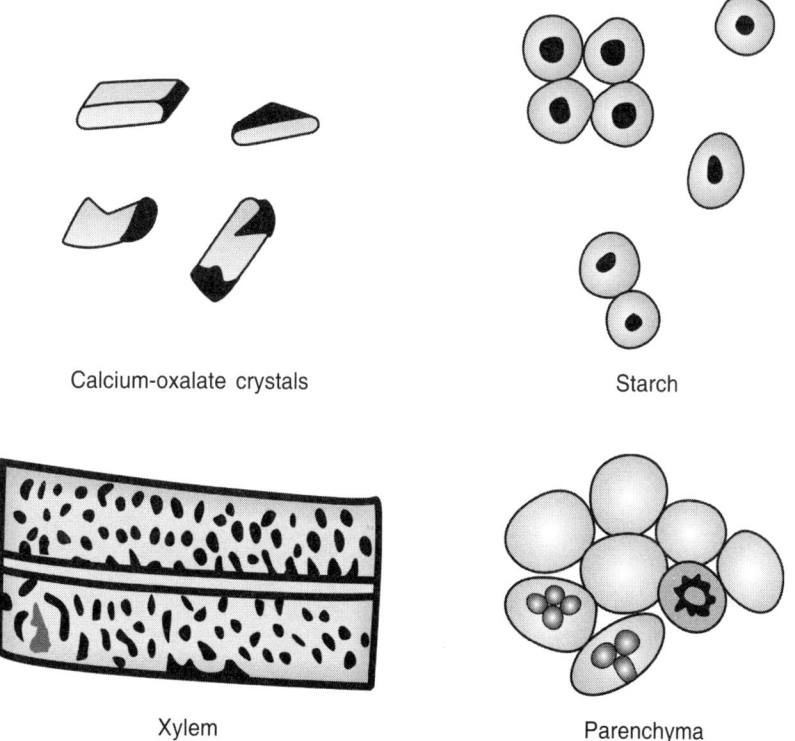

Fig. 2.82: Microscopical characteristics of powdered drugs

EXPERIMENT 33

Aim: To study Powder Characteristics of Indian Squill.

Theory

Biological Source: Indian squill consists of dried slices of the bulb of *Urginea indica* Kunth.

Family: Liliaceae.

Morphology

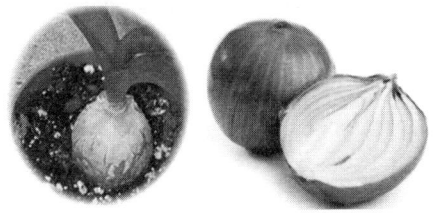

Fig. 2.83: Indian Squill

- *Size:* Length 1 to 5 cm; breadth 5 mm to 10 mm.
- *Shape:* Curved or sickle shaped, slices separate or 4 to 8 slices joined to the axis.
- *Surface:* Fleshy, longitudinally ribbed
- *Fracture:* Brittle in dry drug but tough in moist drug
- *Colour:* Yellowish-white
- *Odour:* Slight
- *Taste:* Bitter and acrid.

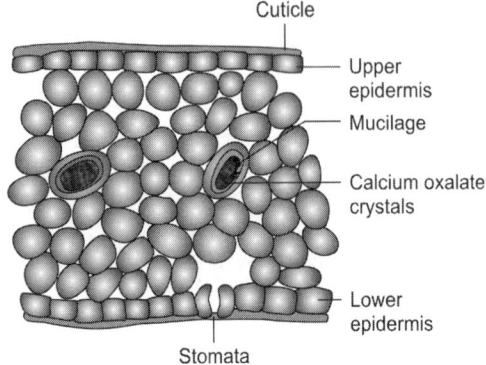

Fig. 2.84: TS of Squill

Microscopical Characteristics of Powdered Drugs

The very abundant acicular crystals of calcium oxalate which are considerably and frequently very large in size they occur in bundles embedded in mucilage in the parenchymatous cells and are scattered throughout the powder in broken groups or as single, much fragmented crystals.

Mucilage cells: Some of them are intact and contain bundle of acicular crystal of calcium

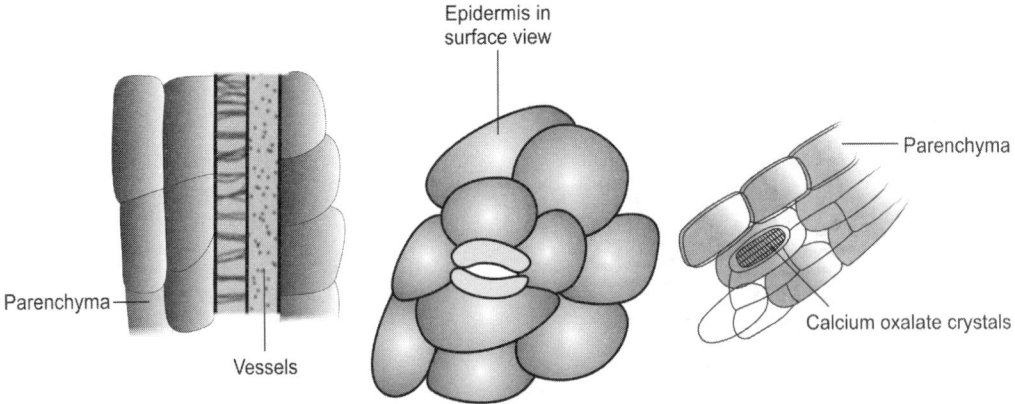

Fig. 2.85: Microscopical characteristics of the powdered drug

oxalate while others are broken, open and show fragment of calcium oxalate crystals or impression left by them.

Vessels: Single or in groups, having spiral or annular thickening.

Parenchyma: The very abundant parenchyma mainly of thin walled, rounded or elongated cells contains spheroidal masses of needle shaped crystal of sinistrin which are pale yellowish in colour.

Stomata: The epidermis composed of thin walled cells, elongated in surface view with infrequent rounded anomocytic stomata.

Chemical Constituents

Cardiac glycosides are present. Mucilage is present in cells of mesophyll, free or with calcium oxalate. Mucilage stains reddish-purple with iodine water. This test distinguishes European scilla and Indian scilla.

Chemical Tests

Place a drop of iodine water on a piece of Indian squill. A reddish purple colour is obtained.

Uses: Cardiotonic.

EXPERIMENT 34

Aim: To identify given unknown Powder mixture (Senna and Squill)

Procedure

Table 2.12: Physical examination

Test	Observation	Inference
Colour	Light yellow	Liquorice, squill may present
	Green	Leaf like senna, digitalis, Datura, Vasaka, Vinca may present
Odour	Odourless	Aromatic drug, Aromatic crude drug may absent
Taste	Bitter	Drug containing alkaloids or bitter glycosids, senna digitalis.

Microscopical Characteristics of Powdered Drugs

SENNA

Epidermal cells: Polygonal, straight walled, epidermal cells with paracytic stomata.

Paracytic stomata: Rubiaceous or parallel celled stomata with two subsidiary cells around the guard cells.

Covering trichomes: Unicellular, thick warty walls, acute apex, bulbous base, narrow lumen, conical shape.

$$\text{Length} = 70\text{–}260\mu$$
$$\text{Width} = 12\text{–}25\mu$$

Xylem vessels: Angular thickening, lignified

Calcium oxalate: Crystal isolated or in parenchymatous cells. Very abundant, occur as prism and also as cluster crystals.'

SQUILL

The very abundant acicular crystals of *calcium oxalate*: which vary considerably in size and are frequently very large; they occur in bundles embedded in mucilage in the parenchymatous cells and are scattered throughout the powder in broken groups or as single, much fragmented crystals.

Mucilage cells: Some of them are intact and contain bundle of acicular crystal of calcium oxalate while others are broken, open and show fragments of calcium oxalate crystals or impression left by them.

Vessels: Single or in groups, having spiral or annular thickening.

Parenchyma: The very abundant parenchyma mainly of thin walled rounded or elongated cells contain spheroidal masses of needle shaped crystal of sinistrin which are pale yellowish in colour.

Stomata: The epidermis composed of thin walled cells, elongated in surface view with infrequent rounded anomocytic stomata.

Result: The given powder mixture is of Senna and Squill.

EXPERIMENT 35

Aim: To identify the given unknown powder mixture (Vasaka and Ipecac).

Procedure

Table 2.13: Physical examination

Test	Observation	Inference
Colour	Light brown, green	Ipecac, unpeeled liquorice, umbelliferous fruits leaf, drug like senna, digitalis, datura, vasaka, etc.
Odour	odourless	Aromatic drug, aromatic crude drug may be absent
Taste	Bitter	Drug containing alkaloids, vasaka, nux vomica, vinca, datura, etc.

Microscopical Characteristics of Powdered Drugs

VASAKA

Epidermal cells: Polygonal thin walled parenchymatous cells with wavy and anticlinal walls.

Stomata: Two subsidiary cells at right angle to stoma (cross-celled stomata).

Covering trichomes: Two to four celled, bent, thick walled, pointed, uniseriate.

Glandular trichome: Sessile with quadra cellular heads.

Xylem vessels: With annular to spiral thickening and lignified.

Cystoliths: Calcium carbonate crystals, dissolves in hydrochloric acids with effervescence.

Calcium oxalate: Crystals in acicular and prismatic form.

IPECAC

Cork: Polygonal, isodiametric cells with granular brown matter.

Parenchyma: Thin walled polyhedral cells with intracellular space and starch grains.

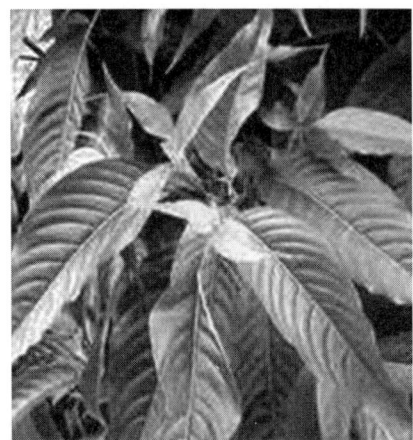
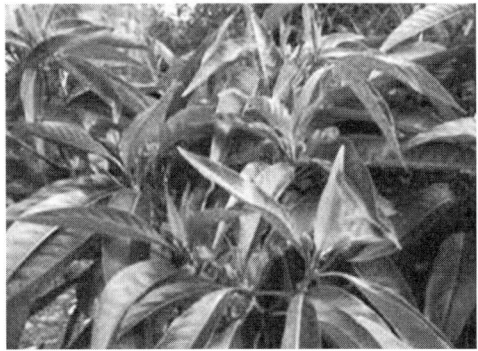

Fig. 2.86: Vasaka leaves

Calcium Oxalate Crystals: Idioblast of acicular raphides of calcium oxalate crystals either in bundles or scattered all over singly.

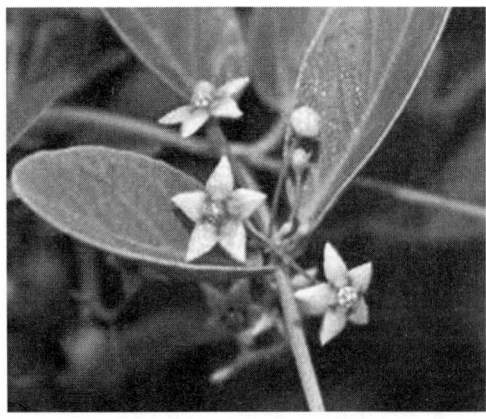

Fig. 2.87: Ipecac plant

Xylem: Tracheids with pitted wall. Mostly pointed and frequently perforated at the ends.

Starch Grains: Single and compound. Individual grain-diameter up to 4 to 10 μ. Few grains show prominent pointed hilum.

Vessels: Sclerenchymatous and fibres are absent.

Result: The given powder Mixture is of Ipecac and Vasaka.

EXPERIMENT 36

Aim: To identify given unknown powder mixture (Digitalis and Liquorice).

Procedure

Table 2.14: Physical examination

Test	Observation	Inference
Colour	Green	Leaf drug like *Senna digitalis*, Datura, Vasaka, Vinca, etc.
Odour	Odourless	Aromatic drug, Aromatic crude drug may be absent
Taste	Bitter	Drug containing alkaloids or bitter glycosides, *Senna digitalis*.

Microscopical Characteristics of Powdered Drugs

DIGITALIS

Stomata: Rananculaceous (irregular celled stomata)

Guard cells are surrounded by irregular number of subsidiary cells.

Epidermal cells: Irregularly beaded, wavy, thick, cuticulized with rananculaceous/anomocytic stomata.

Trichomes: Very rare.

LIQUORICE

Fibres: Lignified, thickened, yellow walls, in bundles of about 10–50, with crystal sheath of parenchymatous cells each containing single prism of calcium oxalate.

Xylem vessels: Large, with numerous boardered pits. Surface is lignified.

Calcium oxalate crystals: Individually prism shaped, 10–15 to 25–35μ long, present in parenchymatous cells and many are scattered in the powder.

Starch grains: Most are simple, oval or rounded, about 2–4 to 10–20 μ long, showing no striations.

Cork: Abundant fragments of orange-brown cork composed of thin walled polygonal cells.

Result: The given powder Mixture is of Digitalis and Liquorice.

EXPERIMENT 37

Aim: To identify given unknown Powder mixture (Cinchona and Vasaka).

Procedure

Table 2.15: Physical examination

Test	Observation	Inference
Colour	Red, Green	Cinchona, arjuna Leaf drug like *Senna digitalis*, datura, vasaka, etc
Odour	Odourless	Arometic drug, Aromatic crude drug may be absent
Taste	Bitter	Drug containing alkaloids, vasaka nux vomica, vinca, datura, etc.

Microscopical Characteristics of Powdered Drugs

CINCHONA

Cork: Thin walled, flat, polygonal cells with reddish brown matter.

Phloem fibres: Numerous large, fusiform, lignified phloem fibres, striated walls having simple pores or branched pores. 30 to 60 μ in width and 500 to 800 μ in length.

Calcium Oxalate Crystals: Microprisms of calcium oxalate crystals, about 2 to 6 μ long, in dark coloured parenchyma.

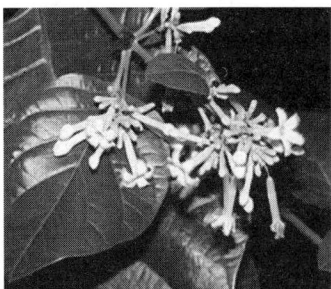

Fig. 2.88: Cinchona plant

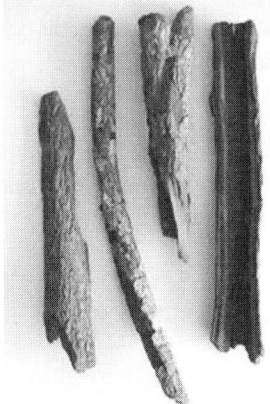

Fig. 2.89: Cinchona bark

Starch Grains: Minute, simple and compound (2 to 5) individual grain, about 2 to 5 μ in diameter. Stone cells and sphaerophides are absent.

VASAKA

Vasaka belongs to the plant family Acanthaceae, its botanical/taxonomic name is *Justicia adhatoda* L. Some of its synonyms are *Adhatoda vasica* and *Adhatoda zeylanica* (Medicus). Additional names for vasaka are malabarnut, Arusa, Vasa, Adhatodai, Basale and Banga. Malabarnut, Arusa, Vasa, Adhatodai, Basak, and Bansa.

Epidermal cells: Polygonal thin walled parenchymatous cells with wavy and anticlinal walls.

Stomata: Two subsidiary cells at right angle to stoma (cross celled stomata).

Covering trichomes: Two to four celled, bent, thick walled, pointed, uniseriate.

Glandular trichome: Sessile with quadra cellular heads.

Xylem vessels: With annular to spiral thickening and lignified.

Cystoliths: Calcium carbonate crystals, dissolves in hydrochloric acids with effervescence.

Fig. 2.90: Vasaka leaves

Calcium oxalate: Crystals in acicular and prismatic form.

Active Principles: Vasaka contains several active ingredients, the main one of which is the alkaloid vasicine, which is responsible for much of the bronchodilating effect. Vasicine is mainly derived from the leaves of the plant, along with the essential oil. Vasicine also known by another name, peganine. Vasicine's ($C_{11}H_{12}N_2O$) systematic name is 1,2,3,9-tetrahydropyrrolo[2,1-b]quinazolin-3-ol. Other important active ingredients contained in the stems and roots include vasicinol and the alkaloid vasicinone. Some other, less active chemicals present in the roots are quinazoline, anisotine, vasicol, vasicinolone, and adhatodine.

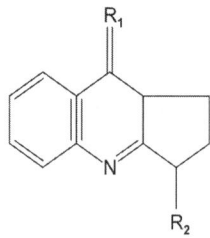

Vasicine (peganine) $R_1 = H_2$; $R_2 = OH$

Vascinone $R_1 = O$; $R_2 = OH$

Deoxyvasicinone $R_1 = O$; $R_2 = H$

Uses: *Vasaka*, a perennial shrub of the family Acanthaceae, is a highly reputed Ayurvedic medicinal plant used in the treatment of cough, bronchitis, asthma, tuberculosis and recommended for other ailments of the respiratory system. Leaves, flowers and roots of this plant are used in herbal drugs against cancer. This plant is also used as antispasmodic, fever reducer, anti-inflammatory, anti-bleeding, brochodilating (opens the breathing passages), antidiabetic, disinfectant, anti-jaundice, assistance in uterine contractions, and expectorant (promotes easier flow of mucous). Most of these attributes fall mainly into the respiratory therapy category for colds, asthma, bronchitis, tuberculosis, etc. The antispasmodic and anti-inflammatory properties apply to diarrhea, arthritis, vomiting, and gingivitis. The leaves are a source of vitamin C as well. The plant is administered orally, locally, or inhaled in various bitter-tasting forms.

Result: The given powder mixture is of Cinchona or Vasaka.

EXPERIMENT 38

Aim: To study Morphology of given drugs:

 i. Ashoka bark
 ii. Arjuna bark
 iii. Tulsi
 iv. Behera
 v. Amla
 vi. Vasaka
 vii. Harad

ASHOKA BARK

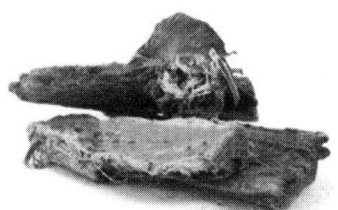

Fig. 2.91: Ashoka bark

Synonym: *Ashoka*.
Biological Source: Asoka is the dried bark of *Saraca indica*.
Family: Leguminosae.

Morphology

Size: In commerce varying but usually occurs in pieces up to 40 cm in length, 3-6 cm wide and 5–8 mm, thick.

Outer surface: Rough with warty protuberances and due to exfoliation rusty brown in colour. Transverse and longitudinal cracks are seen on the outer surface.

Inner surface: Smooth, soft and reddish brown.

Smoothed Transverse surface: Shows radially elongated but irregularly running medullary rays of varying width.

Fracture: Short and fibrous.
Odour: Indistinct.
Taste: Astringent.

Uses

- Popular uterine tonic and sedative
- Bark is used in menorrhagia.

ARJUNA BARK

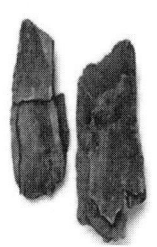 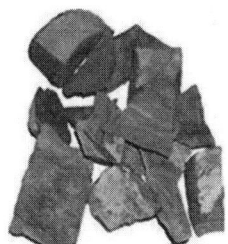

Fig. 2.92: Arjuna bark

Biological Source: Arjuna is the dried bark of *Terminalia arjuna*.
Family: Combretaceae.
Member of this family are characterized by the presense of tannins and are used as tanning agents. Myrobalans and beric fruits belong to this family.
Geographical Source: In India, trees are found in North Gujarat.

Morphology

Size: Pieces of varying sizes upto 15 cm or more in length, 10 cm or more in breadth, and 3 mm to 1 cm thick.

Shape: Flat or slightly curved.

Outer Surface: Smooth and grey-coloured.

Inner Surface: Finely striated, brown.

Fracture: Short, revealing stratified nature of the bark.

Odour: None.

Taste: Astringent.

Active principles: Arjunone; Cerasidin; Friedelin; Terminic acid; Arjunolic acid; Arjunicacid; Arunolone; Arjunglucoside III; Arjunoside I and II Arjunoside III and IV; Arjunglucoside I and II; Arjunetin; Terminoic acid; Arjunic acid and Arjungenin.

Terminoic acid

Uses

- Arjuna is popularly used as a cardiac tonic. Caius, Mhaskar and Isaac found arjuna possessing diuretic property
- Recently mechanism of cardiovascular action of arjuna bark has been reported. Intravenous administration of aqueous extract of dried bark decreases blood pressure and heart rate.
- Extract also inhibits carotid occlusion response.
- In hypotension and bradycardia

Tulsi

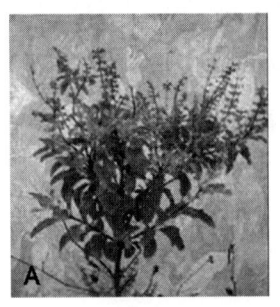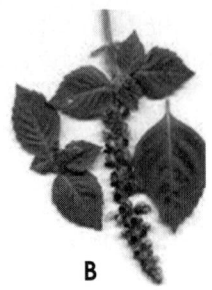

Fig. 2.93: Tulsi (A) Plant (B) Leaves

Biological Source: Tulsi consists of the leaves of *Ocimum sanctum*.

Family: Labiatae.

The plant is found through out India and is considered sacred and worshipped and is grown near Hindu houses and temples.

Morphology

Annual herb 30–60 cm high, much branched stems and branches usually purplish, sub-quadrangular, sometimes woody below, clothed with soft spreading hairs.

Leaves are 2.5–5 cm long and 1.6–3.2 cm broad, elliptical, oblong, obtuse or acute; margin entire or serrate, surface pubescent on both sides, minutely gland-dotted, base obtuse or acute, petioles 1.3–2.5 cm long, slender, hairy. Infloresence verticillate, flowers are in recemes 15–20 cm long in close whorls. Bracts 3 mm, both long and broad, broadly ovate; calyx slender, pubescent, bilabiate, lower lip longer than upper. Corolla 4 mm long, purplish, bilabiate upper lip pubescent on the back. Stamens exserte, filaments slender, the upper pair with a small brached appendage at the base. Nutlets 1.25 mm long broadly ellipsoid, nearly smooth, yellow with small black markings. Seeds are brownish, globose or subglobose, having aromatic and sharp odour and taste.

Active Principles: Cadinene; 1, 8-cineole; eugenol; limonene; melhytchavicol; β-carotene;

ursolic acid; caryophyllene; bornyl acetate; terpinin-4-o1; diacylaldehyde; γ-selinene; β-pinene; camphene and α-pinene.

Uses

- Leaves are anticatarrhal, expectorant and spasmolytic and are used in cold, cough, fever and gastric disorders (Decoction of 10–15 leaves prepared with black pepper, ginger, clove and sugar is given twice a day).
- Also used in aromatic carminative, stimulant and flavouring agent.
- The drug is antiseptic and is used also extremely in skin diseases.
- Recently anti-stress activity of Tulsi and Ashwagantha was determined by estimation of succinic acid. Clinical assessments of these drugs were made in human beings.
- **Pneumonia:** It is an established traditional folklore medicine known for its stimulating effect; aqueous extract of leaves is mixed with equal amount of honey; given 1-teaspoonfull twice a day for three days.

Other Uses

1. **Cough, cold and fever:** Decoction of 10-15 leaves prepared with black pepper, ginger clove and sugar is given twice a day.
2. **Dermal infection:** Leaf paste is applied externally on the affected areas of skin and wounds.

Ocimum canum Sims. (Lamiaceae)

Commonly known as *Van tulsi* in study area.

Active principle: Polysaccharides contained xylose; arabinose; rhamnose; galactose; galacturonic acid; glucuronic acid; ocimin; methylchavicol; linalool; nevadensin; salvigenin; ursolic; oleanolic acid; acidic polysaccharide; camphor; limonene; bergamotene; b-caryophyllene and eugenol.

Uses

1. **Intermittant fever:** Fresh leaves (20), a few black pepper (*Piper nigrum*) and a pinch of common salt are grined and the paste is converted into tablets (about 30). 3 tablets are given thrice a day orally for three days.
2. **Eye infection:** Fresh leaf juice is used as eye drops.
3. **Throat infection:** Decoction of fresh leaves and dried rhizome of ginger is given orally in fever and throat infection.

Ocimum gratissimum Linn. (Lamiaceae)

Commonly known as *"Adak tulsi"*.

Active principle: Eugenol; β-caryophyllene; germacrene; α-copaene; humulene; β-elemene; β-bourbonene; δ-cadinene; gratissimene; ocemene; (–) perillyl alcohol; ocimol and gratissimum.

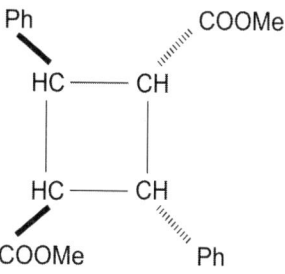

Gratissimum

Uses

1. **Insect repellent:** Leaf juice is used as body lotion as a mosquito repellent.
2. **Leucorrhoea and urinary complaints:** Powdered seeds are mixed with equal amount of crystallized sugar; one tablespoon full is given twice a day with milk for 5 days.
3. **Toothache:** Stem cuttings are used as toothbrush.
4. **Fever:** Aqueous extract of fresh leaves (one teaspoonfull) is given twice a day for 4 day.

BAHERA

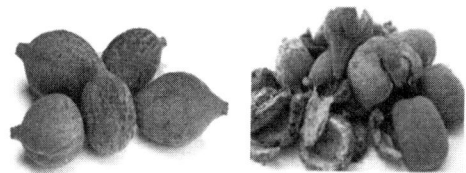

Fig. 2.94: Bahera fruits

Synonym: Baheda, Beleric myrobalans, Bibhitak (Sanskrit).

Biological Source: Baheda consists of dried fruits of *Terminalia belerica*.

Family: Combretaceae.

The plant is a large deciduous tree 60–100 ft. high. It is found wild in hills upto 3000ft, elevation in most parts of India and forests of Burma and Ceylon.

Morphology

Fruit is drupe, 20–26 mm in length and 14–22 mm in diameter, ovoid and grey in colour. Surface is velvety, irregularly wrinkled showing five longitudinal ridges. Upper end of the fruit is depressed while the lower projecting end shows round scar of pedicel up to 5 mm in diameter. Fruit is very hard and when broken exhibits a yellow to dark yellow internal surface with projecting, threads representing the vascular bundles. The hard endocarp occupies the center.

Uses

- Beleric fruit alone or as a constituent of Trifala is used as laxative.
- It is used in cough, bronchitis and bad throat and for correcting the voice.
- Its purgative, diuretic, antidiabetic and antileprotic activity has not been confirmed
- It is useful in dropsy and piles.
- Recently choleretic action has been found and is used in liver diseases.

AMLA

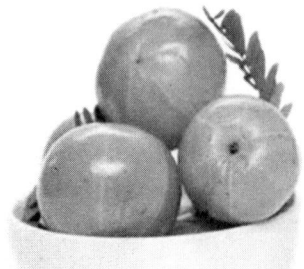

Fig. 2.95: Amla fruits

Biological Source: Amla consists of fresh or dried fruits of *Emblica officinalis* (*Phyllanthus emblica*).

Family: Euphorbiaceae.

Geogrophical Source: The plant is a small or middle sized tree widely distributed throughout tropical and subtropical countries such as India, Ceylon, China and Malaya.

Morphology

Fruit is 1.3 – 1.6 cm in diameter, freshy, globose, with 6 pale vertical furrows. Fruit is smooth, shiny with few prominent but minute light coloured specks. A depression left by the removal of peduncle is seen at one end of the fruit. Colour is green when unripe but light yellow when mature. Taste is sour and slightly bitter and sweet with astringent feelings. On drying the fruits becomes dark brownish to black and longitudinally splitted. Fruit is a drupe and endocarp is stony.

Active principle: It contains Indole acetic acid; four other auxins, a_1, a_3, a_4 and a_5; growth inhibitors–R_1 and R_2; lupeol; linoleic acid; tannin; trigalloylglucose; terchebin; corilagin; ellagic acid and phyllembic acid.

Uses

- Amla is a popular medicine in Ayurveda and Chyavanprash Avaleh is known preparation and is used in cough, bronchitis, haemoptysis, tuberculosis and as rejuvenating tonic and action is attributed to vitamin C.
- It is used in scurvy and as a tonic.
- Amla is used in liver diseases including diabetes often combined with turmeric.
- Amla potentiates the action of adrenalin *in-vivo* and *in-vitro*.

Other Uses

1. **Ulcers:** Powdered bark of the plant is mixed with equal amount of powdered leaves of *Abrus precatorius* and given twice a day with honey in gastric ulcers.
2. **Diabetes:** Powdered seeds are mixed with equal amount of bark of *Syzygium cumini*

and 1-TSF is given twice a day after meal to control blood sugar.
3. **Antiageing and digestion:** One ripe fruit is given twice a day after meal for improve digestion and regular consumption has anti-ageing effects like black hair, skin tone and improved metabolism.
4. **Urinary track infection:** Aqueous extract of fruit pulp is mixed with crystallized sugar and given twice a day for three days.
5. **Laxative:** Dried fruit pulp is powdered and 2-teaspoonfull is given thrice a day to get relief from constipation.
6. Also used in many cosmetic preparations, shampoos and hair oils.

VASAKA

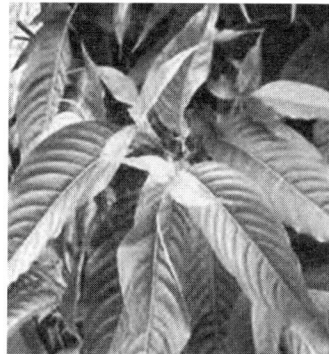

Fig. 2.96: Vasaka leaves

Synonym: Adhatoda, Vasaka folium, Adulasa, Ardushi, Sinhmukhi

Biological Source: Vasaka consists of the fresh or dried leaves of *Adhatoda vasica* Nees.

Family: Acanthaceae.

Geogrophical Source: Vasaca is an evergreen gregarious stiff perennial shrub, 1 to 6 m in height. It is distributed throughout the plains of India and Himalayan ranges upto 1500 m, in Srilanka and Malaysia. The shrub grows onwater lands and in variety of habitats and soil. It is sometime cultivated as a hedge but no systematic cultivation has been undertaken. The shrub is the source of the drug vasaka, well known in the traditional system of medicine.

Morphology

Leaves are elliptica-lanceolate, entire about 5 to 30 cm long and light green coloured. The dried leaves are dull brown on the upper surface and light grayish brown on the lower surface. Flowers are white with red or yellow-barred throats in the spikes with large bracts. The drug has characteristic odour and a bitter taste.

Uses

- Vasaka is mainly used as expectorant and for the treatment of bronchial troubles.
- Vasicine also exhibit an abortifacial effect and also used as oxitosis
- It also shows significant antimicrobial activity against gingival inflammation and pyorrhea.

(7) HARAD

Terminalia chebula (Gaertn.) Retz. (Combretaceae)

Distribution and plant habitat: Present in Kalashwar, Jhadol and in Kumbhalgarh forest. It is a large tree, leaves nearly opposite, shortly petioled, ovate-oblong, obtuse or cordate at base, entire, when young clothed with glossy silky hairs.

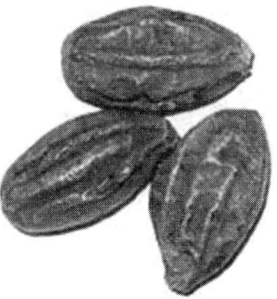

Fig. 2.97: Harad fruits

Flowering and fruiting: Generally occurs from March–April; flowers small whitish arranged in spikes; drupes glabrous.

Chebulinic acid R=H
Chebulagic acid RR=bond

Active principle: Chebulinic acid; chebulagic acid; palmitic acid; stearic acid; oleic acid; arachidic acid; behenic acid and gallic acid.

Uses

- Laxative: Fruit powder (2-teaspoonfull) is given once a day after meal to remove constipation.

- Indigestion and intestinal worms: One-cup decoction of fruit is given once a day.

- Cough: Fruit powder (1-teaspoonfull) is taken with warm water twice a day.

- Weak eyesight: Seeds and fruits are used in weak eye sight, 1-teaspoonfull seed powder or fruit powder is given with milk twice a day.

EXPERIMENT 39

Aim: To study morphology of given drug samples:
- Satavari
- Giloi
- Chhota Gokhru
- Bada Gokhru
- Rasna
- Methi

1. SHATAVARI

Synonym: Shatmuli, Shatavar.
Biological Source: Roots of *Aspargas racemosus*.
Family: Liliaceae.

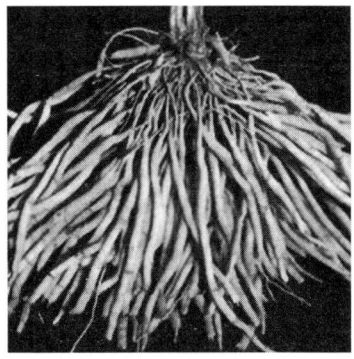

Fig. 2.98: Shatavari roots

Morphology

General Appearance: Drug consists of peeled dried or broken pieces,
Size: 4 to 12 cms long, 6 to 12 mm in thickness.

Roots are cylindrical, straight or slightly curved, white to buff in colour, sometimes pale brownish in colour. Entire roots are tapering on both the ends. Broken pieces show ridges uneven transverse surface. External surface shows deep irregular longitudinal furrows and minute transverse wrinkles. Broken pieces show sometimes hollow cavity. Many times central vascular tissue projects at the cut ends of the pieces. Drug is hard and breaks with uneven fracture and possesses bland taste which becomes bitterish after sometimes. The drug swells considerably when socked in water and becomes soft and flaccid. The smooth transverse surface shows a wide bark and a small central narrow wood.

Active principle: Stigmasterol; saponins of stigmasterol; sarsasapogenin; disogenin; hyperoside; isoquercitrin; kaempferol-3-ol-rhamnoglucoside; cosmosin; rutin; quercetin; oligoglucoside and two kaempferol.

Uses

- Used in Ayurveda in threatened abortion and for safe delivery.
- Galactogogue property.
- Petrol ether extract showed diuretic activity.
- In uterine diseases, as an antacid.
- Dermal disorder: Crushed and fried phyllods are applied on boils, cuts and wounds.
- Lactation: Powdered root is given regularly twice a day, with milk to lactating mother to increase lactation.
- Leucorrhoea and fertility increaser: Root powder is also given orally to get rid off menstruation related problems and to increase fertility of a woman.
- Dysentry: Powdered root is taken orally, 2–3 times a day to get relief in dysentery.

GILOI

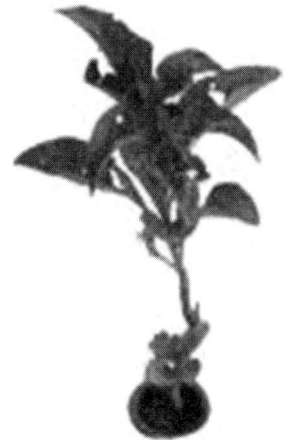

Fig. 2.99: Giloi plant

Biological Source: Dried leaf of *Tinospora cordifolia.*

Family: Menispermaceae. It contain fleshy root.

Geogrophical Source: The plant is found India. Plant is parennial in branching climber with long faciculate. It grows widely in ground as well as hilly area of India upto altitude of 1000 meter. In Bengal, Assam, Odisha, and south India.

Morphology

- Leaves are 5 to 10 cm long, 2.5 to 5.7 cm wide
- Ovate shape and oblong shape.
- Sometimes acute or acuminate, the base is usually cordite, petiole-6 to 13 mm long.
- *Colour:* Yellowish brown.
- *Odour:* None.
- *Taste:* Bitter.

Uses

- Emetic, diaphoretic, expectorant and used in overloaded condition of stomach.
- It is also used in asthma and congestion.
- It is used as bacteriostatic and a good natural preservative in food.

CHHOTA GOKHRU

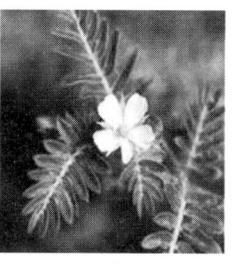 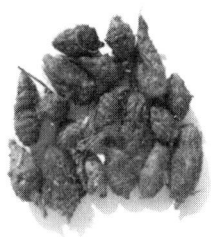

A　　　　　　　　B

Fig. 2.100: Gokhru (A) plant, (B) fruits

Biological Source: Chhota gokhru consists of dried ripe fruits of *Tribulus terrestris.*

Family: Zygophyllaceae.

Geographical Source: *Tribulus terrestris* is a plant that grows in many topical and moderate areas of the world weed of pastures found throughout the farming regions of Australia. The species is also found in Asia, Africa and the United States of America. It is also common throughout India and found especially during the monsoons. It is found upto an altitude of 11000 feet in warm regions of globe.

The plant is annual or perennial herb with woody taproot. Leaves are pinnate with oblong to ovate leaflets. Flowers are bright yellow and solitary in the leaf axils. They mature to form woody, burr-like fruit with conspicuous sharp spines.

Active principle: Diosgenin; ruscogenin; dihydroxy spirosteroidal sapogenin; neo-tigogenin; terrestroside F; saponin C and G; astragalin; trillin; gracillin; dioscin; hecogenin; tribuloside; kaempferol; quercetin; neohecogenin glucoside and tribulosin.

Tribuloside
R=Glu(6"-p-coumaroyl)

Morphology

Fruit is globose, 0.5. inch in diameter and 1/3 inch in thickness. Fruit consists of five densely hairy, woody, often muricate coccii. Each coccus bears two large sharp, pointed, rigid spines directed towards the apex and two smaller, shorter spines directed downwards. Colour is yellowish brown. Seeds several in each coccus with transverse partition between them.

Uses

- Drug has diuretic, cooling, demulcent, aphrodiasic and tonic action.
- It is used in primary nephritis and also in kidney stone.

BADA GOKHRU

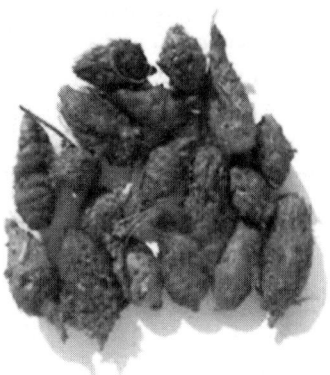

Fig. 2.101: Bada Gokhru fruits

Biological Source: 'Bada' gokhru consists of dried ripe fruits of *Pedalium murex*.

Family: Pedaliaceae.

Geographical Source: The plant is found near the sea-coasts of Saurashtra, Kokan, Deccan peninsula, Shrilanka and tropical Africa. It occurs widely especially after the monsoons in Delhi, Punjab and Rajastan. The plant is an annual, diffuse, succulent herb, 15 to 20 cm high.

Morphology

Fruit is 1.5 to 2 cm long pyramidal ovoid, tapering at the base and apex, 4-sided with stout, and sharp, conical horizontal four spines forming the 4 angles. At the base fruit abruptly tapers into a hollow cylindrical tube. The fresh or dried fruit when briskly shaken with cold water forms a thick mucilage.

Uses

- Drugs are demulcent, diuretic and tonic.
- It is used in dysuria, as an antioxidant, hepatoprotective and as an anti-ulcer agent.
- It is usually used in the form of infusion.
- In Ayurveda it is recommended as tonic and aphrodisiac.

RASNA

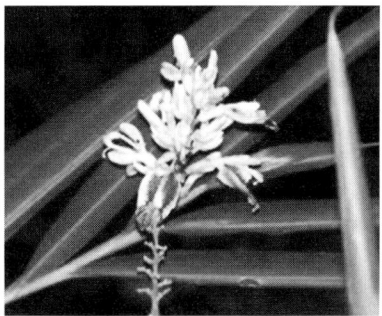

Fig. 2.102: Rasna plant

Synonym: Galangal, East Indian Root or Chinease ginger.

Biological Source: The drug consists of dried as well as fresh rhizomes of *Alpenia officinarum*.

Family: Zingiberaceae.

The drug is obtained from five to ten years old plant. Rhizomes are washed, cut and make into small pieces and carefully dried. This dried material is used for isolation of chemical constituents. The drug contains not less than 0.5% of volatile oil.

Geogrophical Source: The drug is found throughout India, majority in Himalayas and south and west India. The plant is a perinnial herb about 1.0 to 1.5 meter in height. The collection of rhizomes is done between March and April.

Morphology:

- *Colour:* The rhizomes are reddish brown in colour.
- *Odour:* Aromatic.
- *Taste:* Pungent.
- *Size:* The Rhizomes are about 2 to 8 cm in length, and 2 cm in thickness.
- *Shape:* The rhizomes are irregular and branchy and they are marketed with fine fragments.

Uses

- Aromatic, stimulant, carminative.
- Antibacterial, Antifungal.

METHI

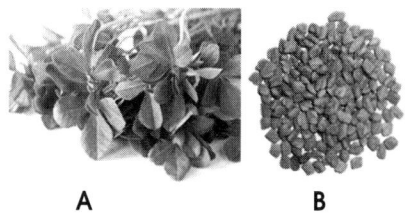

Fig. 2.103: Methi (A) Leaves, (B) Seeds

Trigonella foenum – graecum Linn. (Papilionaceae)

Synonym: Fenugreek (England), Methi (Hindi), Hulba (Arab).

Biological Source: Fenugreek consists of the dried ripe seeds of *Trigonella foenum-graecum* L.

Family: Fabaceae/Papilionaceae

Geogrophical Source: An annual herb, indigenous and originally to the Mediterranean and Western Asia and cultivated and distributed in Southern and Eastern Europe near northern east Africa, India, Pakistan, Morocco, France, Argentina and Egypt.

Morphology

The seeds are rhomboidal; light to dark yellow brown, nearly smooth, 5-7 mm long and about 2 mm thick; on one side runs a diagonal depression, dividing the radical and two yellow accumbent cotyledons. Odor characteristics; taste mucilaginous slightly bitter.

Active Principle

Fenugreek leaves contains 1.5% total lipids (dry weight), 0.9% neutral lipid, 0.38% glycoside, 0.14% phospholipids. The leaf lipid is rich source of essential fatty acids (linolenic, linoleic acid). Leaves also contains α-tocopherol 0.87 mg/gm and α tocopherol 0.37 mg/gm.

Seeds contains sapogenin; diosgenin; tigogenin; gitogenin; neotigogenin; diosgenin; 4-hydroxy iso-lecucine; saponaretin; homoorientin; vitexin; vicenin I and II; yamogenin tetroside; 7-acetoxy-4-methylcoumarin; graecunin A, B, C; graecunins H to N; trigofoenoside A-1 B-1 and E-1

Trigofoenoside E-1
R=Glu [(2→1)Rha](4→1)Xy1

Uses

- It is grown as a condiment, an essential oil being extracted for flavouring different foods and drinks such as cheeses, sweetmeats, pickles and liquors.
- It also used in pharmaceutical and cosmetics industry because of the vast range of chemical products that it contains.
- The plant also has insecticidal properties and is used in stored grains as a repellent.
- Popular medicine attributes tonic and vermifugal properties to its seeds, the mucilaginous components being used to treat stomach ailments.
- In Ayurvedic medicine, the seeds extract is used cardio tonic because of its diuretic, antiphlogistic, hypoglycemic and antihypertensive properties.

Other Uses

1. **Fat reducer:** Seeds grinded; 2-TSF given once a day empty stomach; followed by a glass lemon juice is used subsequently (without salt and sugar).
2. **Dermal disorders:** Paste of seeds is applied externally on wounds, cuts, boils and burns.
3. **Blood purifier:** One cup decoction of seeds is given twice a day for 10 days as blood purifier.
4. **Swellings:** Leaf paste is applied on swellings to get relief.
5. **Stomach cleaner:** Seeds are boiled and given to catters to clean stomach in case of indigestion and after pregnancy.

EXPERIMENT 40

Aim: To study morphology of the given drugs:
- Majith
- Guggal
- Kantakari
- Brahmi
- Punarnava
- Chitrak

MAJITH

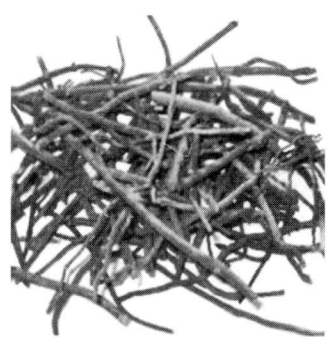

Fig. 2.104: Majith root stocks

Synonym: The Indian Madder.

Biological Source: The drug consists of the dried short rootstock of *Rubia cordifolia* Linn. *Sensu* Hook. F.

Family: Rubia.

Morphology

Size: In commerce varying but, usually occurs in piece 40 cm in length, 3–6 cm wide and 5–8 mm thick.

Outer surface: Rough with warty protuberances and due to exfoliation rusty brown in colour. Transverse and longitudinal cracks are seen on the outer surface.

Inner surface: Smooth, soft and reddish brown.

Smoothed Transverse surface: Shows radially elongated but irregularly running medullary rays of varying width.

Fracture: Short and fibrous.

Odour: Indistinct.

Taste : Astringent.

Uses

- Popular uterine tonic and sedative
- Bark is used in menorrhagia.

GUGGAL

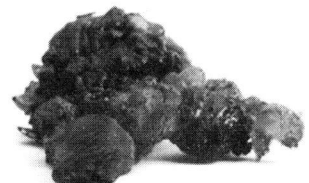

Fig. 2.105: Guggal

Synonym: *Commiphora wightii* (Arn.) Bhandari (Burseraceae)

Commonly known as **Gugul.**

Active principle: Guggulsterol-I, II III and IV; quercetin-3-O-α-L-rhamnoside; ellagic acid; Z-guggulsterol; stigmasterol; 20 β-hydroxy-4-pregnen-3 one; linolic acid; oleic; stearic; palmitic acid; sitosterol; cholesterol; campesterol; α-spinasterol; myricyl alcohol and sitosterol.

Guggulsterol-I R=OH
Guggulsterol-III R=H

Uses

1. **Dermal disorder:** Fresh plant extract (gum resin) is applied externally to remove black heads, pimples, wound, boils and external tumour.
2. **Body pain:** Gum smoke is inhaled to get relief in body pain.
3. **Mouthwash:** Infusion of gum is used as mouthwash in spongy gums and in tonsillitis.
4. **Toothache:** Twigs are used in toothpaste to relieve toothache.
5. **Obesity:** Three drops of fresh extract is mixed with lemon juice taken regularly emply stomach in obesity once a day.
6. Helps in treating leprosy, eczema and menstrual disturbances.
7. As a blood purifiers (used in various skin disorders).

KANTAKARI

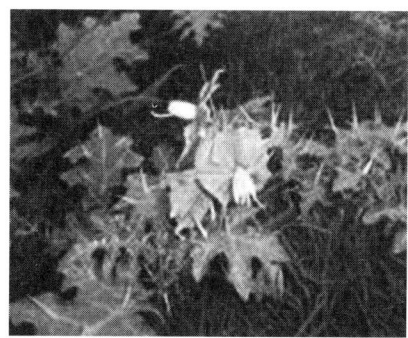

Fig. 2.106: Kantakari plant

Biological Source: The drug consists of the mature, dried whole plant of *Solanum xanthrocarpum* (Schrad and Wendl).

Synonym: *S. surattense* Burm. F. and *S. virginianum* Linn.

Family: Solanaceae.

Geographical Source: *S. xanthocarpum* is a very spiny diffuse herb upto 1.2 m tall. It is commonly found throughout India in the plains and low hills. It grows as a weed along road sides and waste land.

Morphology

The leaves are ovate or elliptic covered with straight spines of about 1 cm long. Stem:

nodes and internodes are prominent. Flowers are purple in few flowered axillary cymes. Fruits are glabrous, globular berries showing green and white stripes when young and yellow to white with green blots when mature. Seeds are smooth, compressed. The roots are almost cylindrical and tapering. Almost all parts shows somewhat bitter taste with no characteristics odour.

Uses

- The power of plants is antitussive and is reported to be beneficial in patient of bronchial asthma and non-specific cough.
- The drug has also shows antipyretic activity.
- The fatty oil of the seed possesses significant antifungal activity.
- Solasodine is reported to have antispermatogenetic, hypocholesterolaemic and antiatherosclelotic effect.

BRAHMI

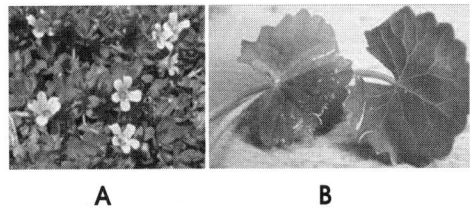

Fig. 2.107: Brahmi (A) Plant (B) Leaves

- **Botanical Name:** *Bacopa monniera*
- **Family:** Scrophulariaceae
- **English Name:** Thyme-leaved Gratiola
- **Common Name:** Brahmi
- **Plant Parts Used:** Whole plant

Biological Source: Two plants known as brahmi in different parts of India:

1. Herb of *Centella asiatica (Hydrocortyl asiatica)* known also as Mandukparni belonging to Umbellifery
2. Herb of *Bacopa monnieri (Herpestis monnieri)* belonging to scrophulariaceae. *Bacopa monnieri* is found in wet, deep and marshy areas and is known as jalbrahmi.

Geographical Source: The plant grows in India, Pakistan, Srilanka and Madagascar, usually in moist places upto an elevation of 6000 ft. There are different varieties or chemical races of the plant.

Morphology

The plant is slender, herbaceous, and creeping. Stems are long and prostrate coming off from the leaf axils of vertical rootstock. Stems are fusiform often reddish and with long internodes, rooting at nodes. Leaves are long petioled, 1.3–6.3 cm in diameter, several from rootstock and 1–3 from each node of stems. Leaves are orbicular, reniform, rather broader than long, more or less cupped, entire, crenate, and glabrous on both sides and with numerous slender nerves from a deeply cordate base. Petioles are variable in length, 7.5–15 cm long, oblong, sessile, glabrous; stipules short, adnate to the petioles forming a sheathing base. Flowers in fasicled umbels, each umbel consisting of 3–4 pink, sessile flowers. Peduncles pubescent or glabrous, short, pink, bracts: ovate, acute concave 2, beneath each umbel. Petals minute, pink, ovate, ciliate. Fruit 8 mm long, mericarps longer than brod, ovoid, hard with thickened pericarp, mericarps reticulate-rugose often crowned and with prominent primary and secondary ridges. Seed compressed laterally.

Chemical Constituents

The herb contains the alkaloids brahmine, herpestine, and a mixture of three bases. It also contains the saponins, monnierin; hersaponin, bacoside A and bacoside B. Other constituents present in the plant are D-mannitol, betulic acid, β-sitosterol, stigmasterol and its esters, heptacosane, octacosane, nonacosane, triacontane, hentriacontane, dotriacontane, nicotine, 3-formyl-4-hydroxy-2 hydroxy-pyran, luteolin and its 7-glucoside. The presence of α-alamine, aspartic acid, glutamic acid and serine is also reported.

Bacogenin-A₃

Bacogenin-A
R=Glu-Ara

Uses

- The drug brahmi has great reputation as brain tonic.
- It is also used in skin diseases, leprosy and syphilis.
- Preliminary pharmacological experiments shows that the drug has tranquilizing, sedative, spasmolytic and antiamoebic properties.
- It has also antianxiety and antistress action.
- It is anabolic and showed improvement in behavioral pattern of retarded children.
- It is used in indigenous systems of medicine for the treatment of asthma, hoarseness, insanity, epilepsy and as a potent nerve tonic, cardiotonic and diuretic.

Other Uses

1. **Fever:** Juice of whole plant (1-teaspoonfull) is given twice a day for three days.
2. **Mental debility:** Leaves are chewed regularly to improve memory, nervous disorders and mental debility.
3. **Mental weakness:** Juice of whole plant or dried powdered leaves (1- Teaspoonfull) is given twice a day with milk to improve memory and mental strength.
4. **Gonorrhoea:** Infusion of leaves is given in empty stomach once a day for 10 days.
5. **Antidote:** One-cup infusion of leaves is applied externally on scorpion sting and insect bite.
6. **Dermal disorder:** Leaf paste is applied on scabies, cuts, and wounds and on itching.
7. **Diarrhoea:** Infusion of whole plant (1-Teaspoonfull) is given thrice a day for relief.
8. **Jaundice:** One-cup of decoction is prepared by leaves with sugar given once a day in empty stomach for 10 days.

PUNARNAVA

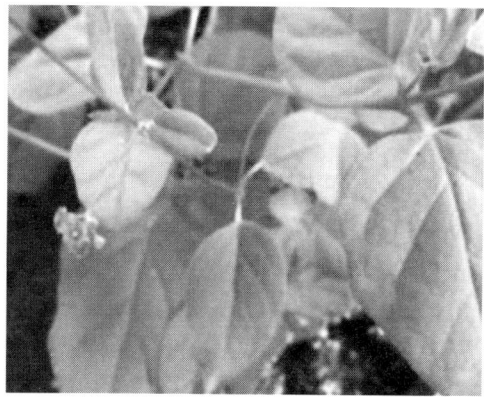

Fig. 2.108: Punarnava plant

Synonym: Spreading hogweed.

Biological Source: Drug consists of dried, mature whole plant of *Boerhavia diffusa* Linn. Syn. *B. repens* Linn.

Family: Nyctaginaceae.

Geographical Source: Punarnava is a veriable, diffusely branched, prostrate herb abundantly occurring as a weed throughout India upto an attitude of 2000 m in the Himalayas. It is cultivated to some extent in West Bengal.

Morphology

The herb consists of the creeping stem often purple coloured and swollen at the nodes. Roots stock is stout, fusiform and woody. Leaves are long petioled, ovate or tarchcordate usually whitish and smooth beneath and rough green on upper surface. Flowers are red, pink or white umbels while fruits are ovate and five-ribbed. The odour is not distinct but the taste is bitter.

Two chief varieties are described based on the flower colour, one with white flowers is "Sweta punarnava" while the other with red flowers is referred to as "Rakta Punarnava".

Uses

- Punarnava posses potent antifibrinolytic, anti-inflammatory and diuretic properties.
- Punarnava is a very useful drug for the treatment of inflammatory renal diseases and nephritic syndrome.
- It is also recommended for the treatment of IUD menorrhagia.
- Plant extract shows hepatoprotective activity and effective in case of oedema and ascites resulting from early cirrhosis of liver and chronic peritonitis.
- Liridodendrin and hypoxanthine-9-arabinofuranoside exhibits, antihypertensive activity, the former being a Ca^{+2} channel antagonist.

6. CHITRAK

- **Botanical Name:** *Plumbago zeylanica*
- **Family:** Plumbaginaceae

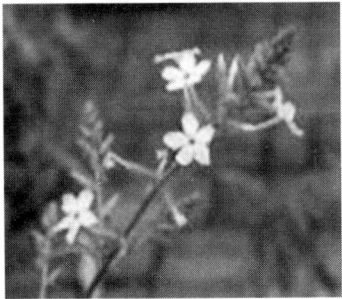

Fig. 2.109: Chitrak plant

- **English Name:** White Leadwort
- **Common Name:** Chitraval or Chitrak
- **Part Used:** Roots

Plumbago zeylanica Linn. (Plumbaginaceae)

Description of *Plumbago zeylanica*: It is a perennial, subscandent shrub. The leaves are ovate and glabrous. The flowers are white, in elongated spikes. The capsules are oblong, pointed, contained in a viscid glandular persistent calyx.

Distribution and plant habitat: Commonly present in wasteland, it is an erect or straggling undershrub. Leaves ovate-lanceolate or oblong, acute, contracted as the base into a petiole, undulate-crispy, glabrous, narrow, amplexicant at the base.

Flowering and fruiting: Generally occurs throughout the year; flowers white in colour, in axillary and terminal, 5-30 cm long racemes combined into leafy panicles. Capsules long, oblong, longitudinally furrowed.

Active principle: Plumbagin; azalein; 3-chloroplumbagin; 3-3'-biplumbagin; binaphthaquinone; chitranone; zeylinone; isozeylinone; elliptinone; droserone; apigenin; luteolin; amyrins; palmitic; β-sitosterol; capansinidin-3-rhamnoside.

Uses

- **Migraine:** One-cup root decoction is given orally twice a day to get relief.
- **Piles:** Root powder is fried with cleared butter and given 1-TSF thrice a day for 5 days.
- **Rheumatism:** One-cup infusion of fresh root (1 root) is given twice a day to get relief; root paste is also applied on affected parts.
- **Dermal disorders:** Root paste is applied externally on wound, cuts, itching, fungal infection, scabies and leprosy.
- **Dyspepsia:** One-cup infusion of root is given twice a day for 2 days.

EXPERIMENT 41

Aim: To study morphology of given drugs:
- Turmeric   • Ajowan   • Black Catechu

TURMERIC

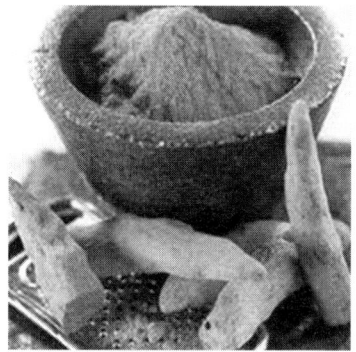

Fig. 2.110: Turmeric powder and rhizomes

Botanical Name: *Curcuma longa*

Family: Zingiberaceae

Hindi Name: Haldi

Part Used: Rhizome

Description

Turmeric (*Curcuma longa*) is a rhizomatous herbaceous perennial plant of the ginger family, Zingiberaceae. The rhizomes are boiled for several hours and then dried in hot ovens, after which they are ground into a deep orange-yellow powder commonly used as a spice, for dyeing, and to impart color to mustard condiments. Its active ingredient is curcumin and it has a distinctly earthy, slightly bitter, slightly hot peppery flavor and a mustardy smell. In medieval Europe, turmeric became known as Indian saffron, since it was widely used as an alternative to the far more expensive saffron spice.

Chemical Constituents

Turmeric contains upto 5% essential oils and upto 5% curcumin, a polyphenol. It is the active substance of turmeric. The chemical name is 1,7-bis (4-hydroxy-3- methoxyphenyl)-1,6-heptadiene-3,5-dione. It can exist at least in two tautomeric forms, keto and enol. The keto form is preferred in solid phase and the enol form in solution. Curcumin is a pH indicator. In acidic solutions (pH <7.4) it turns yellow, whereas in basic (pH > 8.6) solutions it turns bright red.

Uses

It is used as an anti-inflammatory, antiseptic and antibacterial agent, useful in disinfecting cuts and burns; it prevents prostate cancer and stops the growth of existing prostate cancer, when combined with cauliflower. Reduces the risk of childhood leukemia, a natural liver detoxifier, may prevent and slow the progression of Alzheimer's disease by removing amyloyd plaque buildup in the brain. May aid in fat metabolism and help in weight management, because of its anti-inflammatory properties, it is a natural treatment for arthritis and rheumatoid arthritis, Turmeric is currently being investigated for possible benefits in Alzheimer's disease, cancer, arthritis, and other clinical disorders, also used in cosmetics, natural dye.

Curcumin keto form

Curcumin enol form

AJOWAN

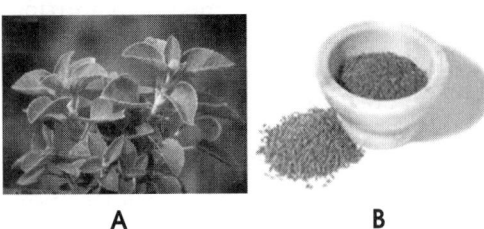

Fig. 2.111: Ajowan (A) Leaves (B) Seeds

Botanical Name: *Trachyspermum ammi/Carum copticum/Ptychotis ajowan*

Family: Umbelliferae

Common Name: Ajwain and Ajmo

Description

An erect, glabrous or minutely pubescent, branched, annual. The stems are striate; the leaves are rather distant, 2–3-pinnately divided, the segments linear. The flowers occur in terminal or seemingly-lateral pedunculate, compound umbels, white and small; the fruits are ovoid, muricate, aromatic cremocarps, covered in grey papillac, the mericarps, which are the components of the fruit, laterally compressed, with distinct ridges and tubercular surface, 1-seeded.

Chemical Constituents

It contains saponin, yellow, crystalline oil known as thymol (mp:291–94°) and a steroidal substance (mp:140–50°). The principal constituents of the essential oil from the fruits are the phenols, mainly thymol and some carvacrol. The Indian Pharmacopoeia requires ajowan oil to contain not less than 40% thymol. Thymene, which constitutes 0.45% of the oil, has the following composition: p-cymene; g-terpinene; α- and β-pinenes and dipentene. Presence of minute amounts of camphene, myrcene and D_3-carene is also reported.

Uses

Ajowan is much valued for its antispasmodic, stimulant, tonic and carminative properties. It is administered in flatulence, atonic dyspepsia and diarrhea, and often recommended for cholera. In the Unani system, ajowan is used as a crude drug to enhance the body's resistance, and is prescribed in amebiasis. It is a potent antimicrobial agent.

Other Uses

1. **Colic complaints and digestive:** Fruit powder is given orally in colic complaints and indigestion.

2. **Galactagogue:** Fruit powder is mixed with dry fruits, jaggary and ghee than fried; 20 gm cake is given once a day for 3 months to a nourishing mother to increase milk production.

3. **Urinary complaints:** Seed powder (1-Teaspoonfull) is given orally thrice a day to cure urinary problem.

4. **Galactagogue and uterus cleaner:** Seed powder (8-10 kg), jaggary (10 kg), edible oil (10 kg) are mixed; 200 gm mixture is given twice a day to cattle after pregnancy.

BLACK CATECHU

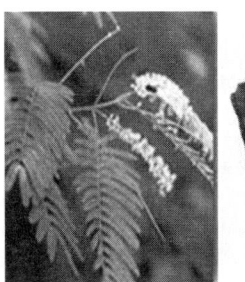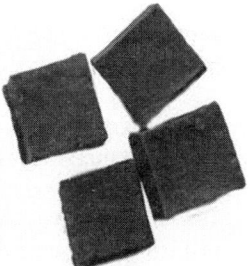

Fig. 2.112: Black catechu

Botanical Name: *Acacia catechu*

Family: Fabaceae – Mimosoideae

Common name: Khadir, Khair, Kattha

Plant Parts Used: Bark

Description: A tree reaching as high as 30 to 40 ft.; branches spreading, armed with strong black spines, downy toward the points. Leaves bipinnate, alternate, from ten to eighteen pinnae; leaflets of pinnae thirty to fifty pairs, linear, auricled at the base, ciliated; petiole angular, grooved above, downy, with orbicular green glands between the bases of the pinnae. Flowers in cylindrical, axillary spikes, on downy stalks, from four to five inches long, numerous, monopetalous, white or whitish yellow, and about twice as long as the tubular, hairy calyx.

Morphology

Colour: Light brown to black

Odour: None

Taste: Very astringent

Size: About 2.5 to 5 cm

Shape: Cube or irregular

Special Features: Cubes as well as brick shaped pieces of catechu show presence vegetable of debris and break with short fracture. Broken pieces are angular with pale annamon – brown colour. It is friable and porous.

Chemical Constituents

It contains catechins 2–12%, phlobatannin 25–33%, gummy matter 20–30%, quercitrin and quercitin.

Uses

In Ayurvedic medicine, Acacia leaves, flowers, and pods have long been used to expel worms, to staunch bleeding, heal wounds, and suppress the coughing up of blood. Its strong astringent action is used to contract and toughen mucous membranes throughout the body.

Black Catechu is used internally for chronic catarrh of the mucous membranes, dysentry, and bleeding. In Chinese medicine, it is used for poorly healing ulcers, weeping skin diseases, oral ulcers with bleeding, and traumatic injuries. A small piece of catechu can be dissolved in the mouth to stop bleeding gums or heal canker sores. In Ayurvedic medicine, decoctions of the bark and heartwood are used for sore throats. Decoctions made from the powdered leaves, stems, and pods are taken for shigella, malaria, dysentery, and diarrhea. An infusion of the flowers and leaves is taken for gastrointestinal inflammations. The flowers are also sedating. It helps soothe mucous membranes from the mouth through the anus, reducing inflammation and attacking microbial infections.

Other Uses

1. **Tonic**
2. **Throat infection and cough:** Dried gum (1-teaspoonfull) is taken orally once a day.
3. **Mouth ulcers:** "Kattha" is obtained from stem. It is applied on ulcers in mouth as a paste.
4. **Leucorrhoea and painful menstrual cycle:** (i) Gum (1-Teaspoonfull) or 1-Teaspoonfull "Kattha" is given with milk once a day to get relief. (ii) Bark powder (1-Teaspoonfull) is also given twice a day for 10 days during menstrual cycle.
5. **Dermal disorder:** Bark paste is applied externally on cuts, wounds, boils and burns.

EXPERIMENT 42

Aim: To study morphology of given drugs:
- Neem
- Aloe
- Lemon grass
- Nirgundi
- Jatropha

NEEM

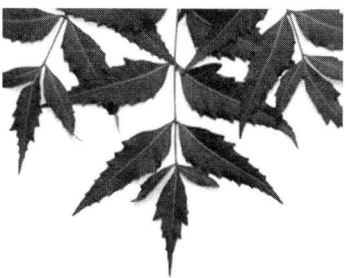

Fig. 2.113: Neem leaves

Botanical Name: *Azadirachta indica Melia azadirachta L*

Family: Meliaceae

Common Name: Neem or Limdo

Part Used: Leaves

Description

Azadirachta indica (neem) is a tree in the Mahogany family Meliaceae. It is one of two species in the genus Azadirachta and is native to India, in tropical and semitropical regions. Neem is a fast growing tree that can reach a height of 15–20 metre. The branches are widespread. The fairly dense crown is roundish or oval.

Chemical Constituents

Meliacine-solanide; nimbin; gedunin; salanin; nimocinol; azadirachtin; nimbocinone; nimocinolide; nimosone; isonimocinolide; isolimbolide; nimbanal; nimbolin A and B; nimbidiol; azadirachtol; 4-epinimbin; 24-methylenelophenol; nimbochalin; azadirachtanin and 2'-3'-dehydrosalannol.

Three bitter compounds are extracted from neem oil, which named nimbin, nimbinin, and nimbidin respectively. The seeds contain a complex secondary metabolite azadirachtin.

Nimbosome

Uses

Anthelmintic, antifungal, antidiabetic, antibacterial, antiviral, contraceptive and sedative. Neem oil is used chewed in order to clean one's teeth, to relieve fever, to treat acne. Neem products are also used in selectively controlling pests in plants. It is considered a major component in Ayurvedic and Unani medicine and is particularly prescribed for skin disease.

Other Uses

1. **Use in eyes ailments:** In *"Chetra"* month fresh 100–150 gm flowers are collected and grinded with "chacha" and taken early in the morning for six days. It increases eyesight and keeps cool and free from eye irritation.

2. **Cooling effect:** Internal heat of body is eliminated by using 1 glass of flower juice in water for three days.

3. **Eye carbon:** Kajal (carbon) prepared from flowers of the plant in "ghee" (cleared butter). It increases eyesight of children and keeps cool the whole year.

4. **Piles:** Paste of seeds (1 kg) after removing seed coat, 2 kg of *"Mava"* and 2 kg crystallized sugar are grinded together and then make cake. 50 gm cake piece is taken twice a day in severe piles. It eliminates the disease. The disease will never come again throughout victim's survival.

5. **Skin disorder:** Seed oil is applied externally in scabies, itch, leprosy and all type of dermal infections.

6. **Fever and malaria:** One cup decoction of bark powder and leaves is given to victim thrice a day for three days in all types of fever.

7. **Blood pressure:** Leaves (10) chewed every morning empty stomach to control high blood pressure.

8. **Ticks removal:** Seed oil is applied externally on the skin of animals to kill lices and ticks. Leaf paste and *"Niboli"* the fruit paste is applied externally on skin to kill ticks and lices.

9. **Foot disease:** The seed oil is poured on feet of domestic animals to kill in *"Khurpaka"* or *"Kharva"* disease.

10. **Intestinal worms:** Ripen fruits "Niboli" and leaves boiled and filtered, ½ liter

filteration is given thrice a day to kill intestinal worms in domestic animals.

11. **Mosquito repellant:** Leaves are burned in cattles residence for its smoke to avoid mosquitos from cattle's residence.

12. **Grain storage:** People used the leaves in storage of grain seeds. A thick layer is spreed on bottom and then randomly mixed with stored grain. Then a top the most layer covered with thick layer of leaves to avoid stored grain pests, insects and fungi.

13. **Insecticide:** Green leaves are mixed with soil in farms to protect crops from soil borne diseases. Leaf and fruit juice is sprayed on vegetable crop to kill insect larvas.

ALOE

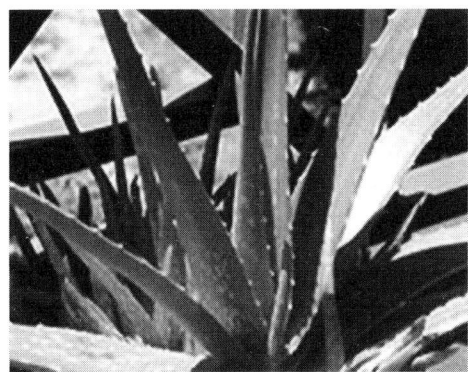

Fig. 2.114: Aloe plant

Botanical Name: *Aloe barbadensis*

Faimly: Liliaceae

Hindi Name: Gawarpata

Part used: Fresh leave, leaf-juice and pulp of leaves

Description

Aloe vera is a stemless or very short-stemmed succulent plant growing to 60–100 cm tall. It is a coarse perennial with short stem and shallow root system; leaves fleshy in rosettes, sessile, often crowded with horny prickles on the margins, convex below, 45 – 60 cm long, tapering to a blunt point, surface pale green with irregular white blotches: flowers yellow or orange in racemes: fruits loculicidal capsule.

Chemical Constituents

The leaves contain barbaloin, chrysophanol glycoside and the aglycone, aloe-emodin. The mucilage of the leaves contains glucose, galactose, mannose and galacturonic acid in addition to an unidentified aldopentose and a protein with 18 amino acids. The plant contains peplic acid; D-galacton; α-glucomannan; tarch acid; malic acid; citric acid; tartaric acid; aloesin; aloesone and a glycoside aloinoside B.

Aloinoside B

Uses

It is helpful in regulating the kapha and pitta dosha. It has anti-inflammatory properties. It is also helpful in normalizing the digestive activities, stimulating liver and spleen for proper activities and functing. It purifies blood. It is helpful in dysurea and other urine related problems. It is also helpful in reducing the impotence and also the mestural problems. Skin related problems are also treated by regular usage of aloe-vera. It reduces geneal body weakness and also helps in reducing the body temperature in case of hyperthermia.

Paste: It is used to apply on the inflammation. It is also used in application on the hepatomegaly. It is used in enhancing the skin texture and complexion.

Juice: it is used in digestive tract problems. It is also helpful in abdominal disturbances like pain in abdomen. It is helpful in reducing inflammation on liver and spleen. It also helps in avoiding chronic constipation. It cures the worm infestation in the body. It helps in preventing piles and rectal disturbances. It is quite effective in urine reated problems.

Other Uses

1. **Stomach troubles:** Juice of leaf pulp (1-TSF) is given orally a day to cure intestinal trouble.
2. **Jaundice:** One-cup juice of leaf pulp is given twice a day to cure the disease.
3. **Fat control:** One small piece (30-40 gm) of pulp is given empty stomach once a day to reduce fat from body.
4. **Dermal disorders:** The pulp is applied externally on boils, cuts, eczema, ringworm, burns and leprosy. It is considered as a good cosmetic, so pulp is used as cosmetic on face.
5. **Swellings:** Leaf-pulp is warmed and tied on affected part and kept (water bottle/warm stone) warmed by external heating source for 1 hour.
6. **Mites repellent property:** It has strong anti-mites property; juice of leaf pulp is dropped into water during irrigation to remove mites.

LEMON GRASS

Botanical Name: *Cymbopogon flexosus*

Family: Poaceae

Hindi Name: Silky heads, citronella grass

Part Used: Leaf

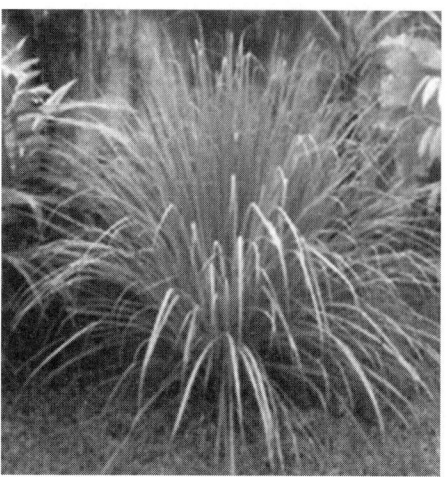

Fig. 2.115: Lemon grass plant

Description

Cymbopogon citratus (lemon grass) is a genus of about 55 species of grasses, native to warm, temperate and tropical regions of the Old World and Oceania. It is a tall perennial grass. It also used as an addition to tea. It has medicinal properties and is used extensively in Ayurvedic medicine. It is supposed to help with relieving cough and nasal congestion.

Chemical Constituents

Citral, Limonene, Citronella, Geraniol and Citronellol

Uses

Antidepressant, antimicrobial, anti pyretic, antiseptic, astringent, bactericidal and carminative properties. For various ailments like headaches, toothaches, etc. Lemon grass is also used as a diuretic agent for fever and as an insect repellent. It is also an excellent antiseptic, rheumatism, circulatory problems, acne. It is added to foot baths and foot talc for smelly, sweaty feet. For any fungal infections of the foot, it can be applied directly to treat ringworm and tinea.

NIRGUNDI

Botanical Name: *Vitex negundo*
Family: Verbenaceae
Sanskrit Name: Sephali
English Name: Five-leaved Chaste tree
Part Used: Whole plant

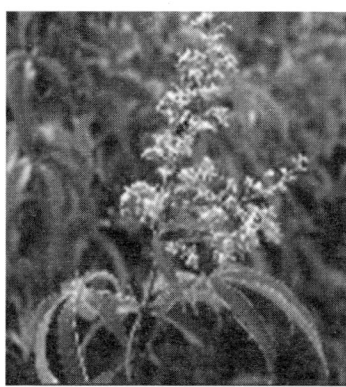

Fig. 2.116: Nirgundi plant

Description

V. negundo is a large, aromatic shrub with quadrangular, densely whitish, tomentose branchlets, or sometimes, a small, slender tree. The bark is thin and grey; the leaves are 3-5-foliolate; leaflets are lanceolate, entire or rarely crenate and the lateral leaflets are smaller than the terminal ones; the flowers are bluish purple, forming large, terminal, often compound, pyramidal panicles; the drupes are globose.

Chemical Constituents

Casticin, isoorientin, chrysophenol D, luteolin, p–hydroxybenzoic acid and D-fructose.

Uses

The leaves are astringent, febrifuge, sedative, tonic and vermifuge. They are useful in dispersing swellings of the joints from acute rheumatism and of the testes from suppressed gonorrhea. The dried fruit is vermifuge and is also used in the treatment of angina, colds, coughs, rheumatic difficulties, etc. The fresh berries are pounded to a pulp and used in the form of a tincture for the relief of paralysis, pains in the limbs, weakness, etc. The root is expectorant, febrifuge and tonic. It is used in the treatment of cold and rheumatic ailments.

JATROPHA

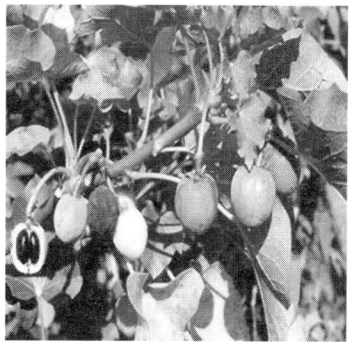

Fig. 2.117: Jatropha plant and fruits

Botanical Name: *Jatropha curcas* L., *Curcas purgans*
Family: Euphorbiaceae
Hindi Name: Ratanjot, Safed Arand
English Name: Purging nut

Description

The drought resistant plant, locally, it is grown as a boundary fence or live hedge and can be used to reclaim eroded areas. Its leaves and stems are toxic to animals. Being rich in nitrogen, the seed cake is also an excellent source of plant nutrient.

Botanical

Small tree or large shrub, up to 8 m tall and with diameter up to 20 cm. Trunk is straight, branching low above the ground; bark is thin and yellowish. Leaves are 6 × 15 cm and lobed. Flowers small and greenish, unisexual with male and female flowers at the same rate.

Fruit: A grey-brown capsule
Seed: Seeds are black (various shades of black)

Chemical Constituents

Macrocyclic diterpenoid jatrophone which co-occurs with the inactive diterpenoids jatropholone A and B. The seeds contain 27–40% oil that can be processed to produce a high-quality biodiesel fuel, usable in a standard diesel engine. The seeds are also a source of the highly poisonous toxalbumin curcin. The latex of *Jatropha curcas* contains an alkaloid known as "jatrophine" which is believed to have anticancerous properties.

Uses

It is used as an external application for skin diseases and rheumatism and for sores on domestic livestock. In addition, the tender twigs of the plant are used for cleaning teeth, while the juice of the leaf is used as an external application for piles. The roots are reported to be used as an antidote for snake-bites. The oil has a strong purgative action and is also widely used for skin diseases and to soothe rheumatic pain. A decoction of leaves is used against cough and as an antiseptic.

Chapter 3

Identification of Crude Drugs

I. CARBOHYDRATES

EXPERIMENT 1

Aim: To identify the given sample of Jaguar gum.

Synonym: Guar flour, Jaguar gum

Biological Source: Guar gum is the powder of the endosperm of the seeds of *Cyamopses tetragonolobus* Linn

Family: Leguminosae

Description: It is a colourless or pale yellowish white coloured powder with characteristic odour and gummy taste. Guar gum swells rapidly in water with a translucent suspension. 0.9% aqueous solution of gum is neutral to limits.

Chemical constituents: The contents of guar gum are divided into water soluble fraction constituting about 85% of the gum is known as guaran, which is a high molecular weight hydro colloidal polysaccharide. Guaran on hydrolysis yields 65% galactose and 35% of mannose, which is combined through glycosidic linkage. Guar gum also contains 5–7% of proteins.

Chemical Test

1. It does not acquire olive green colour with weak solution of iodine.
2. With solution of ruthenium red, the gummy solution does not acquire pink colour.
3. About 2% solution of lead acetate given precipitate with the solution of guar gum.
4. Dissolve 0.9 g of guar gum in 20 ml of water by shaking. To it, add 0.5 ml hydrogen peroxide and 0.5 ml 1% solution of benzidine in alcohol. No blue colour is produced.

Uses: It is used as a protective colloid, a binding and disintegrating agent, bulk laxative, appetite depressant and in peptic ulcer therapy. Guar gum is a good emulsifying agent. Industrially, this is used in paper manufacturing, printing, polishing, textiles and also in food and cosmetic industries. It is extensively used as flocculent in ore dressing and treatment of water.

EXPERIMENT 2

Aim: To identify the given sample of Agar.

Synonym: Agar Agar, Gelose: Japan agar, Bengal isinglass. Ceylon isinglass, Chinese isinglass, Japanese isinglass, vegetable gelatin, kanten.

Biological Source: Agar is a dried, hydrophilic, colloidal polysaccharide complex, extracted from the agaroucytes of algae known as *Gelidium cartil agineum*, Gaillon, *Graularia confervoides* (L), Grev. (Family Sphaerococcaceal) and some other spices of Acanthopletis, Ceramium and Pterocladia (family: Rhodophyceae). Gelidium provides about 35% of the total agar source.

Description: Agar occurs in the form of a transparent or translucent, agglutinated, yellowish white slender, lustrous flattened strips or as front or granulated powder. It is tough in damp, brittle in dried form, odourless or with a slight odour and taste is mucilaginous. Agar is insoluble in cold water and alcohol, slowly soluble in hot water to form a viscous solution and its 1% solution forms a stiff firm jelly on cooling.

Chemical Constituents: Agar is composed of calcium salt of acidic polysaccharides. It can be separated into a natural gelling fraction, agarose and a sulphated nongelling fraction agaropecitin. On hydrolysis, Agar yields galactose and sulphate ions. It is a heterogeneous polysaccharide. Agarose responsible for the gel strength consists of alternate residue of 3,6 anhydro–L-galactose and n-galactose. The viscosity of agar solutions is due to the presence of agaropectin which is a sulphated polysaccharide in which galactose and uronic acid moieties are partly esterified with sulphuric acid.

Chemical Tests

1. Agar responds positively to Fehling solution test. Red precipitate is obtained when agar solution heated with Fehling solution.
2. Agar gives positive test with Molisch's reagent.
3. Pink color is obtained when ruthenium red is added to agar solution.
4. White precipitate is obtained when Barium chloride reagent is added to hot agar solution.
5. Crimson to brown color is obtained when iodine solution is added to agar solution.

Uses: It is used as an emulsifying agent bulk laxative. It is used in preparation of jellies.

EXPERIMENT 3

Aim: To identify the given sample of Acacia.

Synonym: Gum Acacia, Gum Arabic, Indian Gum

Biological Source: Indian gum is the dried gummy exudation obtained from the stem and branches of *Acacia Arabica* wild, belonging to family Leguminosae.

Description

Colour: Powder is light brown in colour

Odour: Odourless

Taste: Bland and Mucilagenous

Sloubility: Soluble in water, the watery solution is viscous and acidic.

Chemical Constituents: It consists principally of arabin, which is a complex mixture of calcium, magnesium and potassium salts of arabic acid. Arabic acid on hydrolysis gives L-arabinose, L-rhamnose, D-galactose and D-glucoronic acid.

Test for purity: To the gum acacia solution, add a drop of hydrogen peroxide and tincture of guar gum. Blue colour is produced with a few drops of 0.1% ferric chloride to 1 ml of solution blue or black colour.

Uses

1. It is a demulscent and suspending agent.
2. It is an emulsifying and binding agent.
3. When it is combined with gelatin, it is used as coacervates for microencapsulation of drugs.

EXPERIMENT 4

Aim: To identify the given sample of Pectin.

Biological Source: Pectin is the purified carbohydrate product obtained by acid hydrolysis from inner portion of the rind of citrus peels, that is *citrus simon* or *Citrus aurantium*.

Family: Rutaceae

Description: It is coarse or fine light powder and hygroscopic in nature.

Colour: Cream or yellowish powder.

Odour: It is odourless.

Taste: Mucilaginous

Sloubility: It is soluble in 20 parts of water, aqueous solution being viscous, opalescent, colloidal and mobile. It is soluble in alcohol and other organic solvents.

Chemical constituents: Total hydrolysis of pectin yields D galacturonic acid, methyl alcohol, small amount of galactose and arabinose.

Pectin should not contain less than 7.0% of methoxy groups and 78.0% of galacturonic acid, calculated with reference to ash free and derived substance.

Identification Tests

1. 10.0% aqueous solution forms stiff gel on cooling.
2. To 5 ml, 1% solution, add 1 ml 2% solution of potassium hydroxide and set aside at room temperature for 15 minutes. A transparent gel or semigel forms. Acidify gel with dilute hydrochloric acid and shake well. A voluminous, colourless, gelatinous precipitate forms which when boiled becomes white and flocculent.

Uses: Pectin is used as an adsorbent in the treatment of diarrhoea and as a homeostasis for internal and external hemorrhage. It is used as an emulsifying agent, a jellying agent in acid medium and as a plasma substitute.

In food industry, it is used as thickening agent for sauces, jams, ketchups, etc. It is extensively used in cosmetic preparations.

EXPERIMENT 5

Aim: To identify the given sample of Honey.
Synonym: Purified honey, Melifere, madhu (Hindi) strained honey, classified honey.
Biological Source: Honey is a sugary secretion deposited by the honey bees, *Apis melifere* Loan and other species of Apis in honey comb.
Family: Apidae
Order: Hymenoptera
Description: It is a thick, syrupy, translucent liquid when fresh.

Colour: Pale yellow or reddish brown

Odour: It posseses pleasant odour and sweet taste which are dependent upon the floral source of the product. The honey obtained from Eucalyptus and Bankisa species has some what unpleasant odour and taste and the honey collected from *Datura stramonium* is poisonous. On storage, it becomes opaque and granular due to crystallization of dextrose.

Chemical Constituents: Honey consists chiefly of glucose (30–40%), fructose (40–50%) and small amount of sucrose (0.1–10%), dextrin, formic acid, volatile oil and pollen grains in addition to these, traces of enzymes, vitamins, proteins, maltose, melezitose, pentosans, gums, trace elements, amino acids and colouring matter are also present in honey.

Chemical Tests: Adulteration in honey is determined by the following tests:

1. *Fiehe's Test for Artificial invert sugar:* Shake 10 ml honey with 5 ml petroleum or solvent ether for 5–10 minutes. Separate upper etherofal layer and evaporate in a China dish. On addition of 1% solution of resorcinol and hydrochloric acid (1 ml), a transient red colour is formed in natural honey while in artificial honey, the colour persists for some time.

2. *Reduction of Fehling's solution:* Add equal mixture of Fehling's solution A and B to an aqueous solution of honey (2 ml) and heat the reaction mixture on a steam bath for 5–10 minutes. A brick red colour is produced due to the presence of reducing sugars.

3. *Limit tests:* The limit tests of chloride, sulphate and ash are compared with the pharmacopoeial specifications.

Uses: Honey shows mild laxative, bactericidal, sedative, antiseptic and alkaline characters. It is used for cold, cough, fever, sore eye and throat, tongue and duodenal ulcers, liver disorders, constipation, diarrhea, kidney and other urinary disorders, pulmonary tuberculosis, marasmus, rickets, scurvy and insomnia. It is applied as a remedy on open wounds after surgery. It prevents infection and promotes healing. Honey works quicker than many antibiotics because it is easily absorbed into the blood stream. It is also useful in healing of carbuncles, chape, scalds, white lows and skin inflammation, as vermicide, locally as an excipient, in the treatment of aphthae and other infection of the oral mucous membrane. It is recommended in the treatment of pre-operative cancer. Honey, mixed with onion juice, is a good remedy for arteriosclerosis in brain. Diet rich in honey is recommended for infant, convalescents, diabetic patients. Honey is an important ingredient of certain lotions cosmetics, soaps, creams, balms, toilet water and inhalation. It is used as a medium in preservation of cornea.

EXPERIMENT 6

Aim: To identify the given sample of Starch.

Synonym: Amylum

Biological Source: Starch consist of polysaccharide granules obtained from the grains of maize (*Zea mays*), rice (*Oryza sativa* Linn), as wheat (*Triticum aestivum* Linn)

Family: Solanaceae

Description

Colour: White

Odour: Odourless

Taste: Mucilaginous

Chemical Constituents: Starch contain chemically two different polysaccharides vis. Amylose and Amylopectin, in the proportion 1:2. Amylose is water soluble and amylopectin is water insoluble but swells in water. Amylose gives blue colour with iodine while amylopectin yields bluish black colouration.

Identification Tests

1. Boil 1 gm of starch with 15 ml of water and cool. A translucent viscous jelly is produced.
2. The above jelly turns deep blue by the addition of solution of iodine. The blue colour disappears on warming and reappears on cooling.

Uses

1. It is used in the preparation of dusting talcum powder for application over the skin.
2. Used as a nutritive, demulcent, protective and as an adsorbent.
3. Used as an antidote in iodine poisoning.
4. It is used as an emollient and a base for suppositories.

EXPERIMENT 7

Aim: To identify the given sample of Tragacanth.

Synonym: Gum tragacanth

Biological Source: It is dried gummy exudation obtained by incision from stems and branches of *Astragalus gummifer* labill and other species of Astragalus.

Family: Leguminosae

Description

Colour: The flakes are white or pale yellowish white

Odour: Odourless

Taste: Mucilagenous

Shape: Tragacanth occurs in the form of thin, flattened ribbon like flakes, more or less curved.

Size: Flakes are approximately $25 \times 12 \times 12$ mm in size.

The gum is horny, translucent with transverse and longitudinal ridges. Fracture of the drug is short. It is partly soluble in water, in which it swells to homogenous, adhesive and gelatinous mass. It is insoluble in alcohol.

Chemical Constituents: Tragacanth contains two fraction, of which one is soluble in water. It is called tragacathion constituting about 8 to 10% of the gum. Water insoluble portion is known as bassorin (60–70%). Tragacanth contains about 19% of methoxy group swells in water. It is the constituent of gum responsible for its high viscosity. The products of hydrolysis of tragalanth are galactouronic acid, D-galactopyranose, L-arabino rhamnose and P-xylo pyranose.

Identification tests

1. When solution of tragacanth is boiled with a few drop of 10% aqueous ferric chloride solution, deep yellow precipitate is formed.
2. A stingy precipitate is formed by dissolving tragacanth and precipitated copper oxide in concentrated ammonium hydroxide.
3. When it is warmed with sodium hydroxide solution, canary yellow colour is developed. With iodine solution, it gives green colour.

Uses

1. It is used as a demulcent and as an emollient in cosmetic.
2. Tragacanth is used as a thickning agent, suspender and as an emulsifying agent.
3. Mucilage tragacanth is used as a binding agent in the tablets and also an excipient in the pills.
4. Tragacanth powder is used as an adhesive.
5. It is used in lotions for external use and also in spermicidal Jellies as a stabilizer for ice cream, also in sauces.

EXPERIMENT 8

Aim: To identify the given sample of Sterculia gum.

Synonym: Indian Tragacanth, Karaya Gum

Biological Source: Gum Karaya is dried gummy exudates obtained from the tree *Stercuilia urens, Sterculica villosa* tragacantha and or other species of Stercuilia.

Description: It is found in the form of irregular tears of vermin form pieces from white to brown in color. It has slight acetous odour and bland mucilaginous taste. Wood fibres and small sand particles may be present in the Gum. It is insoluble in water, but forms a translucent colloidal solution. Powdered gum swells in water.

Chemical Constituents: Karaya gum contains about 8.0% of acetyl group and more than 37% of uronic acid residues. On acid hydrolysis, it gives D-galactose, L-rhamnose, D-galacturonic acid, aldobiuronic acid and an acid trisaccharide.

IdentificationTest: It gives a pink colour with solution of ruthenium red.

Uses: It is a good bulk laxative. It is used as a denture adhesive in dental treatment and in pharmaceutically as an emulsifier, thickener, and stabliser. It is used in large scale in foods such as ice-pops, cheese spread, sherbets and ground meat products. It is also used in paper and textile industries.

EXPERIMENT 9

Aim: To identify the given sample of Isapgol.

Synonym: Ispaghula, Isabgul, Indian psyllium, Isabgol, Flea seed

Biological Source: Isapgol consist of dried seeds of the plant known as *Plantago ovata* forskal.

Family: Plantaginaceae

Description: Isapgol seeds are hard, transparent and smooth with grey or reddish brown oval spot in the center of the convex surface. Concave surface contains the hilum covered with thin membrane having two perforation. The colour of Isapgol is pinkish grey to brown. It poses no odour, it is about 10 to 35 mm in length and 1 to 1.75 mm in width. It is ovate cymbiform.

Chemical Constituents: Isapgol husk and seeds contain mucilage which is present in the epidermis of the seeds. Chemically, it consist of pentosan and aldobionic acid. The products of hydrolysis are xylose, arabinose, galacturonic acid and rhamnose. Fixed oil and proteins are other important constituents of the drug.

Chemical Test

1. Swelling factor is the criterion for purity of the drug. Swelling factor of the drug is a quantitative swelling due to mucilage present on the drug. It is determined by putting 1 gm of the drug in the measuring cylinder of 20 ml. Add water with occasional shaking. The volume occupied by the seeds after 24 hours of wetting is measured. Swelling factor for seeds is 10 to 14.

2. Being the mucilage chemically, isapgol gives pink colour with the solution of ruthenium red.

Uses: The seeds and husks are used as demulcent laxative, emollient and in the treatment of constipation, amoebic and bacillary dysentery. Mucilage of isapgol is used in the preparation of tablets, also as a stabilizer in ice cream industry, in certain cosmetic formulation, etc.

Swelling factor of Isapgol: Take 1 gm of seed in 25 ml stopper cylinder. Add water up to 25 ml marking. Shake occasionally during 23 hours. Keep aside for 1 hour, measure the volume occupied by the swollen seeds.

II. LIPIDS

EXPERIMENT 10

Aim: To identify the given sample of Lipids.

Regional name: Bees Wax, Mom, Min

Biological Sources: Yellow beeswax is purified wax from honey comb of the bee *Apis dorsata*. L. and possible other species of Apis /Bee.

Family: Apidae

Chemical Constituents: The chief constituents are ester of straight chain monohydrate alcohol with straight chain acids. The constituents of beeswax are myricyl palmitate (about–80%) free cerotic acid and melissic acid and aromic substances.

Uses: Preparation of pharmaceutical aid: ointment, plasters, polishes. Also in preparation of lipstick, face creams, etc.

COD LIVER OIL

Synonym: *Oleum morhua*.

Sources: It is processed from fresh liver of cod fish, *Gadus morhua* and other species of Gadus.

Family: Gadidac

Morphology: Pale yellow thin liquid with slightly fishy taste and odour becoming disagreeable on exposure to air, light.

Solubility: It is freely soluble in chloroform, ether, carbon disulphide, petroleum ether, slightly soluble in alcohol.

Chemical Constituents: It has vitamin A and vitamin D groups, 1 g of oil contains not less than 255 mcg of vitamin A and 2.125 mg of vitamin D. The oil contains glyceryl esters of oleic acid, linoleic, gadoleic, myristic, palmitic and other acids.

Uses: Nutritional requirements for polyunsaturates in diet, reduces blood cholesterol.

COCOA BUTTER

Synonym: Theobroma oil, cocoa butter

Biological Sources: It is a fat obtained from roasted seeds of *Theobroma cacao* L.

Family: Sterculiaceae

Morphology: Yellowish-white solid and brittle below 25 °C. It has pleasant chocolate odour and taste, insoluble in water, but soluble in ether, chloroform, benzene, petroleum, etc.

Chemical Constituents: Consists of glycerides of stearic (34%), palmitic (25%), oleic (37%) acid and a small amount of arachidic and linoleic acids. The nongreasiness of the product is due to its glyceride structure.

Uses: It is used as a base for suppositories and ointments, manufactures of creams and toilet soaps.

CASTOR OIL

Synonym: Bherenda, Diveli, Erand

Biological Sources: Castor oil is a fixed oil obtained by cold expression from the seeds of *Ricinus communis*

Family: Euphorbiaceae

Characters

Colour: Colourless or pale yellow

Nature: Viscous liquid

Odour: Faint

Taste: Acrid, nauseating

Solubility: Soluble in alcohol in all proportions.

Active Constituents: Lipids: fixed oils (45-55%), a mixture of triglycerides, triricinolein (75%) which on hydrolysis yields Ricinoleic acid responsible for cathartic effect.

Uses: Cathartic, soap industry, lubricant.

LINSEED

Synonym: Flaxseed, Masina, Alsi

Sources: Linseed is dried ripe seed oil *Linum usitatissimum* L, contains not less than 25% of fixed oil.

Family: Linaceae

Morphology:

Shape: Ovoid or oblong–lanceolate flattened obliquely pointed to one side

Size: 4–6 mm (lenght) 2–3 mm (width)

Colour: Brown

Hilum and micropyle in slight depression below pointed end.

Active constituents: Fixed oils (30–40%)
1. Mucilage (6%), yields on hydrolysis galactose (8–12%), arabinose (9–12%), rhamnose (13–29%), xylose (25–27%) Galacturonic acid: mannuronic acid (30%).

2. Protein (25%): cyanogenetic glycoside, glycosides. Linamanin (1–5%) – Lotaustralin.

Uses: Externally as a poultice

Internally as a demulcent,

laxative and in case of hemorrhoids

RICE BRAN OIL

Synonym: Rice oil

Biological Sources: Rice bran is the cuticle existing between the rice and the husk of the paddy and consists of embryo and endosperm of the seeds of *Oryza sativa*.

Family: Gramineae

Morphology: Golden yellow oil difficult to bleach and not affected by temporary heating to 160°C. Insoluble in water but soluble in common fat solvents

Chemical Constituents: Rice bran oil contain 20–25% of saturated and 80–85% of unsaturated fatty acids as glycerides. Mainly fatty acids are oleic (40–50%), linoleic (30–40%), palmitic acid (12–18%).

Uses: It contains antioxidants, used in manufacture of cosmetics and as an emollient, it is an edible oil and used in preparation of vegetable ghee.

HYDROUS WOOL FAT

Synonym: Lanolin

Sources: Hydrous wool fat is the purified fat like substance obtained from wool of the sheep *Ovis aries* Linn.

Family: Bovidae

Chemical Constituents: It's a complex miniature form of ester and polyster of 33 high molecular weight with alcohols and 36 fatty acids. It also contains ester of cholesterol and isocholesterol with carnaubic, oleic, myristic, palmitic, lanoceric and lanopalmitic acids.

Description

Colour: Whitish yellow

Odour: Faint and characteristic odour.

Taste: Bland.

Solubility: Insoluble in water and soluble in chloroform and solvent ether with separation of water.

Uses: Water absorbable ointment base, common ingredient and base for water soluble cream and cosmetic preparations.

LARD

Synonym: Adeps

Biological Sources: It is the purified internal fat obtained from abdomen of the hog *Sus scrofa* Linn

Family: Suidae

Descripiton: It is a white, homogenous fatty mass unctuous to touch. Lard has slight odour and bland taste. It is insoluble in alcohol and soluble in benzene, carbon disulphide, ether and chloroform

Chemical Constituents: Chemically it contains about 60% olein and 40% of stearin and palmitin

Uses: Used as an ointment base and in formulations where more effective absorption is desired. Benzoinated lard contains benezoin resin as preservative.

SHARK LIVER OIL

Synonym: *Oleum selachoids*

Biological Sources: Shark liver oil, is a fixed oil obtained from the fresh and carefully preserved livers of various species of the shark, mainly *Hypoprion brevirostris* and *Galeorhinus zyopterus*.

Description

Colour: Pale yellow to brownish yellow

Odour: Characteristic fishy but not rancid

Taste: Bland or fishy

Solubility: Soluble in solvent ether, chloroform and light petroleum, insoluble in water and slightly soluble in ethyl alcohol.

Chemical Constituents: Contains vitamin A. The concentration of vitamin A in oil varies from 15000 to 30000 IU. Other constituents of oil are the glycerides of the saturated and unsaturated fatty acids.

Uses: Used in deficiency of vitamin A. It is known as antixeropthalmic factor. It is nutritive, shark liver oil with vitamin D, is used in burn and sun burn ointments.

SANDALWOOD OIL

Synonym: Chandan oil, Sandal oil, Yellow sandal wood oil lignum.

Biological Sources: Sandalwood oil is obtained by distillation of sandalwood, *santalum album* Linn.

Family: Santalaceae

Description: Sandalwood oil is a viscous, yellowish, liquid having a peculiar honey, sweet and very lasting odour. It has specific gravity 0.97–0.98, viscosity 1.5 and acid value 0.5–0.8.

Chemical Constituents: The main odour and medicinal constituent of sandalwood is santalol ($C_{15}H_{24}O$). This primary sesquiterpene alcohol forms more than 90% of the oil and is present as a mixture of two isomers, α-santalol and β-santalol, the former predicating the other constituents reported are hydrocarbons santene, nontricycloe kasantalere α and β santalenes, the alcohols santerol and faresantalol, the aldehyde or tricycloersentalal and isovaleraldehyde, the ketones l-sintalone and sintalone and the acids terisantalic acid and α and β santalic acids.

Uses: Sandalwood oil is highly used in perfumery creations and finds an important place in soaps, face cream, toilet powder, etc.

III. RESIN AND RESIN COMBINATION

EXPERIMENT 11

Aim: To perform morphological and chemical tests of Asafoetida.

Synonym: Devil's dung, Regional Name: Hindi: Heeng: Tamil: Perungayam, Sankrit: Hinguka

Source: Asafoetida is the oleo-gum-resin obtained by incising the living rhizomes and roots of *Ferula asafoetida*.

Family: Umbelliferae

Morphology: Asafoetida occurs in 2 forms.

1. Tears either in round or flattened forms.

   Size: 1 to 3 cm

   Colour: Dull yellow, grayish white or reddish brown.

2. Masses which are the most common form when tears agglutinate to form masses and also contain impurities like fruit, root, etc.

   Surface: Rough in general

   Fracture: Brittle

   Odour: Strong, alliaeceous (gastric smell)

   Taste: Alliaceous, bitter, acrid

Active Constituents

Volatile isobutyl propanyl disulphide (4–20%), also responsible for the smell.

Resins (40–65%) tree as a resinotannol and as well in combination with ferulic acid gum (25%).

Uses

1. As a carminative (relieves excessive collection of gas in stomach)
2. As expectorant (promotes removal of catarrhal discharge and phlegm from bronchial tubes)
3. As antispasmodic (counteracts sudden, violent, involuntary muscle contraction)
4. As a laxative (induce active movement of bowels)

Tests

1. A yellowish-orange emulsion turning to greenish yellow on addition of alkali, when asafoetida is triturated with water.
2. When fragment of asafoetida is treated with dil. H_2SO_4, a reddish brown solution results. On diluting this with water, filtering and on neutralising the filtrate, a purplish-blue fluorescence is produced.
3. A pink colour is produced on adding a few drops each of phloroglucinol and concentrated HCl to 10 ml of alcoholic extract of drug.
4. Drug does not contain free umbelliferone but a blue fluorescence is produced due to presence of combined umbelliferone.
5. Triturate the drug with sand. Boil drug with dilute HCl and filter into ammonia. Blue flourescence is produced.

EXPERIMENT 12

Aim: To perform morphological and chemical tests of Balsam of Tolu.

Source: Tolu Balsam is a solid or semi-solid balsam obtained by incision from trunk of *Myroxylon balsamum*. It contains not less than 35% and not more than 50% of total balsamic acids.

Family: Leguminoseae

Characters

Colour: Brownish yellow to brown

Odour: Aromatic (ranilla smell)

Solubility: Insoluble in water, soluble in alcohol, ether, chloroform, etc.

Active Constituents

Resins (80%) – Resin alcohols combined with cinnamic and benzoic acids.
Volatile Oil (7.8%) – Benzyl benzoate.
Free organic acids – Cinnamic acids (2–15%), Benzoic acid (8%)

Uses

1. As an expectorant
2. Flavouring agent
3. As an antiseptic

Chemical Tests

1. Alcoholic solution of drug is acidic.
2. Green colouration obtained by adding ferric chloride solution to alcoholic solution of Tolu.
3. Bring to boil 1 g of Tolu balsam in 5 ml. water, filter and heat the filtrate with 30 mg $KMnO_4$ Benzaldehyde, odour is noted.

EXPERIMENT 13

Aim: To perform morphological and chemical tests of Balsam of Peru.

Synonym: Peru balsam, Indian black balsam, percevian balsam

Source: Obtained from trunk of the free, *Myroxylon balsam* after the bark has been beaten and scorched.

Family: Leguminoseae

Morphology

Colour: Dark brown to reddish brown viscous liquid and transparent thin layers

Odour: Aromatic vanila like

Taste: Bitter acrid

Solubility: Insoluble in water, soluble in alcohol, glacial acetic acid, partly soluble in ether and petroleum ether.

Chemical Test: 50–65% high boiling volatile oil with cinnamein and 25–28% resin, traces of styrene, vanillin and coumarin.

Volatile oil contains esters of cinnamic acid and benzoic acid like, cinnamyl cinnamate, cinnayml benzoate, benzyl benzoate and benzyl cinnamate, with small amount of free benzyl alcohol, free benzoic and cinnamic acids.

Uses

1. Use in tropical preparations for scabies, treatment of wounds ulcers and bedsores, in feminine hygiene sprays soaps and cosmetics.
2. As flavouring agent and for masking
3. As fixative of flavours

EXPERIMENT 14

Aim: To perform morphological and chemical tests of Benzoin.

Synonym: Gum benzoin

Regional name: Hindi : Loban, Malayalam : Sambrani, Sanskrit: Sriloban

Source: Benzoin is a balsamic resin obtained from *Styrax benzoin*. It contains not less than 25% of total balsamic acids calculated with reference to dry alcohol soluble matter.

Family: Styraceae

Morphology:

Form: Appears as hard masses consisting of tears embedded in a translucent, reddish brown matrix.

Size: Varies

Surface: Rough but smooth tears

Fracture: Brittle

Odour: Aromatic, Balsamic, Pleasant

Taste: Slightly acrid

Active Constituents

a. Sumatra benzoin

Balsamic acids: Cinnamic acid 20%, Benzoic acid 10%

Triterpenoid acids: Siaresinolic acid (19 hydroxyo leanolic acid), Sumaresinolic acid (10 hydroxy oleanotlic acid), Alcohol soluble extractive (not less than 70%).

b. Siam benzoin

Balsamic acids: Cinnamic acid in traces, Benzoic acid 10%, Coniferyl benzoate 70%,

Vanillin and some triterpenoid acids, alcohol soluble extracture (not less than 90%).

Uses

1. Expectorant
2. Antiseptic
3. Tincture is used in cosmetic solution and as inhalation aid in respiratory diseases.

Tests

1. Heat 0.5 g slowly in a dry test tube, it melts and evolves irritating whitish flame which crystalize to form whitish crystalline sublimate in upper part of tube.
2. Warm gently 1 g of powder with 5 ml $KMnO_4$ solution in test tube: Distinct odour of benzaldehyde is produced
3. Triturate 0.1 g of powder with 5 ml alcohol, filter and to the filtrate add 0.5 ml of 5% w/v solution of ferric chloride in alcohol. No bright green colour is produced (distinction from Siam benzoin).
4. Digest 0.2g benzoin with 5 ml ether for 5 min pour 1 ml of ethereal solution in a porcelain dish containing 2–3 drops of conc H_2SO_4 and rotate the dish. Reddish–brown colour is obtained.

EXPERIMENT 15

Aim: To perform morphological and chemical tests of Colophony.

Source: Colophony is the solid residence obtained after distilling the oleo-resin from various spices of *Tinus*

Family: Pinaceae

Synonym: Long needle pine,

Regional name: Hindi: Chir: Sanskrit: Sarala, Tamil: Simai Devadari

Morphology:

Form: Angular masses, glassy, irregular
Colour: Pale brownish yellow
Size: Varies
Surface: Smooth

Fracture: Brittle
Odour and Taste: Bitter
Solubility: Insoluble in water, soluble in alcohol, ether, benzene, glacial acetic acid and light petroleum.

Active Constituents

Resin Acids: Resin acid or diterpene acids like abietic acid (90%). Nutral pinest substances, ester of fully acids.

Uses

1. In ointments and medicinal plasters
2. Manufacturing of varnishes and disinfectant liquids.

Chemical Test

1. Dissolve 0.1 g in 10 ml of acetic anhydride by means of gentle heat, cool and add a drop of conc H_2SO_4. A bright purplish red colour rapidly changing to violet.
2. Dissolve 0.1 g in light petroleum and fiter. To this, add 2–3 drops of dil. Copper acetate solution. Petroleum layers show emerald green colour (green for abietic acid)
3. Alcoholic solution of colophony shows acidic to litmus paper.

EXPERIMENT 16

Aim: To perform morphological and chemical tests of Cannabis.

Synonym: Indian Hemp, Hashis, Marijuana.

Regional name:

Malyalam: Kanchavu: Hindi–Bhang, Ganja: Tamil – Kanja

Source: Cannabis consists of the dried flowering tops of the cultivated pistillate plants of *Cannabis sativus*.

Family: Cannabinaceae

Morphology

Form: Compound rough dusky green masses consisting of branched upper part of stem bearing leaves and pistillate flower of fruit matted together by recinous secretion. Upper leaves simple, alternate, lower leaves opposite and digitate consisting of 5–7 linear lanceolate leaflets, fruits are single seeded, supported by ovate – lanceolate tract

Odour: Strong and Characteristic (narcotic)
Taste: Acrid and pungent.

Active Constituents

Resin (2.5% – 15%) – Tetrahydrocannabinol/ (THC) Cannabidiolic acid (CBDA)

Uses

1. Sedative (calms down excitement)
2. Analgesic (pain killer)
3. Hypnotic (include sleep)
4. Psychotropic (exciting effect on mind)
5. Antibacterial agent

EXPERIMENT 17

Aim: To perform morphological and chemical tests of Capsicum.
Synonym: Chilli, Red pepper, Spanish pepper.

Regional names

Malyalam: Mulagu, Sanskrit: Marichiphalam, Tamil: Pachemolaga

Source: Capsicum consists of dried ripe fruit of *Capsicum frutescens*. It contains not less than 12% non-volatile ether extractive
Family: Solanaceae

Morphology

Form: Oblong conical, obtuse, and 2-celled
Colour: Full orange red to brownish red
Size: 1.2–2.5 mm and upto 7mm maximum attached to 5 toothed inferior calyx and straight slender pedicel. Pericarp some what shriveled, glabrous and leathery containing about 10–20 brownish yellow, flat, subrein form seeds.
Seeds: 3–4 mm, loose or attached to thin reddish dissepiments.

Colour: Characterstic
Taste: Pungent

Active Constituents

Pungent phenolic compounds, Capsaicinoids, a mixture of 5 isomeric acid amides, Capsaicin (70%), Homocapsaicin, Dihydrocapsaicin – Homodi hydrocapsaicin – Norhydrocapsaicin

Carotenoids: (0.12%–0.35%)
Ascorbic acid: (0% – 0.5%)
Fixed oil
Flavonoids

Uses

1. Carminative
2. Nerve stimulant
3. Increase the capillarity of blood vessels
4. Source of vitamin C
5. In galenic to treat cases of Rheumatoid arthritis (rheumatism of joints)

EXPERIMENT 18

Aim: To perform morphological and chemical tests of Jalap.
Synonym: Mexican Jalap
Regional name: Hindi:Mirchai, Gujarat: Gurayo
Source: Jalap consists of dried tuberous roots or tubercles of *Ipomea purga*
Family: Convolvualaceae

Morphology

Form: Irregularly oblong, napiform or fusiform
Colour: Dark brown
Size: 3–15 cm, 3–8 cm
Surface: Longitudinal wrinkles with transverse lenticels
Odour: Slightly smoky
Taste: First sweet and then acrid

Active Constituents:

Resins: Glycosidal resins (8–20%), convolvulin, jalapin

Uses

A hydrogogue cathartic (drug which discharge watery fluid)

EXPERIMENT 19

Aim: To perform morphological and chemical tests of Ginger.

Regional name

Hindi: Adrak, Malyalam: Inchi, Sanskrit: Adrakam

Source: Ginger is the rhizome of *Zingiber officinale* Rosioe scraped to remove dark outer skin, and dried in sun.

Family: Zingiberaceae

Morphology:

Form: Irregularly branched, laterally compressed, branches known as fingers arise obliquely from rhizome which terminate in depressed scars or undeveloped buds. Nodes, internodes and scalar, conspicuous features of fresh ginger, samples are not clearly seen in dried ones.

Colour: Buff

Size: 7 to 15 cm

Surface: Longitudinal striations seen

Fracture: Short, mealy and fibrous, fractural surface show projecting fitness

Odour: Agreeable and aromatic

Taste: Pungent

Active Constituents

Volatile oil (0.6. to 3%), Sesquiterpene, Zingiberene, Alcohol, Zingiberol, Borneol, Linalool, Geraniol, etc. – Aldehyde citral. Pungent Principles (5 to 8%) – Gingerol, Shogaol, Zingerone. Resinous matter: starch–mucilage.

Uses:

1. Carminative
2. Stimulant
3. Flavouring agent

EXPERIMENT 20

Aim: To perform morphological and chemical tests of Myrrh.

Synonym: Myrrh, Arabian or Somali Myrrh

Regional name

Tamil: Vellaippapolam, Sanskrit: Vola

Source: Myrrh is the oleo-gum resin obtained by incision from stem of *Commiphora molmol*.

Family: Burseraceae

Morphology

Form: Irregularly rounded tears or lumps of agglutinated tears

Colour: Reddish yellow or reddish brown

Size: Variable

Surface: Rough, covered with fine yellow powder

Fracture: Brittle, fractured surface brown, shining, oily and with whitish marks.

Odour: Aromatic

Taste: Bitter

Active Constituents

Volatile oil (2.5. to 8%)–Phenol-eugenol, cuminic aldehyde, α-pinene, limonene and sesquiterpenes

Resin–(25–40%) Resin acids like α, β, γ commiphoric acids

Gums (60%)–yield on hydrolysis arabinose, galactose, 4-0-methyl glucuronic acid and aldobiuronic acid

Uses

1. Antiseptic
2. Stimulant

3. Used in mouthwash, toothpaste.
4. In perfume industry

Chemical Test

1. Yellowish brown emulsion obtained when myrrh is triturated with water.
2. An ethereal solution of drug attains reddish colour when treated with Br_2 vapour, whereas purple colour when moistened with nitric acid. These 2 distinguishing tests are not answered by Bdellium (a species of commiphora)

EXPERIMENT 21

Aim: To perform morphological and chemical tests of Podophyllum.

Regional name:

Hindi: Popra, Malyalam: Padwal, Sanskrit: Vakra
Source: Indian podophyllum consists of dried rhizomes and roots of *Podophyllum hexandrum*.
Family: Berberidaceae

Morphology:

Form: Irregular, knotty dorsiventrally flattened contorted and tortuous pieces.
Colour: Yellowish brown to earthy brown
Size: 2–4 Cm
Surface: On upper side 3–4 cup shaped scars of aerial stems and leaves seen, on other sides numerous stout roots seen.
Fracture: Short and fractured surface – pale brown, starchy
Odour: slight and characteristic
Taste: Bitter acrid

Active Constituents

Resin – (10-18%) hignon resin, podophyllin, a mixture containing – podophyllotoxin (40%) -α-peltatin – B- Peltatin in trace.
Flavonoid: Quercetin derivatives

Uses

1. Highly toxic
2. In treatment of condylomata acuminatum
3. Antimitotic effect – in case of certain types of cancer
4. A new synthetic derivative of podophyllotoxin – Etoposide now used to care small cell and testicular cancer.

Characters

Indian podophyllum

Surface – Wooly fibres absent
Fracture – Starchy
Taste – Bitter, acrid
Trichomes absent, resin cells abundant

Chemical Test

Macerate 0.5 g of powdered drug in 10 ml 90% alcohol for 10 min and fitter. A brown precipitate is obtained by adding 0.5 ml concentrated solution of copper acetate to filtrate. American podophyllum gives a green colour instead of brown precipitate.

EXPERIMENT 22

Aim: To perform morphological and chemical tests of Turmeric.

Synonym: curcuma, Indian saffron

Regional name:

Hindi: Haldi, Sanskrit: Haldi, Tamil: Manjal
Source: Turmeric consists of dried rhizomes of *Curcuma longa*
Family: Zingiberaceae

Morphology:

Form: Primary rhizomes ovate, oblong or pyriform and are called as 'bulb' or 'round turmeric' whereas the branched rhizomes are more cylindrical and often short, branched and they are called 'long turmeric'.
Colour: Yellow to Yellowish brown externally, yellow to yellow orange internally.
Size: The round form is about half as broad as Long forms are about 4 to 7 cm.

Surface: Root scars and annulations are seen
Fracture: Horny
Odour: Aromatic
Taste: Aromatic, bitter

Active Constituents

Curcuminoids (nonvolatile colouring matter–5%)-Curcumin, a diferuloylmethane–desmethoxy curcumin dicinnamoylmethane–bidesmethoxy curcumin.

Volatile Oils (5%)– Sesquiterpenes (60%) like 1-cycloisoprenmyrcene-Zingiberene (25%), tumerone

Xatlantone, r-attantone, phellandrene, sabinene, and also cineole, bornool and curcumone.

Sugars: Arabinose (1%), fructose (12%), glucose (28%), Billersustitence, fixed oil, acids.

Uses

Choleretic and cholagogue, anti-inflammatory agent, aromatic, stimulant, tonic and carminative, anti-fertility agent, in respiratory diseases to lower blood cholesterol, externally applied in pains and bruises, As colouring agent, in cosmetics, and is antimicrobial.

Chemical Test

1. Mix concentrated H_2SO_4 and the drug with alcohol, imparts a deep crimson colour to turmeric.
2. Boric acid colours to reddish brown which on addition of alkalis become greenish blue.

IV. TANNIN AND TANNIN CONTAINING DRUGS

EXPERIMENT 23

Aim: To perform morphological and chemical tests of Black catechu.
Synonym: Kattha, Cutch, Khadir, Catechu, Catechee

Regional name

Sanskrit: Khadira, Tamil: Karangalli, Hindi: Khayir

Biological Sources: It consists of dried aqueous extract prepared from the heart wood of *Acacia catechu* wild and *Acacia chandra* wild.

Family: Leguminosae

Morphology

Colour: Light brown to black
Odour: None
Taste: Astringent
Size: About 2.5 to 5 cm
Shape: Cube or irregular
Special features: Cubes as well as brick shaped pieces of catechu show presence of vegetable debris and break with short fracture. Broken pieces are angular with pale brown colour. It is friable and porous.

Chemical Constituents: Black catechu contains about 10% acacatechin. It is also known as *Acacia catechin*. Acacatechin undergoes oxidation to catechutannic acid in presence of water and the latter constitutes 30% of the drug. Other contents are catechured, quercetin, gum and quercitrin. It does not contain chlorophyll and the fluorescent substance present in pale catechu.

Chemical Tests

1. Because of the presence of catechin, black catechu gives pink or red colour with ranillin and hydrochloric acid.
2. Catechin when treated with HCl produces phlouroglucinol, which burns along with lignin to give purple or magenta colour. For this purpose, tannin extract is taken on match stick dipped in HCl acid and heated near the flame.
3. Lime water when added to aqueous extract of black catechu gives brown

colour, which turns to red precipitate on standing for some time.

4. Green colour is produced when ferric ammonium sulphate is added to dilute solution of black catechu. By addition of NaOH, green colour turns to purple.

Uses

Catechu is used as an astringent externally for boils, skin eruptions, and ulcers and it is also used in cough and diarrhea.

Catechu is also used medicinally for other purposes like dyeing and colouring, water softening, reducing viscosity of mud mercaptans from gasoline, protective for fishing nets and in manufacture of ion exchange resins.

EXPERIMENT 24

Aim: To perform morphological and chemical tests of Myrobalan.

Synonym: Chebulic myrobalan, Harad, Haritaki

Regional name

Hindi: Harad, Sanskrit: Haritaki, Tamil: Kadukki

Biological Sources: It consists of dried ripe, and fully matured fruits of *Terminalia chebula* Relzr

Family: Combretaceae

Morphology

Colour: Fruits yellowish brown

Odour: Odourless

Taste: Astringent, slightly bitter and sweetish at the end

Size: 20 to 25 mm long and 15 to 25 mm wide

Shape: Ovate and wrinkled longitudinally

Extra features: Fruits are hard and strong with single seed which is light yellow in colour and 15 to 320 mm in length. Purple of the fruit is nonadherent to the seed.

Chemical Constituents: Myrobalan fruits are important source of Tannin. Depending on geographical source, they vary in tannin content. Approximate analysis of the fruit is as follows:

Moisture: 10%

Tannin: 25 to 32 %

Water soluble matter: 40 to 50%

Tannins of myrobalan are pyrogallol type, which on hydrolysis yield chebulic acid and d-falloyl glucose. Chebulagic, chebulinic, ellagic and gallicacids are the other content of myrobalan. It also contains glucose and sorbitol.

Uses

Myrobablan is mainly used as an astringent, laxative, stomachic, and tonic. Laxative property of myrobalan is due to anthracene derivative present in the pericarp. It is also an anthelmintic agent. Fruit pulp is used to cure bleedings. It's an ingredient of ayurvedic preparation. 'Triphala' used for treatment of variety of aliments. It's used in dyeing and tanning industry and in treatment of water used for locomotives. It's used in treatment of piles and external ulcers.

V. CHEMICAL EVALUATION OF POWDERED DRUGS

EXPERIMENT 25

Aim: To perform chemical tests of Digitalis, Datura, Senna, Cinchona, Aloe, Rauwolfia, Nux Vomica.

DIGITALIS

Biological Source: It consists of dried leaves of *Digitalis purpurea*

Family: Scrophulariaceae

Chemical Tests

1. **Keller–Kiliani Test:** Boil about 1 gm finely powdered digitalis with 10 ml of 70% alcohol for 2–3 minutes. The extract is filtered. To the filtrate, add 5 ml water and 0–5 ml strong solution of lead acetate. Shake well and filter. The clear filtrate is treated with equal volume of chloroform and evaporated to yield the extractive. The extractive is dissolved in glacial acetic acid and after cooling, 2 drops ferric chloride solution is added to it. These contents are transferred to a test tube containing 2 ml concentrated sulphuric acid. A reddish brown layer acquiring bluish green colour after standing is observed due to presence of digitoxose.

2. **Legal test:** The extract is dissolved in pyridine, sodium nitroprusside solution is added to it and made alkaline–pink or red colour is produced.

3. **Baljet test:** To a section of digitalis, sodium picrate solution is added. It shows yellow/orange colour.

Use: Cardiotonic

DATURA

Biological Source: It consists of dried leaves and flowering tops of *Datura metal*.
Family: Solanaceae

Chemical Tests

Vitali–Morin Reaction: Drug is treated with fuming nitric acid, followed by evaporation to dryness. To the nitrate residue, add acetone solution and further add methanolic potassium hydroxide to this solution. Violet colouration takes place due to tropone derivative.

Use: Central nervous system depressant

SENNA

Biological Source: It consists of dried leaflets of *Cassia acutifolia* (Alexandrian senna) and *Cassia angustifolia* (Tinnevelly Senna)
Family: Leguminosae

Chemical Test

Borntrager's Test: The powdered drug is boiled with dilute sulphuric acid, filtered and to the filtrate organic solvent is added and shaken well. Using separating funnel, the organic layer is separated to which ammonia solution is added slowly. The ammoniacal layer shows pink to red colour due to the presence of anthraquinone glycosides.

Use: Purgative

CINCHONA

Biological Source: It is the dried bark of the cultivated trees of *Cinchona calisaya*, *C. officinalis*, *C. ledgeriana*, *C. succirubra*
Family: Rubiaceae.

Chemical Test

1. **Thalleoquin Test:** The powdered drug extract treated with one drop dilute sulphuric acid and 1 ml water. Add bromine water dropwise till a permanent yellow tinge is obtained. Add dilute ammonia solution, emerald green colour is obtained.

2. Heat the powdered drug in a dried test tube with little glacial acetic acid, purple vapours are produced at the upper part of test tube.

Use: Antimalarial drug.

ALOE

Biological Source: It is the dried juice of the leaves of *Aloe barbadensis* (Curacao aloes) or of *Aloe perryi*, known as *Socotrine aloes* or of *Aloe ferox* and hybrids of this species with *Aloe africana* and *Aloe spicata* known as *Cape aloes*.

Family: Liliaceae

Chemical Tests: Boil 1 gm Aloe powder with 10 ml water, filter. The filtrate is used for bromine test and Schoenteten's reaction.

1. **Bromine Test:** Add freshly prepared bromine solution to the filtrate gives pale yellow precipitate of tetrabromalin.

2. **Schoesteten's Reaction (Borax Test):** Treat filtrate with borax and shake well till borax dissolves. Add a few drops of this solution to a test tube, nearly filled with water, a green fluorescence appears.
3. **Nitrous Acid Test:** To an aquous solution of Aloe a small amount of sodium nitrite and a few ml of acetic acid are added, pink colour is developed.

Use: Purgative, protective

RAUWOLFIA

Biological Source: It consists of dried roots of the plant known as *Rauwolfia serpentina*

Family: Apocynaceae

Chemical Tests

1. Powdered drug is treated with concentrated nitric acid gives red colour.
2. Powdered drug treated with solution of vanillin in acetic acid gives violet red colour due to the presence of reserpine.

Uses: Antihypertensive drug

NUX VOMICA

Biological Source: It consists of dried ripe seeds of *Strychonos nux vomica*

Family: Loganiaceae

Chemical Tests

1. Powdered drug treated with Ammonium Vanadate and concentrated Sulphuric Acid shows purple colour due to strychnine.
2. Powdered drug is treated with concentrated nitric acid gives orange colour due to brucine.

Use: Respiratory and cardiac stimulant, bitter tonic.

4
Chapter

Fibres

EXPERIMENT 1

Aim: To identify the given samples of natural fibres (cotton and jute).

Theory: Fibres are obtained from natural sources or prepared artificially. They are used for preparing surgical dressing (absorbent cotton, viscose rayon), absorbing blood, pus and mucus (absorbent cotton), manufacture of ropes and yarns (jute, hemp) and filtration and straining (wool).

Classification of fibres:

a. Natural fibres
   1. Vegetable sources (cotton, hemp, jute)
   2. Animal sources (wool, silk)
b. Artificial fibres
   1. Regenerated sources (viscose rayon, acetate rayon)
   2. Synthetic sources (nylon, terylene)

Identification Tests:

Table 4.1: Types of fibre

Vegetable and regenerated sources	Animal sources
Do not produce foul smell when ignited Dissolve in cuoxam* (ammonical copper oxide)	Burns with an unpleasant smell when ignited Soluble in 50% potassium hydroxide
Produces a blue colour with iodine and sulphuric acid	Stained permanently with picric acid
Produce a violet colour with alpha napthol and sulpuric acid (Molisch test).	Produce a red stain with Millon's reagent

Contd.

*****Cuoxam:** Triturate 2.5 gm of copper carbonate with 50 ml of distilled water in a pestle mortar. Add 50 ml of strong ammonia solution. This reagent should be prepared afresh.

ABSORBENT COTTON

Nonabsorbent cotton consists of the epidermal trichomes of the seeds of *Gossypium herabaceum* Linn. and other cultivated species of *Gossypium*. The trichomes as removed from the seeds containing about 0–6% of wax and oil renders them nonabsorbent when this has been removed by treatment with sodium hydroxide solution under pressure and the alkali removed by washing, absorbent or prepared cotton is produced. Single trichomes are unicellular and flattened with thickened edges and bluntly pointed apices. They are from 2 to 4 cm in length and from 15 to 20 µ wide. Each fibre exhibits 50–120 twists to the length and apart from the small cell contents and any waxy cuticle, consists entirely of cellulose.

Synonym: Purified cotton.

Source: Absorbent cotton consists of epidermal hairs of the following seeds:

1. Cultivated species of *Gossypium herabaceum*
2. Other cultivated species of Gossypium (Family: Malvaceae). These hairs are freed

from impurities and fatty material. Later they are bleached and dried.

Characters: Absorbent cotton is a loose mass of filament like hairs. They are very soft and white in colour, they are odourless and tasteless.

Constituents: Absorbent cotton almost entirely consists of cellulose. The cellulose molecule is made of glucose residues. These glucose residues are united by glycosidic linkage.

Identification Tests

1. **Cuoxam test:** A few threads of cotton wool is moistened with alcohol and mounted in water. The preparation is irrigated with ammoniacal solution of copper oxide (cuoxam). The appearance is examined under high power microscope. It can be seen that absorbent cotton swells uniformly and dissolves ultimately. But raw cotton develops balloon like swelling which are separated by ring shaped constrictions.
2. **Absorbency test:** One gram of absorbent cotton wool compressed to a volume of about 20 ml and placed lightly on the surface of water at 20°C, sinks or gets saturated within 10 seconds.
3. Mount several strands in glycerin solution, examine under high power magnification and draw representative filaments.
4. Mount in iodine solution, irrigate with dilute sulphuric acid and note any colouration formed.
5. Boil in picric acid solution for 2 minutes, leave for 5 minutes; wash with water and determine whether the fibres are stained yellow.
6. Mount in 5% sodium hydroxide solution and warm gently. Acertain whether cotton is soluble in this reagent.
7. Mount in dilute sulphuric acid and note whether cotton is soluble in this reagent.

Uses: Used in surgical dressing, filtering medium, absorption of blood, mucus and pus and as an insulating material.

JUTE

This is obtained from the bark of the stem of *Corchorus olitorus* Linn. and other species of Corchorus grown chiefly in Bengal. The phloem fibres are loosened from the bark by fermentation in water and then separated by suitable treatment. Tow consists of strands of jute made into cheese rolls. Each strands may be from 1 to 3 metres long and consists of a large number of fibres. Individual fibres are up to 5 mm in length and from 10 to 25 µ in diameter. The ends are mostly rounded and the walls exhibit no transverse lines. The cell cavity is not uniform throughout the length of the fibre and may disappear in some places. The fibres give positive tests for lignin.

Synonym: Gunny

Source: Jute consists of strands of phloem removed from the stem bark of:

1. *Corchorus capsularis*
2. *Corchorus olitorius*
3. *Other species of Corchorus* (Fam. Tiliaceae)

Characters: Individual jute has a length of about 0.8 to 5 mm. They are yellowish brown in colour and somewhat coarse in texture. They are hygroscopic and have a good tensile strength.

Identification Tests

1. Mount a little tow in chloral hydrate solution, warm gently; examine under low power magnification and draw several bundles of fibres.
2. Macerate some tow in warm dilute nitric acid to which sufficient potassium chlorate has been added to maintain gentle effervescence. Wash well, a piece of the material will easily separate; tease out and mount in glycerin solution, examine under high power magnification and draw representative.
3. Mount in phloroglucinol and hydrochloric acid; examine and note any staining.
4. Mount in cuoxam and iodine solution followed by dilute sulphuric acid.

Uses: Used in manufacture of yarns, ropes and gunny bags, as a filtering and straining media, making medicated tows.

EXPERIMENT 2

Aim: To identify the given samples of animal fibres (wool, silk).

Theory:

Wool: This is prepared from the fleece of the sheep *Ovis aries* Linn By scouring with soap and sodium carbonate solution to remove the wool fat, followed by washing and drying. Individual hairs are subcylindrical and solid and vary from 15 to 60 µ in width. They consists of a pith (medulla) of polyhedral or rounded cells, a cortex of spindle-shaped with nuclei and an epithelium of imbricated scales, the free edge of which point towards the apex of the hairs and give rise to the characteristic transverse markings of the wool, which gives positive reaction when tested for protein.

Synonym: Sheep's wool, animal wool.

Source: Wool consists of hairs from the fleece of sheep *Ovis aries*

Family: Bovidae, Ungulata

Characteristics:

1. Wool occurs as a loose mass of elastic, lustrous and curly hairs. It is smooth and slippery.
2. Wool is soluble in alkali. It is insoluble in hot or cold concentrated hydrochloric acid or 66% sulphuric acid.
3. Wool is hygroscopic so it absorbs moisture.

Constituents: Wool contains keratin (a protein) which is rich in sulphur containing amino acids. A black colour is produced with lead acetate and alkali due to the presence of these amino acids.

Identification Tests

1. Mount several fibres in glycerin solution, examine under high power magnification and draw representative filaments.
2. Mount several fibres in cuoxam solution, leave for 3 minutes, examine and note the effect.
3. Mount in iodine solution, examine and note any staining.
4. Boil in picric acid solution for 2 minutes; leave for 5 minutes, wash with water and note whether the fibres are stained permanently yellow.
5. Mount in 5% sodium hydroxide solution, warm gently and note whether solution takes place.
6. Mount in dilute sulphuric acid and note whether solution takes place.
7. Mount in Millon's reagent and warm gently, note the colouration produced.

Uses: Used as a medium for filtering and straining, for the manufacture of crepe bandages and dressings.

SILK

This is the dried secretion of the larva of the silkworm *Bombyx mori* Linn. and obtained from the cocoon of varying thickness. During the process of manufacture, the sericin is more or less removed and the threads separated from each other. Individual threads appear solid, structureless, and nonceluller when examined microscopically. They vary from 5 to 65 µ in diameter and externally are smooth or finely striated. They are composed of protein.

Source: Silk is the prepared fibre obtained from:

1. The cocoons of *Bombyx mori*, called as mulberry silk worm.
2. Other species of *Bombyx* and *Antherae* (order: Lepidopteria).

Characters

1. Silk are soft, smooth, fine and yellow in colour. They have considerable soft texture.
2. Silk is soluble in concentrated hydrochloric acid and 66% sulphuric acid.

Constituents

1. Silk contains a protein called fibroin. The main amino acids of fibroin are alanine and glycine.
2. Sulphur containing amino acids are absent in silk. So it does not give a black colour with lead acetate and alkali.

Identification Tests:

1. Mount several filaments of silk in lactophenol, examine under high power magnification and make a drawing of representative filaments.
2. Mount in Millon's reagent, warm gently and note the colouration produced.
3. Mount in hydrochloric acid and note whether the fibre dissolves.
4. Mount in iodine solution and note the staining produced.
5. Mount in 5% sodium hydroxide solution, warm gently and note whether the fibre dissolves.
6. Boil in picric acid solution for 2 minutes, leave for 5 minutes, wash with water and note whether the filament are permanently stained yellow.
7. Burn a few threads, hold a piece of moistened red litmus paper in the fumes and note their reaction.

Uses: Silk is used for making ligatures, oil, silk and sieves.

EXPERIMENT 3

Aim: To identify the given samples of artificial regenerated fibres (viscose rayon, acetate rayon)

VICOSE RAYON

Source: Viscose rayon is a regenerated fibre. It is prepared from wood cellulose of bleached cotton linters.

Characters: The viscose rayons are white and highly lustrous. The tensile strength may be more or less than that of cotton, depending on the finishing treatment. When wetted with water, it loses 60 % of its tensile strength.

Constituents: Viscose rayon consists of cellulose only.

Identification tests:

1. With N/50 iodine and 80% sulphuric acid, it gives a blue colour.
2. It dissolves in 60% cold sulphuric acid.

Uses: For making lint, gauze, net and other surgical dressings.

ACETATE RAYON (CELLULOSE ACETATE)

This is made from timber, usually pine, by delignifying, bleaching and disintegrating. It consists of delignified xylem elements; vessels are generally absent but tracheids exhibiting bordered pits, often in single row, are characteristically present. It gives positive tests for cellulose and therefore may only be distinguished from cotton by its macroscopical and microscopical appearance. It should give negative tests for lignin.

Characters: The filaments of acetate rayon are lustrous, grooved and slightly twisted. In all aspects, it resembles viscose rayon.

Constituents: It contains cellulose chains which are shortened as a result of partial hydrolysis.

Identification tests:

1. It is soluble in cold 60% sulphuric acid and warm concentrated hydrochloric acid.
2. It is insoluble in 5N hydrochloric acid and 4% potassium hydroxide.
3. It is soluble in acetone and 90% phenol.
4. It gives a yellowish brown colour with iodine and sulphuric acid.

Uses: For making cellulose acetate films.

EXPERIMENT 4

Aim: To identify the given samples of artificial synthetic fibres (nylon, terylene)

NYLON

Nylon is a synthetic fibre. It is a polymer of adipic acid and hexamethylene diamine.

Characters: Nylon occurs as cylindrical, solid and smooth filaments. They are available in various diameters. The filaments may be lustrous or dull white or coloured. Nylon filaments are very strong both when dry and wet.

Identification tests

1. When heated in a flame, nylon melts forming a bead.
2. Nylon is soluble in 5M hydrochloric acid and insoluble in acetone (this distinguishes from acetate rayon).
3. It is soluble in 90% formic acid and 90% phenol (this distinguishes from vegetables and animal fibres).

Uses

1. For preparing filter cloths, sieves and nonabsorbable sutures.
2. For making nylon syringes.
3. For the preparation of polyamide.

TERYLENE (DACRON)

Terylene is a synthetic polyester fibre. It is obtained by the condensation of ethylene glycol and terephthalic acid.

Characters:

Terylene occurs as soft, smooth and solid filaments of various diameters. The fibres may be lustrous, dull or coloured. They are very strong irrespective of whether they are wet or dry.

Table 4.2: Summary of chemical tests

Reagent	Cotton (raw) and cellulose wadding	Wool	Silk	Jute
5% Sodium hydroxide	Insoluble	Soluble	Slowly soluble	Insoluble
50% Sulphuric acid	Soluble	Insoluble	Soluble in the cold	Insoluble
Iodine solution	No permanent stain	Stained yellow	Stained yellow	Stained yellow
Iodine followed by sulphuric acid	Bluish-violet colour	No blue colouration	No blue colouration	No blue colouration
Picric acid solution	No permanent staining	Stained yellow	Stained yellow	No permanent staining
Millon's reagent	No brick-red colour	Brick-red colouration produced on warming	Brick-red colouration produced on warming	No brick-red colour
Cuoxam. (ammoniacal copper oxide)	Soluble with uniform swelling /soluble with characteristic balloon-like swelling (raw cotton)	Insoluble	Slowly soluble	Insoluble
Phloroglucinol and hydrochloric acid	Does not stain red	Does not stain red	Does not stain red	Stains red
Hydrochloric acid	Insoluble	Insoluble	Dissolves readily	Insoluble

Identification tests: Terylene retains its structure when boiled with 90% phosphoric acid for one minute.

Uses: Used for making filter cloths, sieves and nonabsorbable suture manufacturing fabrics.

EXPERIMENT 5

Aim: To examine a fabric used as a surgical dressing (crepe bandage)

Procedure:
1. Examine the bandage and determine whether it is composed of yarns of good uniform grade, the material of which is clean and reasonably free from weaving defects.
2. Remove a 20-inch length from the bandage; extend it as far as possible and measure the extended length. Keep it fully extended for 1 minute, then release it, shake lightly, and again measure the length. Record these results.
3. Take about 4 inches of the bandage and soak it in picric acid solution for 5 minutes; wash well with water and examine the fabric with a linen tester. Examine the weft for stained fibres and determine whether the wrap consists of two stained threads (wool) one unstained thread (cotton), and so on. Remove two adjacent cotton threads from the wrap and untwist them. Confirm that one is right twist and the other reverse twist.
4. Stain a second piece of bandage in picric acid solution and count the number of threads to the inch in the wrap. Record the results in terms of cotton and wool for a bandage 3 inches wide.
5. Stretch a piece of bandage fully and with the aid of a linen tester count the number of weft threads to the inch in the stretched condition.
6. Take about 10 inches of bandage, fray out and separate the cotton and wool from the wrap. Measure about 250 inches of each (fully extended) and determine the weight of the measured lengths. Hence calculate the count of the wool and the cotton yarns.
7. Remove a similar length of weft threads; determine the weight of a measured length and calculate the count.
8. Determine the moisture content of the bandage using 5 gm of the bandage.
9. Determine the foreign matter by the following process: Boil the dried bandage obtained from the moisture determination with water; decant and repeat the boiling with water; agitate repeatedly with sufficient quantities of water; remove and dry at 100°C until of constant weight and weigh. The loss in weight is the foreign matter.

Tabulate the result and compare them with the specification.

EXPERIMENT 6

Aim: To examine surgical dressings.

Theory:

Surgical dressings are materials which are used for wound dressings, wound and blood swapping/cleaning and bandages in order to protect a wound and favour its healing.

Requirements of surgical dressings:
1. They should protect the wound from environment and from infection.
2. They should effectively absorb exudations of wounds.
3. They should give mechanical support for the damaged and surrounding tissues.
4. They should be durable, sterilizable and also easy to handle.

Wound dressings: They are materials placed over the surface of wound to absorb the secretion. The materials which are used as wound dressings are:

1.**Absorbent materials** like gauze, muslin and lint. These materials adhere to wound and cause pain when removed.

2. **Nonabsorbent materials** like paraffin gauze and petrolatum gauze. They do not adhere to wound. So they can be safely removed without pain.

Absorbents: They are used for absorbing the exudations from wounds. They include:
1. Nonwoven materials like cotton wool and rayon wool.
2. Woven materials like gauzes.
3. Specific absorbent dressings like laparotomy sponges. Sanitary napkins and eye pads.

Bandages: They are used to hold the dressings in position and also to support the injured tissues. They include:
1. Nonelastic bandages like plain bandage and Plaster of Paris bandage.
2. Elastic bandages like crepe bandage and conforming bandage.
3. Adhesives like zinc oxide adhesive tapes.

SUTURES

A **suture** is a string or fibre which is used for sewing or stitching tissues like skin, muscle and tendon with the help of a needle.

A **ligature** is also a suture but it is used without a needle for tying injured blood vessels to prevent bleeding.

Classification of sutures: Sutures can be classified as:
1. **Absorbable sutures:** Which are absorbed and digested in the tissue of the body, e.g. surgical catgut, kangaroo tendon, synthetic absorbable polymers.
2. **Nonabsorbable sutures:** Which are not absorbed and remain as such in the body, e.g. silk, cotton, nylon, stainless steel wire.
3. **Surgical catgut:** Surgical catgut consists of strands prepared from collagen of healthy animals. The collagen is usually obtained from the submucosal layer of small intestine of sheep.

Preparation: The intestine of freshly killed sheep is cleaned. It is split longitudinally into ribbons. Now, the inner most mucosal layer and outer muscular and serous layers are removed mechanically. The ribbons now contain the submucosal layer only. One to five such ribbons are woven, spun and dried, all under tension. They are then polished, cut into suitable sizes and sterilized.

Kangaroo tendon: It is obtained from the tail of kangaroo and processed like catgut. It is used in hernia and bone repairs.

Synthetic absorbable sutures: They include:
1. Glycolides which are cyclic derivatives of glycolic acid.
2. Lactides which are cyclic derivatives of lactic acid.

These sutures have high tensile strength and are easily hydrolysed and absorbed by tissues.

Nonabsorbable sutures: These sutures are not absorbed and remain unchanged in tissues. Silk, cotton, nylon and metals are used as non-absorbable sutures.

Silk: Strands of silk are available in various diameters. They are used in the plaited or braided form, silk sutures are strong and smooth.

Cotton: Cotton sutures are relatively non-reactive. But they do not maintain durable strength. This is a disadvantage.

Nylon: Nylon sutures are available as monofilament or multifilament. Nylon sutures are strong and water resistant. They are used for skin and plastic surgery.

Metals: Metallic sutures are made of wires of metals like silver or stainless steel.

EXPERIMENT 7

Aim: To determine crude fibres by Dutch method.

Requirement: Ginger powder, 10% nitric acid, 2.5% sodium hydroxide, muslin cloth, etc.

Theory:

Fibres are thick walled, spindle shaped or elongated cells with pointed ends. Fibres are best differentiated on the basis of the tissue in which they occur, e.g. cortical fibres, pericyclic fibres, xylem fibres, phloem fibres, etc.

Procedure

1. Take ginger powder and add 50 ml of 10% nitric acid to it.
2. Heat it to boiling with constant stirring and strain it through muslin cloth. Wash the residue with hot water.
3. To the residue add 50 ml of 2.5% v/v NaOH. Strain again through muslin cloth and wash again with hot water.
4. Perform identification tests.
5. Calculate the percentage of fibres present.

Identification Tests

Take the residue and add water or 70% alcohol followed by addition of fluoroglucinol. Development of pink color shows presence of fibres.

Calculation

% fibres

$$= \frac{\text{Total amount of fibres obtained}}{\text{Total amount of drug taken}} \times 100$$

Result: _____

Chapter 5

Plant Tissue Culture

Tissue culture is *in vitro* cultivation of plant cell or tissue under aseptic and controlled environmental conditions, in liquid or on semisolid well defined nutrient medium for the production of primary and secondary metabolites or to regenerate plant. This technique affords alternative solution to problems arising due to current rate of extinction and decimation of flora and ecosystem. BOD incubator required to maintain the culture condition should have the following characteristics:

- Temperature range, 2–40°C
- Temperature control 0.5°C
- Adjustable fluorescent lighting up to 10,000 lux
- Relative humidity range 20–98%
- Relative humidity control ± 3%
- pH 6

General Procedure Involved in Plant Tissue Culture

In vitro culturing of plant tissue involves the following steps:

- Sterilization of glassware tool vessels
- Preparation and sterilization of explant
- Production of callus from explant
- Proliferation of cultured callus
- Subculturing of callus
- Suspension culture

Handling of Laminar Airflow Hood

1. Switch on light and blower motor for 20 minutes before taking any aseptic transfer.
2. Check the ideal requirements of the laminar flow like the sterile air coming out of the filter uniformly make and sure that no paper or obstacle blocking the flow of air.
3. Use savlon or 95% ethanol use to wipe the working surface area of the laminar air flow hood.
4. Put only sterile instruments, glasswares, appliances like petri dishes, culture tubes or other required articles for experiment in the hood.
5. During wiping or flame sterilization of the hood sprit lamp or Bunsen burner be kept at a sufficient distance from the inflammable substances like alcohol to avoid fire in the aseptic room.
6. Now the laminar hood is suitable for working.
7. After using the hood, don't forget to rewipe its surface with ethanol and remove all material from the laminar hood and switch off the light and blower.
8. Cover the hood with an airtight screen.

Cleaning and Disinfection

Cleaning and disinfection are essential elements in the operation of clean and aseptic areas. This process is used to remove microbial and particulate contamination that arise in the area during the handling of culture in aseptic areas. Aseptic areas require additional procedure for cleaning, e.g. fumigation of room with formaldehyde vapour at high relative humidity for a period of 12 hours is undertaken on monthly basis depending upon the use of room. Cleaning agents are used like nonionic surfactants, disinfectants, etc.

Table 5.1: Disinfectants for sterilization of plant material

Disinfectants	Concentration (%)	Exposure (min)
Benzalkonium chloride	0.01–0.1%	5–20
Bromine water	1–2%	2–10
Calcium hypochlorite	9–10%	5–30
Ethyl alcohol and isopropanol	75–95%	–
Hydrogen peroxide	3–12%	5–15
Mercuric chloride	0.1–1.0%	2–10
Silver nitrate	1.0%	5–30
Sodium hypochlorite	0.5–5%	5–30
Quaternary ammonium compounds	0.1–0.2%	5–20
Formaldehyde	1.0%	2–5
Cetrimide or chlorhexidine	70.0%	2–10

All materials entering into the aseptic areas must be sterile. Entry of the materials in the aseptic room preferably through a double ended interlocked autoclave or air sterilize or sterilized double wrapped materials can be passed into the aseptic room through a double ended interlocked exchange hatch.

Sterilization of Culture Room and Transfer Area

- Washing gently all floors and walls with detergent soap solution.
- Wiping with 2% sodium hypochlorite solution or 95% ethyl alcohol
- Commercially available lysol, zephiran and roccal disinfectant for sterilization of surface and culture rooms
- Sterilization required regularly and repeatedly
- Antifungal spirochete is used for sterilization of transfer area
- Large room is sterilized by UV light
- Install HEPA filter into the ventilation units.

Culture Media

Several culture media developed by scientists to culture diverse tissues and organs are Gautheret (1942), White (1943), Haberblanot et al (1956), Murashige and Skoog (1962), Eriksson (1965) and B_5 (Gamberg et al 1968).

Murashige and Skoog medium (MS) is a plant growth medium used in the laboratories for cultivation of plant cell culture. MS medium was invented by plant scientists *Toshio Murashige* and *Folke K Skoog* during Murashige's search for a new plant growth regulator. It is the most commonly used medium in plant tissue culture experiments in laboratories. One of the most important factors governing the growth and morphogenesis of plant tissues in culture is the composition of the culture medium. The basic nutrient requirements of cultured plant cells are very similar to those of whole plants.

Plant tissue and cell culture media are generally made up of some or all of the following components: macronutrients, micronutrients, vitamins, amino acids or other nitrogen supplements, sugar(s), other undefined organic supplements, solidifying agents or support systems, and growth regulators. Several media formulations are commonly used for the majority of all cell and tissue culture work. These media formulations include those described by White, Murashige and Skoog, Gamborg et al, Schenk and Hilderbrandt, Nitsch and Nitsch, and Lloyd and McCown. Murashige and Skoog's MS medium, Schenk and Hildebrand's SH medium, and Gamborg's B5 medium are all high in macronutrients, while the other media formulations contain considerably less of the macronutrients.

Table 5.2: Composition of Murashige and Skoog(MS), and Gambourg medium (B5)

Chemicals	Murashige and Skoog's medium (MS)*	Gambourg Medium (B5)*
Macronutrients (Inorganic Nutrients)		
Ammonium nitrate (NH_4NO_3)	1.65 g	–
Potassium nitrate (KNO_3)	1.9g	2.5g
Calcium chloride ($CaCl_2 \cdot 2H_2O$)	0.44 g	0.15 g
Magnesium sulphate ($MgSO_4 \cdot 7H_2O$)	0.37g	0.25g
Potassium dihydrogen phosphate (KH_2PO_4)	0.17g	–
Ammonium sulphate ($(NH_4)_2SO_4$)	–	13.4g
Sodium dihydrogen phosphate ($NaH_2PO_4 \cdot H_2O$)	–	0.15g
Micronutrients (Inorganic Nutrients)		
Sodium ethylene diamine tetra acetic acid ($Na_2 EDTA \cdot 2H_2O$)	33.6 mg	40.0 mg
Boric acid (H_3BO_3)	6.2 mg	3.0 mg
Manganese sulphate ($MnSO_4 \cdot 4H_2O$)	22.3 mg	10.0 mg
Zinc sulphate ($ZnSO_4 \cdot 7H_2O$)	8.6 mg	2.0 mg
Potassium iodine (KI)	0.83 mg	0.75 mg
Sodium molybdate (Na_2MoO_4)	0.25 mg	0.25 mg
Ferrous sulphate ($FeSO_4 \cdot 7H_2O$)	27.8 mg	43.0 mg (ferric salt)
Copper sulphate ($CuSO_4 \cdot 5H_2O$)	0.025 mg	0.025 mg
Cobalt choloride ($CoCl_2 \cdot 6H_2O$)	0.025 mg	0.025 mg
Vitamins (Organic Suppliments)		
Nicotinic Acid	0.50 mg	1.0 mg
Thiamine HCl	0.10 mg	10.0 mg
Pyridoxine HCl	0.50 mg	1.0 mg
Glycine	2.0 mg	–
Hormones (Growth Regulators)		
Inositol	0.1 g	0.1 g
Glutamine	0.1 g	0.1 g
BAP (6-benzylamino purine)	0.25 mg	0.25 mg
GA_3 (Gibererllic acid)	0.1 mg	–
Carbon source		
Sucrose	20.0 g	20.0 g
Gelling/Solidifying Agent		
Agar	8.0 g	8.0 g
pH	5.7	5.7

*Quantities of chemicals are in g/l or mg/l.
Ref: Murashige T and Skoog F (1962), A revised medium for rapid growth and bioassays with tobacco tissue cultures, *Physiol Plant*, 15 (3): 473–497.

Sterilization of Culture Media

Culture media packed in glass containers or vessels are sealed with cotton plugs and covered with aluminum foils and are autoclaved at pressure of 15 psi at 121°C for 15–45 minutes (time to be fixed from the time when temperature reaches the required temperature). The exposure time depends on the volume of the liquid to be sterilized as given below.

Table 5.3: Autoclave sterilization conditions		
Temperature (Pressure)	Volume (ml)	Sterilization time (min)
121°C	<50	15
(15 psi)	75	20
	250–500	25
	500–1000	30
	1000–2000	40

Sterilization of Culture Vessels and Instruments

1. Hot air oven (glass culture vials, metal instruments, aluminium foils, etc. 160–180 °C for 2–4 hrs)
2. Autoclave (Plastic labware, e.g. propylene, polymethyl pentene, polyallomer, ETPE, reflon, etc.)

Table 5.4: Dry heat sterilization conditions			
Sl. No.	Temperature (°C)	Heating time (min.)	Sterilization time (min.)
1	160	60	45
2	170	60	18
3	180	60	7.5
4	190	60	1.5

Sterilization of Plant Tissues

Heavily contaminated plant tissues, particularly those covered with dirt and debris should be washed in a weak detergent solution and rinsed many times with distilled water prior to sterilization. Some buds twigs, wets and spreads are cleaned by different concentration of ethanol solution. Some materials which are commonly used for sterilization of plant tissues are:

- Chemical agents : 0.025 – 0.256 sodium hypochlorite (NaOCl)
- Surface sterilizers : 3–10% hydrogen peroxide (H_2O_2) solution

   1 – 2% Bromine water

   1% Silver nitrate ($AgNO_3$)

   0.1 – 1% Magnesium chloride ($MgCl_2$)
- Surfactants : Tween-20 or Triton x –100 (0.05%)
- Ultrasonic bath : Useful for sterilization of buds and woody tissues.

After surface sterilization, a minimum of three sequential rinses with sterile distilled water to remove excess of chemical agents.

Preparation of explant

Explant can be defined as a portion of plant body, which has been taken from the plant to establish a culture. Explant can be obtained from plants, which are grown in controlled environmental condition. Such plants will be usually free from pathogens and are homozygous in nature. Explant may be taken from any part of the plant like root, stem, leaf, or meristematic tissue like cambium, floral parts like anthers, stamens, etc.

A suitable portion from the plant is removed with the help of a sharp knife and the dried and mature portions are separated from young tissue. When seeds and grains are used for explant preparation, they are directly sterilized and put in nutrient medium, after germination, the obtained seedlings are to be used for explant preparation.

Surface sterilization of explant

For the surface sterilization of the explant, chromic acid, mercuric chloride (0.11%), calcium hypochlorite, sodium hypochlorite

(1-2%) and alcohol (70%) are used. Usually the tissue is immersed in the solution of sterilizing agent for 10 seconds to 15 minutes and then they are washed with distilled water. Repeat the treatment with sodium hypochlorite for 20 minutes and the tissue is finally washed with sterile water to remove sodium hypochlorite. Such tissue is used for inoculation.

In the case of leaf or green fresh stem the explant needs pretreatment with wetting agent (70–90% ethyl alcohol, Tween 20), 5–20 drops in 100 ml of purified water or some other mild detergent to be added directly into the sterilization solution to reduce the explants. We can use different surface sterilizing agent mentioned above.

Production of callus from explant

The sterilized explant is transferred aseptically into defined medium contained in flasks. The flasks are transferred to BOD incubator for maintenance of culture. Temperature is adjusted to 25 ± 2°C. Some amount of light is necessary for callus (undifferentiated amorphous cell mass) production. Usually sufficient amount of callus is produced within 3–8 days of incubation.

Proliferation of callus

If callus is well developed, if should be cut into small pieces and transferred to another fresh medium containing an altered composition of hormones, which supports growth. The medium used for production of more amount of callus is called proliferation medium.

Subculturing of callus

After sufficient growth of callus, it should be periodically transferred to fresh medium to maintain the viability of cells. This subculturing will be done at an interval of 4–6 weeks.

Suspension culture

Suspension culture contains a uniform suspension of separate cells in liquid medium. For the preparation of suspension culture, callus is transferred to liquid medium, which is agitated continuously to keep the cells separate. Agitation can be achieved by rotary shaker system attached within the incubator at a rate of 50–150rpm. After the production of sufficient number of cells sub- culturing can be done.

EXPERIMENT 1

Aim: To prepare and sterilize given tissue culture medium.

Requirement: Autoclave, culture tube, MS-media, cotton plugs, brown paper, beaker, glass rod, etc.

Theory: Tissue culture is an experimental technique through which mass of cell is produced from the explant tissue. Callus culture and suspension culture are the basic technique used to produce the desired metabolites of plants. Tissue culture is an alternative way for the production of phytochemical of therapeutic importance. Latest techniques like hairy root culture, biotransformation, immobilization and elicitations are used to increase production of secondary metabolites. Through plant tissue culture the totipotent characteristics of cell can be used for the *in vitro* regeneration of plant. It is a technique offering the prospect of absolutely uniform plant material obtainable at all times and manageable under regulated and reproducible conditions rarely possible in entire living plants.

Murashige and Skoog medium (MS) is a plant growth medium used in the laboratories for cultivation of plant cell culture. MS medium was invented by plant scientists *Toshio Murashige* and *Folke K Skoog* during Murashige's search for a new plant growth regulator. It is the most commonly used medium in plant tissue culture experiments in laboratories. One of the most important factors governing the growth and morphogenesis of plant tissues in culture is the composition of the culture medium. The basic nutrient requirements of cultured plant cells are very similar to those of whole plants.

Plant tissue and cell culture media are generally made up of some or all of the following components: macronutrients, micronutrients, vitamins, amino acids or other nitrogen supplements, sugar(s), other undefined organic supplements, solidifying agents or support systems, and growth regulators. Several media formulations are commonly used for the majority of all cell and tissue culture work. These media formulations include those described by White, Murashige and Skoog, Gamborg et al, Schenk and Hilderbrandt, Nitsch and Nitsch, and Lloyd and McCown. Murashige and Skoog's MS medium, Schenk and Hildebrand's SH medium, and Gamborg's B5 medium are all high in macronutrients, while the other media formulations contain considerably less of the macronutrients.

Table 5.5: Composition of Murashige and Skoog medium (MS), and Gambourg medium (B5)

Chemicals	Murashige and Skoog's medium(MS)*	Gambourg Medium (B5)*
Macronutrients (Inorganic Nutrients)		
Ammonium nitrate (NH_4NO_3)	1.65 g	–
Potassium nitrate (KNO_3)	1.9g	2.5g
Calcium choloride ($CaCl_2 2H_2O$)	0.44 g	0.15 g
Magnesium sulphate ($MgSO_4 7H_2O$)	0.37g	0.25g
Potassium dihydrogen phosphate (KH_2PO_4)	0.17g	-
Ammonium sulphate ($(NH_4)_2SO_4$)	–	13.4g
Sodium dihydrogen phosphate ($NaH_2PO_4H_2O$)	–	0.15g
Micronutrients (Inorganic Nutrients)		
Sodium ethylene diaminetetraacetic acid (Na_2 $EDTA.2H_2O$)	33.6 mg	40.0 mg
Boric acid (H_3BO_3)	6.2 mg	3.0 mg
Manganese sulphate ($MnSO_4.4H_2O$)	22.3 mg	10.0 mg
Zinc sulphate ($ZnSO_4.7H_2O$)	8.6 mg	2.0 mg
Potassium iodine (KI)	0.83 mg	0.75 mg
Sodium molybdate (Na_2MoO_4)	0.25 mg	0.25 mg
Ferrous sulphate ($FeSO_4 7H_2O$)	27.8 mg	43.0 mg (ferric salt)
Copper sulphate ($CuSO_4.5H_2O$)	0.025 mg	0.025 mg
Cobalt choloride ($CoCl_2 6H_2O$)	0.025 mg	0.025 mg
Vitamins (Organic Suppliments)		
Nicotinic Acid	0.50 mg	1.0 mg
Thiamine HCl	0.10 mg	10.0 mg
Pyridoxine HCl	0.50 mg	1.0 mg
Glycine	2.0 mg	–

Table 5.5: Composition of Murashige and Skoog medium (MS), and Gambourg medium (B_5) (*Contd.*)

Chemicals	Murashige and Skoog's medium(MS)*	Gambourg Medium (B5)*
Hormones (Growth Regulators)		
Inositol	0.1 g	0.1 g
Glutamine	0.1 g	0.1 g
BAP (6-benzyl-amino purine)	0.25 mg	0.25 mg
GA_3 (Gibbererllic acid)	0.1 mg	–
Carbon Source		
Sucrose	20.0 g	20.0 g
Gelling/Solidifying Agent		
Agar	8.0 g	8.0 g
pH	5.7	5.7

*Quantities of Chemicals are in g/l or mg/l.

Ref: Murashige T and Skoog F (1962), A revised medium for rapid growth and bioassays with tobacco tissue cultures. *Physiol Plant 15(3): 473–497.*

Procedure

1. Weigh accurately the required amounts of ingredients of MS medium.
2. Dissolve the ingredients in 100 ml of double distilled water in increasing order of their weights (except agar).
3. Heat the solution if necessary to dissolve the contents.
4. Add agar powder in small quantities at a time to the hot solution with constant stirring.
5. Boil to affect the solution.
6. Adjust the pH of the solution by the addition of 0.1M NaOH/0.1M KOH solution.
7. Make up the volume to 1000 ml with distilled water.
8. Transfer 10 ml of this solution to culture tube or 25 ml in 100 ml conical flasks, plug the tubes/flasks with cotton plugs and wrap the cotton plug with aluminium foil or brown paper.
9. Autoclave the tubes in an autoclave at 15 lb for 15–20 min.

Result: _____

EXPERIMENT 2

Aim: To carry out aseptic germination of given seeds.

Requirement: Laminar flow bench, autoclave, petri plates, cotton, forceps, alcohol, etc.

Theory: Tissue culture is an experimental technique through which mass of cells is produced from the explant tissue. It is a technique offering the prospect of absolutely uniform plant material obtainable at all times and manageable under regulated and reproducible conditions rarely possible in entire living plants. Through plant tissue culture the totipotent characteristics of cell can be used for the *in vitro* regeneration of plant. It is a technique offering the prospect of absolutely uniform plant material obtainable at all times and manageable under regulated and reproducible conditions rarely possible in entire living plants.

Procedure

1. Wash the given seeds with mild detergent and rinse thrice with distilled water.
2. Immerse the seeds in 70% ethanol for two minutes and rinse thrice with sterile distilled water.
3. Carry out surface sterilization of seeds by immersing them in 2% v/v mercuric chloride solution or 2% v/v solution of sodium hypochlorite. Wash the seeds thrice with sterile distilled water to remove any traces of sterilizing agent.
4. Germinate the seeds in dark for 4–5 days on sterile filter paper or cotton wool, previously moistened with sterile distilled water in petri plates at 26 ± 2°C.
5. Transfer the germinated seeds in the previously sterilized culture tubes containing MS medium on the laminar flow bench.
6. Keep the transferred culture tubes on the tissue culture rack, provided photoperiodic light in air conditioned tissue culture lab.

Result: Germinated seedlings were obtained after _____ days.

EXPERIMENT 3

Aim: To perform *in vitro* callus induction of aseptically germinated seedlings/given plant.

Requirement: Aseptically germinated seedlings, sterile culture medium, scalpel, forceps, spatula, incubator, laminar flow bench, etc.

Theory: Tissue culture is an experimental technique through which mass of cell is produced from the explants tissue. Callus culture and suspension culture are the basic techniques used to produce the desired metabolites of plants. Tissue culture is an alternative way for the production of phytochemical of therapeutic importance. Latest techniques like hairy root culture, biotransformation, immobilization and elicitations are used to increase production of secondary metabolites. Through plant tissue culture the totipotent characteristics of cell can be used for the *in vitro* regeneration of plants.

Procedure

1. Take the germinated seedlings; remove the cotyledon portion by cutting with sterile scalpel.
2. Transfer the explant portion into sterile medium in culture tubes/flasks.
3. Incubate the culture at 26 ± 2°C in darkness for three weeks. Transfer the cultures aseptically on sterile fresh medium at an interval of 4 weeks.
4. Calculate the growth rate in terms of growth index.

Calculation:

$$\text{Growth Index} = \frac{\text{Final weight of callus}}{\text{Initial weight of callus}}$$

Result: _____

EXPERIMENT 4

Aim: To develop callus culture from carrot combine explants.

Requirement:

Chemical/Reagent:

Callus induction medium, Ethanol 70% solution, Sodium hypochlorite solution (NaOCl solution), Sterile distilled water.

Apparatus: Sterile petri plates, Sterile BF culture vessels, forceps and scalpel, vegetable scrapes, carrot taproot.

Theory: Carrot (*D carota* L, Apiaceae) is one of the most commonly used vegetables for human nutrition. It is a tall robust biennial spiny-fruited herb growing in dried-out fields or meadows. Carrots are cultivated worldwide. Their juices and blends are among the most popular nonalcoholic beverages. It is regarded as a healthy food item because of its high vitamin and fiber content.

To develop *in vitro* method for rapid propagation root, stem, leaf and nodal explants of *Daucus carota* L. can be cultured on MS medium supplemented with different concentration and combinations of hormones [0.5 mg/l of 6-benzylaminopurine (BAP) or 2 mg/l of BAP and 1 mg/l of α-nephthalene acetic acid (NAA)]. Differentiation of shoot initiated after one week of culture, and after eight weeks of primary culture, an average of six plantlets can develop from a single shoot. The shoots when subcultured in the medium supplemented with 1 mg/l NAA produced roots after five weeks of subculture. Root and leaf explants induced roots and callus when cultured on MS medium with NAA at the rate of 1 mg/l and 2 mg/l. Similarly, stem explants also induced roots and callus in the same concentration of hormones whereas few multiple shoot can induce when cultured on MS supplemented with 2 mg/l of BAP and 1 mg/l of NAA. This result suggests that this methodology can be applied for the rapid and mass propagation of this species.

Procedure:

1. Wash the taproot with tap water for three times. Remove the outermost two millimeter of tissue from a carrot taproot using a vegetable scraper.
2. Slice the taproot crosswise into 10 mm wide disc. Handle discs with a flame-sterilized forceps.
3. Wash these discs with detergent water and then wash with sterilized distilled water for 3–5 times and surface sterilized by immersing them in 1% solution of sodium hypochlorite for 15 min, 70% ethanol for 1 min and finally by rinsing three times with sterilized distilled water.
4. Transfer this sterile disc into a sterile vessel using a pair of flame sterilized forceps and add enough sterile distilled water and wash three to four times.
5. Swirl the vessel slowly every minute to remove the remaining sterilized solution.
6. Using flame sterilized forceps, transfer the discs to a sterile petri plate. By a flame sterilized scalpel, slice the discs and periodically sterilizes the forceps and scalpel to reduce the possibility of contamination.
7. Aseptically transfer small piece of root disc to an individual culture tube containing callus induction culture medium (MS medium supplemented with 3% sucrose and solidified with 0.8% agar. Adjust pH of the medium to 5.8 before autoclaving).
8. Prepare at least 10 carrot taproot cultures as instructed above.
9. Put a water proof cable or grease pencil or water proof marker which has following information like name, date, sterilization treatment.
10. Incubate the jars or tubes (cultures) under a cool white florescent light at 25 °C ± 2 °C and expose to 16 hours light per day.

Result: _____

EXPERIMENT 5

Aim: To determine antimicrobial activity of crude drugs.

Theory: Herbs have been used for pain relieving and healing properties and today we still rely on the curative properties of plants in about three-fourth of our medicine. In the present time, the people more often depends on allopathic drugs but the microorganisms are becoming resistant against such drugs. So the time is shifting towards the use of natural products and medicinal plants, which were mainly used in ancient time in Ayurveda. Antimicrobial screening is used to find new therapeutic agents of infection and infectious diseases because microbes are very sensitive to natural drugs and react at very fast rate, so result comes in very short time. The plant species are selected on the basis of the ethnic claims for a particular disease. So, the causing agents were taken for screening, since it is essential to certify the ethnic claims. This idea led us for screening of antimicrobial agents of plant origin. The crude plant extract may be helpful in the isolation of new therapeutic drugs and active principle.

Microorganisms used as experimental organism: Various microorganisms can be taken as experimental organism, these are as follows:

a. *Mycobacterium tuberculosis*: It is a causative agent of tuberculosis. Tuberculosis is still one of the most widespread diseases. The mammalian tubercles, both bovine and human varieties, are pathogenic for man. The bacterium infects the respiratory tract and gets established in lung tissues. After being phagocytosed by macrophages the bacteria are enclosed into the small and hard tubercles, which are the characteristics feature of the disease. It is a gram-positive straight or slightly curved rod shaped, having 3 μm × 0.3 μm, occurring singly and in pairs.

b. *Escherichia coli*: It forms a part of normal intestinal flora of humans and animals. It causes urinary track infection, diarrhoea, pyrogenic infections and septicemia. These are gram-negative bacilli exhibit considerably variation in their morphology. The usual dimensions observed from 2μ to 4μ in length and from 0.4μ to 0.7μ in breadth. Two types of virulent factors have been recognized in *E coli* – surface antigens and toxins. This pathogen produces two kinds of exotoxins; *hemolysins* and *enterotoxins*. *Hemolysins* do not appear to be relevant in pathogenesis but *enterotoxins* are important in the pathogenesis of diarrhoea.

c. *Bacillus subtilis*: It is occasionally responsible for infection particularly of eyes and rarely may produce septicemia in juvenile and young animals. The pathogenicity of these forms is very slight.

d. *Candida albicans*: Mycosis caused by *Candida albicans* is called candidiasis. It is an acute or chronic superficial mycosis. It is one of the most frequently encountered fungal diseases. It is a part of normal flora of oral cavity, large intestine and vagina. It is ovoid or spherical budding yeast like fungus, 2.5 × 4 × 6 μm in dimension.

e. *Aspergillus fumigatus*: It causes the disease Aspergillosis and highly pathogenic for birds, animals and man as well. Aspergillosis is important in patients with the malignant disease particularly with leukemia and lymphoma. Human cases of Aspergillosis are most frequently in infections of external ear called Otomycosis. Pulmonary infection is relatively uncommon in man.

Materials and Methods

Culture media:

Overnight grown cultures in nutrient broth for bacterial culture and Sabouraud's dextrose broth for fungal culture at 37°C are used for the preparation of bacterial lawn.

a. **Nutrient broth:** It contains 3 gm meat extract; 5 gm peptic digest of animal tissue in 1000 ml-distilled water and pH is adjusted to 6.8 ± 0.2. The broth is dispensed in 10 ml amount in each tube and autoclaved at 121°C and 15 lbs for 15 minutes. The test culture are grown overnight in broth for the development of bacterial lawn.

b. **Nutrient agar:** It is prepared by addition of 2% agar powder in nutrient broth. The medium is autoclaved at 121°C and 15 lbs for 15 minutes. Then it is poured onto the sterilized glass petridishes. Each petridish contained 30–35 ml medium having 3–4 mm depth.

c. **Sabouraud's dextrose broth:** The broth contains dextrose 40 g, peptone 10 g per liter in distilled water and pH is adjusted to 5.4 ± 0.2.

d. **Sabouraud's dextrose agar:** The agar is prepared by addition of 2.0% agar powder in broth. The medium is autoclaved at 115°C and 15 lbs for 10 minutes.

Method of Screening

a. **Disc diffusion method:** The discs of Whatman filter paper no. 2 are cut in 5 mm diameter and sterilized in hot air oven. Then the discs are placed on to the agar medium keeping proper distance among discs. The stock solution 5 gm/50 ml methanolic concentrations are made and 10 µl of stock solution is poured on to the discs. Ciprofloxacin is taken as control under bacterial screening.

b. **Cup-well method:** The cup-well is prepared by using 6 mm sterile steel borer. The stock solution 10 gm/50 ml methanolic concentrations are made and 30ml of stock solution is poured in each well. The methanolic extracts is dissolved in DMF (*n, n*-dimethyl formamide).

c. **Statistical criteria for indication of efficacy:** A statistical presentation of crude extract is classified on the basis of inhibition zone. The effectiveness of microorganisms is further divided into 4 categories, viz., traces, weak, normal and excellent. 1–3 mm is included under traces, more than 3 to 6 mm is included under weak, more than 6 to 9 mm is included under normal, more than 9 to 12 or more included in excellent category. The criterion is as follows:

Table 5.6: Indication of efficacy on the basis of inhibition zone

S.No.	Number of plant extract on the basis of inhibition zone	Indication of efficacy
1.	1–3 mm inhibition zone	Traces
2.	More than 3 to 6 mm inhibition zone	Weak
3.	More than 6 to 9 mm inhibition zone	Normal
4.	More than 9 to 12 mm or more inhibition zone	Excellent

Procedure

a. **Antimicrobial tests against *Mycobacterium tuberculosis*:** 5 gm of the plant materials used are extracted in 50 ml of methanol and the extracts prepared are used to perform disc diffusion test. The diameter of disc are measured in mm.

b. **Antimicrobial tests against *Escherichia coli*:** Methanol and Ciprofloxacin was taken as control. 5 gm of the plant materials used are extracted in 50 ml of methanol and the extracts prepared are used to perform disc diffusion test. The diameter of disc are measured in mm.

c. **Antimicrobial tests against *Bacillus subtilis*:** Methanol is used as control; 5 gm of the plant materials used can be extracted in 50 ml of methanol and the extracts prepared are used to perform disc diffusion test.

d. **Antimicrobial tests against *Candida albicans*:** The methanolic extracts are dissolved in DMF. 10 gm of the plant materials used are extracted in 50 ml of methanol and the extracts prepared are used to perform Cup-well method. 30 ml extract can be taken to perform tests.

e. **Antimicrobial tests against *Aspergillus fumigatus*:** The methanolic extracts are dissolved in DMF. 10 gm of the plant materials used are extracted in 50ml of methanol and the extracts prepared are used to perform cup-well method. 30 ml extract can be taken to perform tests.

Observations

Table 5.7: Zone of inhibition

S. No.	Name of microorganisms	Zone of Inhibition (in mm)
1.	M tuberculosis	
2.	E coli	
3.	B subtilis	
4.	C albicans	
5.	A fumigatus	

Result:

The observations are made after 24 and 48 hours of aerobic incubation at 37°C for bacteria and fungi. The zone of inhibition produced by plant extracts, as taken in millimeters.

6
Chapter

Extraction, Isolation, Identification and Estimation of Phytoconstituents

EXPERIMENT 1

Aim: To carry out isolation of *starch* from potatoes.

Requirement: Potatoes, mixer/blender, centrifuge, stirrer, muslin cloth, oven, distilled water.

Theory: Starch is a polysaccharide obtained commercially from wheat, maize, potato and rice. It is present in the form of grains, in different parts of the plants and chemically consists of amylopectin and starch. The yield of starch is approximately 10%. Starch is made up of glucose repeat units known as polysaccharides. **Polysaccharides** are carbohydrate polymers consisting of tenth to hundreds to several thousand monosaccharide units. Most of the polysaccharides contain glucose as the monosaccharide unit. Polysaccharides are synthesized by plants, animals, and humans to be stored for food, structural support, or metabolized for energy. Plants store glucose as the polysaccharide starch. A naturally abundant nutrient carbohydrate $(C_6H_{10}O_5)_n$, is found in cereal grains (wheat, rice, corn, oats, barley) as well as in tubers such as potatoes are rich in starch.

Pure starch is a white, tasteless and odourless powder that is insoluble in cold water or alcohol. It consists of two types of molecules: Linear and helical starch and the branched amylopectin. Depending on the plant, starch generally contains 20 to 25% starch and 75 to 80% amylopectin.

Modified Starches

A modified food starch is a starch that has been chemically modified to allow the starch to function properly under conditions frequently encountered during processing or storage, such as high heat, high shear, low pH, and freeze/thaw and cooling.

The **potato** is a starchy, tuberous crop perennial *Solanum tuberosum* of the Solanaceae family. **Potato starch** is extracted from potatoes. The cells of the root tubers of the

Starch-Amylose

m > 1000

potato plant contain starch grains (leucoplasts). Potato contains about 15% starch. To extract the starch, the potatoes are crushed; the starch grains are released from the destroyed cells. The starch is then washed out and dried to powder. Potato starch contains typical large oval spherical granules; their size ranges between 5 and 100 μm. Potato starch is a very refined starch, containing minimal protein or fat. This gives the powder with a clear white colour, while the cooked starch of typical characteristics with neutral taste, good clarity, high binding strength, long texture and a minimal tendency to foaming or yellowing of the solution.

Procedure

1. Wash potatoes thoroughly with water to remove adhering soil and earthy matter, cut into small pieces and reduce to fine slurry with water in a mixer/blender.
2. Pass the slurry through muslin cloth in order to remove the cell debris and other impurities.
3. Allow the suspension to settle down.
4. Decant the supernatant liquid.
5. Wash starch 2–3 times with distilled water with constant stirring.
4. Centrifuge the suspension, dry it in oven at a low temperature and powder it.

Chemical Test:

It gives blue colour with weak iodine solution which disappears on heating and reappears on cooling.

EXPERIMENT 2

Aim: To carry out extraction of *solanine* from potatoes.

Requirement: Potatoes, water bath, centrifuge, acetic acid, ammonium hydroxide, methanol.

Theory: Solanine is a sterioidal glycoalkaloid found in species of the nightshade family (Solanaceae), such as the potato (*Solanum tuberosum*). Potatoes naturally produce solanine and chaconine, a related glycoalkaloid. It can occur naturally in any part of the plant, including the leaves, fruit, and tubers. When potato tubers are exposed to light, they turn green and increase glycoalkaloid production. The green colour is cause of chlorophyll, and is itself harmless. However, it is an indication that high level of solanine and chaconine may be present. Commercial varieties of potatoes are screened for solanine and most varieties have solanine content of less than 0.2 mg/g. However, potatoes that have been exposed to light, become started to green can show concentrations of 1 mg/g or more. In these situations a single unpeeled potato can result in a dangerous dose. Solanine has fungicidal and pesticidal properties, and it is one of the plant's natural defense.

Procedure

1. Wash potatoes thoroughly with water to remove adhering soil and earthy matter, cut into small pieces.
2. Macerate the pieces of potatoes with twenty parts of 5% acetic acid for 24 hours.
3. Warm to 70°C and add concentrated ammonium hydroxide solution drop wise to adjust pH 10.
4. Centrifuge, wash the precipitate thrice with sufficient quantity of 1% ammonium hydroxide and recentrifuge.
5. Discard the supernatant liquid and then wash.
6. Dry and weigh the crude solanine.
7. Purify it by dissolving in boiling methanol, then filter and concentrate until the solanine starts crystallizing out.

Solvent System for TLC of Solanine:

Toluene: Ethyl acetate:Diethyl amine (70:20:10)

Ethyl acetate: Formic acid: Glacial acetic acid: Water (100:11:11:26)

Detection

Dragendroff reagent

EXPERIMENT 3

Aim: To carry out isolation of *citric acid* from lemon.

Requirement: Lemons, sodium hydroxide, sulfuric acid, calcium chloride, distilled water.

Theory

Scientific Name: *Citrus limon* (L.) Burm. f. [*medica × aurantifolia*] Family: Rutaceae

Common Name: Lemon

Citrus fruits in general contain sugars, polysaccharides, organic acids, lipids, carotenoid (pigment), vitamins, minerals, flavonoids, bitter limonoids, and volatile components. Lemon is a good source of potassium (0.15%), bioflavonoids and vitamin C (0.04–0.5%). Calcium (0.06%) is also present, along with vitamins A, B_1, B_2, and B_3. The fruit is also with low calories (27 Kcal/100 g).

Other constituents of lemon include volatile oil (2.5% of the peel), limonene, α-terpinene, α-pinene, citral, coumarins, mucilage, pectins, and bioflavonoids (mostly from pith and peel). Flavonoids eriocitrin and hesperidin have been evaluated. Low-cost powdered lemon and other citrus fruit peel contains only 1% to 2% flavonoids; however, standardized products contain 10% to 90% flavonoids.

Lemon is primarily important for its vitamin C nutritional value and for its potassium content. Epidemiological studies associate the intake of citrus fruit with a reduction in the risk of various diseases. Lemon investigated for its antioxidant and anticancer properties and also suggested for hypocitraturic calcium nephrolithiasis. Lemon shows some antimicrobial activity also, lemon juice has been used as an astringent, diaphoretic, diuretic, gargle, lotion and tonic. Lemon also has been used externally for acne, fungus (ringworm and athlete's foot), sunburn, and warts. 120 ml of lemon juice, contain 5.9 g of citric acid diluted and consumed daily. It is also used in the treatment of scurvy and gum deterioration.

Citric acid is a weak organic acid. Citric acid exists in a variety of fruits and vegetables, most notably citrus fruits. Lemons and limes have particularly high concentrations of the acid; it can constitute as much as 8% of dry weight of these fruits (about 47 g/L in the juices). The concentrations of citric acid in citrus fruits range from 0.005 mol/L for oranges and grapefruits to 0.30 mol/L in lemons and limes. It is a natural preservative/conservative and is also used in foods and soft drinks for sour and acidic taste. In biochemistry, the conjugate base of citric acid, citrate, is important as an intermediate in the citric acid cycle, and therefore occurs in the metabolism of virtually all living things. It can also be used as a cleaning agent. Citrate is a critical component of bone, helping to regulate the size of calcium crystals. Citrate is an inhibitor of phosphofructokinase, which helps to regulate the rate of glycolysis in the cell.

$$\begin{array}{c} H_2C-COOH \\ | \\ HO-C-COOH \\ | \\ H_2C-COOH \end{array}$$

Citric acid

The lemon is important for it's nutritional value. Vitamin C is necessary to sustain the body's resistance to infection and heal wounds. It is also used in the treatment of scurvy and gum deterioration.

Procedure

1. Concentrate 90 ml of lemon juice into beaker.
2. Add 10% sodium hydroxide solution carefully with constant stirring until the solution is slightly alkaline (a distinct color change occurs at this point).
3. Strain the solution through muslin cloth to remove large particles of pulp and then filter through filter paper in a buchner funnel.
4. Place the filtrate in a beaker and add 5 ml of calcium chloride solution for each 10 ml of filtrate with constant stirring.

5. Heat to boiling and filter off the copious precipitate of calcium citrate, from the hot solution using a Buchner funnel.
6. Wash the precipitate with a small quantity of boiling distilled water.
7. Suspend it in a minimum quantity of distilled water.
8. Heat to boil and collect the insoluble calcium citrate by filtration.
9. Allow it to air dry.
10. Citric acid may be prepared from the calcium citrate salt by adding sufficient 1N sulfuric acid required to convert the salt to acid. Allow the mixture to stand for a few minutes.
11. Filter off the insoluble $CaSO_4$ and concentrate the filtrate to a small volume on a water bath.
12. Citric acid crystalizes out then filter and dry.

EXPERIMENT 4

Aim: To isolate *calcium citrate* from lemon juice.

Requirements: Conical flask, Beaker, Funnel, Measuring cylinder, Glass rod, pH strip, lemon.

Theory: Calcium is the most abundant mineral in the human body and is vital to proper funtioning in the body. Calcium supplements exist in different compounds: calcium citrate, calcium carbonate, calcium gluconate, calcium lactate and calcium pyruvate. Calcium citrate has 21% elemental calcium, one of the highly concentrated compound of calcium and has the best absorption rate of calcium supplements.

Calcium citrate is a salt of calcium and citric acid, forming a somewhat sour-tasting food grade nutritional product. Beyond its use as a dietary supplement, calcium citrate is also frequently used as a food additive to impart a sour taste to foods, as a food preservative and as a water softener because the citrate ions can chelate unwanted metal ions. Aside from maintaining strong bones and teeth, calcium is required for muscle contraction, nerve conduction, heart functioning, blood coagulation, glandular secretion, energy production and immune function.

Calcium citrate is 2-Hydroxy-1,2,3-propanetricarboxylic acid calcium salt (2:3) tetrahydrate; Tricalcium citrate tetrahydrate

Molecular Formula: $C_{12}H_{10}Ca_3O_{14} \cdot 4H_2O$

Molecular Weight: 570.49

Procedure

1. Take 25 ml of lemon juice and add NaOH till slightly alkaline, indicated on pH strip or by colour change of solution from yellow to brown.
2. Filter the mixture through cotton, remove the fluffy material by staining material.
3. Neutralize the filtrate with dilute HCl.
4. Add $CaCl_2$ till the precipitates of calcium citrate are obtained.
5. Filter the precipitate of calcium citrate, wash with slightly warm distilled water.
6. Dry the precipitates of calcium citrate, calculate the % yield. Take melting point.

EXPERIMENT 5

Aim: To carry out extraction of *pectin* from fresh orange peels.

Requirement: Fresh orange peels, vacuum drier, distillation unit, thermometer, muslin cloth, distilled water, isopronanol, acetone, citric acid, pH paper.

Theory: Orange peel consists of cellulose, essential oils, proteins and some simple carbohydrates. Pectin is a polysaccharide component in the cell walls of fruits and vegetables. Polysaccharides are polymers made up of many simple carbohydrates (sugars) linked together into long, continuous molecules.

Pectin is obtained from orange peels, lemon peels, sunflower-head and raw papaya. Chemically, it is a mixture of polymers of uronic acid and their methyl esters. The yield of pectin from fresh orange peel is 4 to 5% w/w. It is yellowish white powder with mucilaginous taste.

Pectin is currently valued for use as a gelling and thickening agent, beverage stabilizer, and fat substitute. Most commercial pectin is obtained by extraction from citrus peels, but sugar beet pulp is also rich source of pectin.

Procedure

1. Cut fresh orange peels into smaller pieces.
2. Weigh about 50 g of the peels, wash thoroughly with water and immerse in 200 ml of distilled water.
3. Adjust the pH to 4 with addition of citric or tartaric acid or by addition of H_2SO_4.
4. Heat at 50–85°C with stirring for about half an hour and filter immediately while solution is hot.
5. Cool the filtrate and pour it slowly into three volumes of acidic isopropanol/ ethanol/acetone.
6. Stir the solution thoroughly for precipitation of pectin.
7. Filter through muslin cloth and wash it several times with small volumes of 70% isopropanol/ acetone in order to make it free from acidic ions.
8. Dry the product in vacuum drier, weigh and store in well closed container.

Chemical Test: Dissolve 1 g in 9 ml of water by heating. On cooling, it forms a stiff jelly.

EXPERIMENT 6

Aim: To isolate *hesperidin* from orange peel.

Requirements: orange peel powder, petroleum ether, methanol, dilute acetic acid, round bottom flask and condensor.

Theory: Hesperidin (Hesperitin 7-rhamnoglucoside, Hesperitin-7-rutinoside) is a flavanone glycosides found abundantly in citrus fruits (orange, tangerine, orange and lemon peel). The peel and membranous parts of lemon and oranges have highest hesperidin concentration. Its aglycone form is known as hesperetin. It is yellow to white crystalline powder. Orange peel is the dried pericarp of ripe fruits of *Citrus aurantium* (Rutaceae). It contains volatile oil and various flavonoids like hesperidin, levohesperidin (isomer of hesperidin), rutin, nariogin, narirutin. Hesperidin is believed to play a role in plant defense.

Hesperidin is insoluble in ether, benzene, acetone and chloroform. Slightly soluble in ethanol, methanol, soluble in pyridine, glycerol, and dilute alkali solution. Solvent extraction, alkaline extraction and acid precipitation, extraction, microwave extraction and enzymatic hydrolysis are commonly used extraction methods, where the solvent extraction, alkaline extraction and acid precipitation method are simple and economical with high rate of extraction.

Hesperidin has antioxidant, anti-inflammatory, vasoprotective anticarcinogenic and cholesterol lowering actions. It increases the strength of blood capillaries and regulates their permeability.

Principle

Hesperidin is isolated by steam distillation. Defatting the dry peel by successively extracting with petroleum ether. Extraction with petroleum ether removes the essential oil, resins and other waxy substances yielding a defatted marc. After drying, the marc is further extracted with methanol which extracts out the hesperidin bringing it out into the methanol. Hesperidin precipitates out from the extract after acidification.

Procedure

1. Place 20 gm of dried orange peel powder in round bottom flask fitted with a reflux condenser.

2. Add petroleum ether (40–60°C) to RBF and heat on a water bath for 1 hour.
3. Filter the contents while hot and dry the powder at room temperature to remove the petroleum ether.
4. The dry powder is further extracted with methanol for 3 hours. Filter it while hot and wash the marc with hot methanol.
5. Concentrate the combined filtrate, to a syrupy mass.
6. Add dilute acetic acid solution to the concentrate, hesperidin crystallizes as white needles.

Identification Tests:

- *Melting point:* 252°–254°C
- With $FeCl_3$ solution hesperidin produces wine red colour.
- *Shinoda's tests:* To the ethanolic solution add Mg turnings and then add drop wise conc. hydrochloric acid, a bright violet color develops.

EXPERIMENT 7

Aim: To prepare TLC plates.

Requirement: Silica Gel, TLC plates, Oven, Glass rods, Pestle mortar, Capillary tubes, Sprayer, TLC Chamber, Wax, Beaker (500 ml), Measuring cylinder.

Theory: TLC is the method of analysis in which the stationary phase is a finely divided solid spread as a thin layer on the rigid supporting plate, and mobile phase, is a liquid, which is allowed to migrate across the surface of the plate. It differs from the rest of chromatographic techniques in that the separation does not take place in a closed column, but rather on a planer surface and the mobile phase does not flow under the influence of gravity at high pressure but is drawn across the plate by capillary action. This method has the advantages of speed, versatility and simplicity.

A wide variety of stationary phase are available based on particle size ranges. Silica gel, the most frequently used material stationary phase is employed as such for adsorption TLC modified for reversed phase separation by coating with a thin layer of a non polar functional group to it such as Silicone oil or by binding an nonpolar functional group to it such as Octadecylnilyl. The surface of the silica is acidic due the presence of many Silanol hydroxyl groups; therefore it is best suited to the analysis of acidic compounds such as amino acids and sugar. Alumina has a basic surface and is chosen over silica gel for the separation of basic and weakly polar compounds. The selection of the optimum solvent or mixture for use as mobile phase depends also on the nature of the solutes and stationary phase.

Procedure

- Take silica and make slurry with the help of water.
- Pour slurry on glass plate.

Hesperitin-7-rhamnoglucoside

- Dry the plate at room temperature.
- Activate the plate in oven for 15–20 min at 60°C.
- Now work on the plate.

EXPERIMENT 8

Aim: To isolate *caffeine* from tea leaves.

Requirements: Tea leaves, lead acetate, muslin cloth, sulphuric acid, charcoal, conical flask, beaker, funnel, measuring cylinder, glass-rod, separating funnel and filter paper.

Principle: Caffeine is a member of the class of organic compounds called *alkaloids*. Alkaloids are nitrogen containing basic compounds that are found in plants. Caffeine is a very common substance and is found in coffee, tea, soft drinks, chocolate, and "stay-awake" pills such as Vivarin. It can be synthesized or isolated from natural sources. Caffeine constitutes approximately 4% of tea and coffee leaves, and is also found in cola nuts and cocoa beans.

Tea leaves consist mostly of *cellulose*, a water-insoluble polymer of *glucose*, which is a simple sugar (a *monosaccharide*). Along with cellulose, tea leaves also contain number of other things including caffeine, tannins (phenolic compounds, compounds that have an –OH directly bonded to an aromatic ring) and a small amount of chlorophyll.

Caffeine

Caffeine is a purine alkaloid. It is obtained from the leaves of *Thea sinensis*, (Theaceae); seeds of *Coffea arabica* (Rubiaceae) and *Coca nitida* (Sterculiaceae).

Caffeine is closely related to theophylline and theobromine. Caffeine occurs as a white crystalline powder and bitter in taste. It has a melting point of 235 °C–238 °C, and a molecular weight of 194.19. It is freely soluble in chloroform and in boiling water; sparingly soluble in water and in ethanol, slightly soluble in ether. Caffeine has the chemical name 3,7-dihydro-1,3,7-trimethyl-1H-purine-2, 6-dione and the molecular formula $C_8H_{10}N_4O_2$.

Caffeine acts as a CNS stimulant. It stimulates the heart, respiration, central nervous system, and is a diuretic. It is physically addictive. Caffeine is extracted by boiling tea leaves with water. Basic lead acetate is added to the filtrate to precipitate out tannins and albuminoids. The excess of lead is removed from filtrate by adding sulphuric acid as a lead sulphate. The solution is decolourises by adding charcoal and caffeine is extracted from the filtrate using chloroform.

Procedure:

1. Boil 25 gm of tea leaves powder with 200 ml of distilled water for 15 minutes with constant stirring. Strain the hot solution through a muslin cloth.
2. To the filtrate add 10% lead acetate solution till the formation of precipitate ceases.
3. Heat the mixture to boiling and filter. Rapidly wash the residue with 50 ml of hot water twice.
4. Heat the filtrate to boiling and add dilute sulphuric acid until no more precipitate is formed.
5. Filter it then add 1 gm charcoal to the filtrate and boil till the volume reaches 50 ml.
6. Filter hot solution, cool and transfer it to separating funnel and extract it with 3 successive 10 ml of chloroform.
7. Combine the chloroform extract and add a little quantity of anhydrous sodium

sulphate. Stir well and filter it and allow to stand for overnight.

8. Weigh the product, take M.P. Calculate % yield and carry out TLC study.

Identification Tests:
- Melting Point: 235°C
- Murexide Test: Place caffeine in a china dish and to it add HCl and potassium chlorate. Heat the mixture to dryness cautiously. Expose the residue to vapours of dilute ammonia. Purple colour is produced and it disappears on addition of fixed alkali.
- Caffeine with tannic acid produces white precipitate.
- TLC:
    1. Solvent system: Ethyl acetate: Methanol: Acetic acid (80:10:10)
       Detection: Iodine vapours
    2. Solvent system: Ethyl acetate: Formic acid: Glacial Acetic acid: Water (100 : 11 : 11 : 2)
       Detection: UV 254 nm (fluorescent zone at 0.6 R_f)

EXPERIMENT 9

Aim: To carry out isolation of *nicotine picarate* from tobacco leaves.

Requirement:

Reagents: Tobacco leaves powder, alcoholic potassium hydroxide solution, dilute sulphuric acid, dilute sodium hydroxide solution, solvent ether, picric acid, separating funnel, oven.

Glasswares: Conical flask, Beaker, Funnel, Measuring cylinder, Glass-rod.

Theory: There are many species of tobacco in the genus *Nicotiana*. It is part of the nightshade family (Solanaceae). Many plants contain nicotine, a powerful neurotoxin to insects. However, tobaccos contain a higher concentration of nicotine than most other plants. Unlike many other Solanaceae, they do not contain tropane alkaloids, which are often poisonous to humans and other animals. Along with nicotine tobaco contains other compounds such as germacrene, anabasine and other piperidine alkaloids.

Nicotine is a colorless, and volatile liquid alkaloid that naturally exists in the *Nicotiana tobacum* plants. The alkaloid is water-soluble and forms water-soluble salts. It has a bitter taste and a sharp odour. Lower concentrations of soluble phenolics were found in lamina from tobacco (*Nicotiana tobacum L*) Nicotine ($C_{10}H_{14}N_2$) content is highest in Beedi Tobacco (6.5% – 8.25%). Nicotine is also called 3-(1-methyl-2-pyrrolidinyl) pyridine. It is a bicyclic compound with a pyridine cycle and a pyrrolidine cycle. Melting point of nicotine is 218°C.

Nicotine

Nicotine can be rapidly absorbed into the bloodstream, especially under a high pH environment and/or during combustion which releases nicotine. Nicotine is highly addictive.

A. Isolation of Nicotine Picrate

Procedure

1. Moisten 20 g of powdered tobacco leaves with sufficient quantity of 20% alcoholic potassium hydroxide to liberate alkaloidal base.
2. Dry it in oven below 60°C.
3. Place the powder in conical flask, add 50 ml of solvent ether, put a cotton plug, heat on a water-bath till it boils, shake for 2 minutes, boil again and repeat this process for 5 minutes.
4. Filter and concentrate the filtrate to 20 ml.
5. Treat ethereal extract with 25 ml of 1% sulphuric acid twice in a separating funnel.

6. To aqueous layer, add sufficient quantity of 5% sodium hydroxide solution.
7. Extract free base with 20 ml of solvent ether twice.
8. Concentrate ethereal extract and dissolve residue in about 3–5 ml of distilled water, filter, and to the filtrate, add saturated solution of picric acid dropwise till complete precipitation of nicotine picrate takes place.
9. Keep the solution in refrigerator for half an hour.
10. Remove supernatant liquid by decantation.
11. Dry the product, weigh and determine the melting point and carry out TLC study.
12. Calculate R_f values and % yield.

Chemical Test: Nicotine with iodine solution in dry ether gives red crystals of iodo-derivative.

B. TLC of Nicotine

Stationary phase : Silica gel G
Mobile phase : Toluene: Ethylacetate: Diethylamine (70:20:10)
Detection : Dragendorff's reagent
UV 254 nm (0.75 R_f)

EXPERIMENT 10

Aim: To carry out isolation of *curcumin* from *Curcuma longa*.

Requirement: Conical flask, Beaker, Funnel, Measuring cylinder, Glass-rode, Water bath, Refrigerator, Centrifuge tubes.

Reagent: Powder *Curcuma longa*, NaOH solution, H_2SO_4.

Theory: Curcumin (Curcuma) is a water soluble yellow-orange polyphenol. In its usual form it is a dry yellow powder that is oil-soluble. Curcumin is without flavor and aroma. Curcumin is derived from the root of the *Curcuma longa* by drying and powdering, to create the spice called Turmeric, then by a solvent extraction. The resulting powder is 18 times stronger in the essential ingredients than the common spice. Curcumin is one of three curcuminoids of turmeric. The other two curcuminoids are demethoxycurcumin and bisdemethoxycurcumin.

- Chemical formula: $C_{21}H_{20}O_6$
- Molecular weight: 368.38
- Three Molecular Forms: Curcumin, demethoxycurcumin and bisdemethoxycurcumin.
- Molecular structure: It is a dimer of vanillin (2 molecules of vanillin conjoined).

1,7-Bis(4-hydroxy-3-methoxyphenyl)-1,6-heptadiene-3,5-dione

Curcuma longa extract has significant effects on arthritis, amyloid-beta (Alzheimer's polymers), cancer and diabetes. It is used as strong antioxidant and anti-inflammatory; antiarthritis; antialzheimer's; antiplatelet; anticancer; antiviral, antifungal, antibacterial; antidiabetic.

Procedure

1. Reflux 20 gm of *Curcuma longa* powder in a conical flask with addition of 50 ml methanol on water bath for 40–50 minutes.
2. Cool the mixture; filter the supernant with cotton or filter cloth.
3. Transfer the filtrate to a china dish and evaporate on water bath.
4. Extract the residue with 50 ml of aq. NaOH solution by stirring with glass rod.
5. Filter the supernant.
6. Neutralize the filtrate with aq. H_2SO_4, till precipitates will form.
7. Filter the precipitates and dissolve it in about 15 ml of methanol.
8. Stoppered it properly and keep it overnight in freeze.
9. Collect the crystals, dry and then weigh them and calculate the yield and perform TLC.

Result:

Practical yield = ——— gm.
% Practical yield = ——— % w/w.

TLC of Curcumin:

Type 1

Stationary Phase: Silica gel G.

Mobile Phase: Ethyl acetate : benzene or hexane (20 : 80).

Detection: Yellow spot in visible range.

Type 2

Stationary Phase: Silica gel G.

Mobile Phase: Chloroform : Ethanol : Glacial acetic acid (94:5:1).

Detection: Vanillin sulphuric acid.

EXPERIMENT 11

Aim: To carry out isolation of *calcium sennoside* from Senna leaf powder.

Theory:

Calcium Sennosides (Senna extracts)

- **Scientific name** : *Cassia angustifolia*
- **Family** : Leguminosal
- **Common name** : Senna, Indian Senna, Cassia Senna
- **Plant part used** : Pods, Stems and Leaves.
- **Standardized for** : Upto 60% Calcium Sennoside

Sennosides are hydroxyanthracene glycosides derived from Senna leaves.

Anthraquinone Glycosides: In the leaf, sennosides A and B have aglycones sennidin A and B, Sennosides C and D which are glycosides of heterodianthrones of aloe-emodin and rhein. Others include palmidin A, rhein anthrone and aloe-emodin glycosides, some free anthraquinones and some potent, novel compounds of undetermined structure. Cassia senna usually contains more of the Sennosides.

Naphthalene Glycosides: tinnevellin glycoside and 6-hydroxmusizin glycoside, Miscellaneous: Mucilage, flavonoids, volatile oil, sugars, resins, etc.

Main effective constituents: Sennosides C, Sennosides D, Rhein, Chrysophanol, aloe-acid, isorhamnetin, barbaloin, kaempferol, etc.

Senna leaf contains 1.5–3% hydroxyanthracene glycosides, mainly Sennosides A and B, which are rhein-dianthrones and smaller amounts of Sennosides C and D, which are rhein-aloe-emodin-heterodianthrones, naphthalene glycosides, flavonoids (derivatives of kaempferol and isorhamnetin), 10–12% mineral matter, 7–10% mucilage (galactose, arabinose, rhamnose and galacturonic acid), about 8% polyol (pinitol), sugars (glucose, fructose and sucrose) and resins.

Calcium Sennosides (Senna extract) is one of the best known **herbal medicines.** Leaves of the Senna plant are used for extraction of Calcium Sennoside. The leaves and pods of this plant contain the commercially important laxative sennoside B. They have been used as natural, safe time-tested antidysentric, laxatives in traditional as well as modern systems of medicine. It is very effective laxative. It is slightly bitter. Senna has always being specially used for constipation.

Procedure

1. Weigh accurately about 20 gm of senna powder. Add 250 ml of alcohol and 2.5 ml

Molecular structure of curcumin

of conc. HCl and warm it on water bath at 50°C with continuous stirring for about 1 hour.

2. Filter it and to the filtrate add 25 ml of alcohol.
3. Basify the filtrate with 5 ml of NH_3 in 20 ml ethanol (pH is adjusted to 8.2 to 8.5). Stir for 10 minutes.
4. Add 1.5 gm of $CaCl_2$ in 25 ml of ethanolic extract slowly with stirring. After addition of $CaCl_2$ mixture continuously stirr for 20 minutes.
5. Filter the precipitates and wash it with alcohol. Dry, weigh and find out the % yield.

TLC of Senna:

Stationary phase: Silica gel G
Mobile Phase: n-propanol:ethylacetate:water:glacial acetic acid (40:40:29.1)
Spray: After spraying with conc. HNO_3, heat at 120°C for 20 minutes and spray with 10% KOH

EXPERIMENT 12

Aim: To carry out isolation of *lawsone* from Heena powder.

Requirement: Conical flask, Beaker, Funnel, Measuring cylinder, Glass rod.

Reagent: Powder Heena, 20% $NaHCO_3$, 20% HCl, Benzene.

Theory: The leaves of *Lawsonia inermis* have been used since ancient times in the Indian Subcontinent for decorating and dyeing hands, soles, beard and hair and to impart beautiful shades of dark red color. An aqueous mixture is often used for medicinal purposes focusing various skin ailments. For centuries, henna leaves were renowned as the most extensively used natural hair dying and tattooing agent in many civilizations and cultures. The word henna which means "to become queen" is indicative of something highly elegant. The plant has got several vernacular names, e.g. *Ligusturum egypticum* which is the Latinized English synonym for henna.

Seven compounds are isolated from the methanolic extract of henna (*Lawsonia inermis* L.) leaves. [*p*-coumaric acid, lawsone, apigenin, luteolin and 2-methoxy-3-methyl-1,4-naphthoquinone, cosmosiin and apiin] Dried leaves of henna contains 1–1.4% brown colouring material Lawsone (2-hydroxy-1,4-naphthoquinone, $C_{10}H_6O_3$, mp:190° C)

Lawsone

Lawsone is used for decorating and dyeing hands, soles, beard and hair and to impart beautiful shades of dark red color. The plant extract or its purified compounds exhibit a variety of biological activities such as antimicrobial activity, antisickling, hepatoprotective activity, cytotoxic activity, anti-inflammatory, antipyretic, and analgesic activities.

Procedure

1. Take 25 gm of Heena powder in a beaker with 100 ml of 20% $NaHCO_3$.
2. Keep it on water bath for heating with constant shaking for 1 hour.
3. Filter it and wash the marc with 150 ml of $NaHCO_3$ solution.
4. Treat the filtrate to neutralization with diute HCl till no more precipitation or effervescence comes.
5. Filter and collect the precipitates of Lawsone on filter paper.
6. Dry them in oven below 100°C.
7. Recrystallize them by dissolving in benzene.
8. Boil on a water bath and then cool it.
9. Weigh, recrystallized product and take its melting point and calculate % yield.

Result:
Practical yield = ──── gm.
% practical yield = ──── % w/w.

EXPERIMENT 13

Aim: Isolation of *vasicine* in Vasaka leaf powder.

Requirement: Conical flask, Beaker, Funnel, Measuring cylinder, Glass-rod.

Reagent: Powder vasaka, dil ammonia, chloroform.

Theory: Vasaka belongs to the plant family Acanthaceae, its botanical/taxonomic name is *Justicia adhatoda* L. Some of its synonyms are *Adhatoda vasica* and *Adhatoda zeylanica* (Medicus). Vasaka appears to be the most common name for this plant; but additional names, to name a few are: Malabar nut, Arusa, Vasa, Adhatodai, Basak, and Bansa.

Vasaka contains several active ingredients, the main one of which is the alkaloid vasicine, which is responsible for much of the bronchodilating effect of Vasaka. Vasicine is mainly derives from the leaves of the plant, along with an essentail oil as well. Vasicine also goes by another name, peganine. Vasicine's ($C_{11}H_{12}N_2O$) systematic name is 1,2,3,9-tetrahydropyrrolo[2,1-b]quinazolin-3-ol, other important active ingredients contained in the stems and roots include vasicinol and the alkaloid vasicinone. Some other, less active chemicals present in the roots are quinazoline, anisotine, vasicol, vasicinolone, and adhatodine.

Vasicine (peganine) $R_1=H_2; =R_2=OH$
Vascinone $R_1=O; R_2=OH$
Deoxyvasicinone $R_1=O; R_2=OH$

Vasaka a perennial shrub of the family Acanthaceae, is a highly reputed Ayurvedic medicinal plant used in the treatment of cough, bronchitis, asthma, tuberculosis and recommended for other ailments of the respiratory system. Leaves, flowers and roots of this plant are used in herbal drugs against cancer. This plant is also used as antispasmodic, fever reducer, anti-inflammatory, antibleeding, brochodilating (opens the breathing passages), antidiabetic, disinfectant, antijaundice, assistance in uterine contractions, and expectorant (promotes easier flow of mucous). Most of these attributes fall mainly into the repiratory therapy category for colds, asthma, bronchitis, tuberculosis, etc. The antispasmodic and antiinflammatory properties apply to diarrhea, arthritis, vomiting, and gingivitis. The leaves are a source of Vitamin C as well. The plant is administered orally, locally, or inhaled in various bitter-tasting forms.

TLC Analysis

Thin layer chromatographic analysis of the extracts is performed on silica gel 60 F 254 TLC plates. Aliquots (10 µL) of the extracts is applied on the plates as bands. Plates are developed in TLC chamber previously saturated (30 min) with the mobile phase, chloroform: methanol (9:1 v/v). The plates are visualized under UV 254 and 365 nm and then sprayed with Dragendorff's reagent.

Procedure

1. Take 15 gm vasaka powder in a conical flask.
2. Basify with dilute ammonia solution till pH 9.
3. It is further extracted with 15 ml chloroform with 3 times in a separating funnel.
4. Combine the total chloroform layer and again extract with 50 ml water.
5. Collect the chloroform layer.
6. The solvent is evaporate to get the total alkaloid extract contain in vasicine as a major alkaloid.

7. Vasicine can be further purified from the dry extract by crystallization.

Result:

Practical yield = ——— gm.
% practical yield = ——— % w/w.

B. TLC of Vasaka:

Stationary Phase: Silica gel G
Mobile Phase: Toluene : Methanol:Dioxane: Ammonia (1:1:2.5:0.5)
Detection: Dragendoff's reagent

EXPERIMENT 14

Aim: To carry out isolation of *diosgenin* from Fenugreek seeds.

Reagent: Powder fenugreek seeds, Acetone, 2M H_2SO_4, 10% Na_2CO_3 Solution. Borosil Conical flask, Beaker, Funnel, Measuring cylinder, Glass-rod, Water bath, Hot air oven, china dish.

Theory:

Fenugreek

Scientific Name: *Trigonella foenum-graecum* L.

Family: Fabaceae

Common Name: Fenugreek, methi

The leaves contain at least 7 saponins, known as graecunins. These compounds are glycosides of diosgenin. Seeds contain 0.1% to 0.9% diosgenin and are extracted on a commercial basis. Plant tissue cultures from seeds grown under optimal conditions have been found to produce as much as 2% diosgenin with smaller amounts of gitongenin and trigogenin. The seeds also contain the saponin fenugrin B. Several coumarin compounds have been identified in fenugreek seeds as well as a number of alkaloids (e.g. trigonelline, gentianine, carpaine). A large proportion of the trigonelline is degraded to nicotinic acid and related pyridines during roasting. These degradation products are, responsible for the flavor of the seed. The seeds also yield as much as 8% of fixed, foul-smelling oil.

Diosgenin

The C-glycoside flavones vitexin, vitexin glycoside, and the arabinoside isoorientin have been isolated from the plant. Three minor steroidal sapogenins also have been found in the seeds: smilagenin, sarsapogenin, and yuccagenin.

The mucilages of the seeds of several plants, including fenugreek, have been determined and their hydrolysates analyzed. Fenugreek gel consists chiefly of galactomannans characterized by their high water-holding capacity. These galactomannans have a unique structure and may be responsible for some of the characteristic therapeutic properties attributed to fenugreek.

The herb has been used for centuries as a cooking spice in Europe and remains a popular ingredient in pickles, curry powders, and spice mixtures in India and Asia. In folk medicine, fenugreek has been used in the treatment of boils, cellulitis and tuberculosis and has cholesterol-lowering effects. It also has been recommended for the promotion of lactation. Fenugreek seeds have been used as an oral insulin substitute, and seed extracts have been reported to lower blood glucose levels. The maple aroma and flavor of fenugreek has led to its use in imitation maple syrup.

Procedure

1. Weigh about 20 gm of coarse fenugreek seeds and extract it with 40-50 ml of acetone by refluxing it on water bath. Filter

the solution, take the marc and hydrolyze the marc with 2 M H_2SO_4 at 120°C and 15 psi pressure.

2. Filter it again then collect the marc. Wash it thoroughly with water and then neutralize it with 10 % Na_2CO_3 solution.

3. Again wash the material with water to remove extra alkaline solution. Dry the hydrolyzed seeds in oven at 80–100°C. Collect the dried seeds and powder it and pass through 40 # sieve.

4. This dry powder is reflux with 30 ml petroleum ether twice and extracts whole hot solution and filter through filter paper. Combine filtrate and evaporate to 15 to 20 ml over water bath. Cool the solution wash with petroleum ether and keep it for crystallization.

5. Group of needle crystal are seen in the part.

Result:

Practical yield = ——— gm.
% practical yield = ——— % w/w.

EXPERIMENT 15

Aim: To carry out isolation of *aloin* from Aloe powder.
Requirement: Conical flask, Beaker, Funnel, Measuring cylinder, Glass-rod.
Reagent: Powder aloe, Sulphuric acid, Ammonia.

Theory:

Aloin from *Aloe vera*

Aloe barbadensis Mill. (Liliaceae)

Commonly known as **"Gwarpatha"**

Chemical Name: Aloin

Synonyms: Aloin: Aloin B; Aloin A; Barbaloin; Aloe Powder; Aloins A and B; Barbaloin std.; Aloin/Barbaloin.

Molecular Formula: $C_{21}H_{22}O_9$
Weight: 418.39

Distribution and plant habit: Common in waste places, usually forming clumps. It is now cultivated in waste land. It is a scapigerous perennial. Leaves in rossette, erect, upto 60 cm long, lanceolate, truncate as base, spine tipped.

Flowering and fruiting: Generally occurs in February to May. Flowers in long racemes, on a stout shape upto 1 m high, tinged with yellow fruits trigonous, oblong, loculicidally 3-valved.

Active principle: Peplic acid; D-galacton; α-glucomannan; arabian acid; malic acid; citric acid; tartaric acid; aloesin; aloesone and α-glycoside aloinoside B.

Aloin

Aloin A

Aloin B

The species in *Aloe* L. have been used as ethnic medicines in many different countries for centuries, possessing functions, such as anticancer, anti-inflammatory, antivirus, evacuating, protecting liver, and increasing immunity. *Aloevera* L. has been most commonly used as medicine, healthy foods, and cosmetics nowadays. The active components of aloe include anthraquinones, chromones, polysaccharides, enzymes and, so on. It is reported that anthraquinones and chromones are responsible for the anticancer activity, anti-inflammatory, and evacuating.

Uses

1. **Stomach troubles:** Juice of leaf pulp (1-TSF) is given orally a day to cure intestinal trouble.
2. **Jaundice:** One-cup juice of leaf pulp is given twice a day to cure jaundice.
3. **Fat control:** One small piece (30-40 gm) of pulp is given empty stomach once a day to reduce fat from body.
4. **Dermal disorders:** The pulp is applied externally on boils, cuts, eczema, ringworm, burns and leprosy. It is considered as a good cosmetic, so pulp is used as cosmetic on face.
5. **Swellings:** Leaf-pulp is warmed and tied on affected part and kept (water bottle/warm stone) warmed by external heating source for 1 hour.

Procedure

1. Dissolve 20 gms of powdered aloe in 10 times of boiling water.
2. Extract it for 10–15 minutes. Filter by decantation.
3. Acidify the filtrate with sulphuric acid, in order to precipitates resinous matter, remove the precipitates by filtration.
4. Neutralize the filtrate with sufficient quantity of ammonia; allow it to stand for few hours for slow crystallization of aloin.
5. Filter the precipitates; dissolve in 50% alcohol for recrystallization.
6. Calculate practical and % yields.

TLC

Solvent System:
Ethyl acetate:Methanol:Water (100:13.5:10)

Detection:
UV-365 nm/ UV-254 nm/10% ethanolic KOH reagent.

Result:
Practical yield = ——— gm.
% practical yield = ——— % w/w.

EXPERIMENT 16

Aim: To carry out isolation of *quinine sulphate* from cinchona bark powder.

Requirements: Cinchona bark powder, chloroform, ammonia, sulphuric acid, activated charcoal, ammonia solution, benzene, etc.

Theory:

Quinine from Cinchona bark

Family: Rubiaceae

Genus: *Cinchona*

Species: *officinalis, ledgeriana, succirubra, calisaya*

Synonyms: *Quinaquina officinalis, Quinaquina lancifolia, Quinaquina coccinea*

Common Names: Quinine bark, quina, quinine, kinakina, China bark, cinchona bark, yellow cinchona, red cinchona, Peruvian bark, Jesuit's bark, quina-quina, calisaya bark, fever tree

Parts Used: Bark, wood

It is also called as *Jesuit's bark*. Cinchona bark has slight, characteristic odour and astringent and intensely bitter taste. It is available in the form of quills and curved pieces. Cinchona bark consists of alkaloids which belong to quinoline group. The important alkaloids are quinine, quinidine, cinchonine and cinchonidine, quinicine, cinchonicine hydroquinine, hydrocinchonidine and homocinchonidine. Quinine and quinidine form many salts, among their salts, sulphates are more significant. Quinine and quinidine are stereoisomers of each other. Cinchonine and cinchonidine are also isomers of each other. Cinchona also contains quinic acid and cinchotannic acid. It also contains a glycoside called quinovin, tannins and bitter essential oil.

Quinine is a natural white crystalline alkaloid having antipyretic (fever-reducing), antimalarial, analgesic (painkilling), anti-inflammatory properties and have bitter taste. It is a stereoisomer of quinidine which, unlike quinine, it is an anti-arrhythmic. Quinine contains two major fused-ring systems: the aromatic quinoline and the bicyclic quinuclidine. The bark of the cinchona tree is the only known natural source of quinine. Quinine was the first effective treatment for malaria caused by *Plasmodium falciparum*, appearing in the 17th century. It remained the antimalarial drug of choice until the 1940s, after that other drugs replaced it. Since then, many effective antimalarials have been introduced, although quinine is still used to treat the disease in certain critical situations. Quinine is an effective muscle relaxant.

Quinine Sulfate

Molecular Formula: $(C_{20}H_{24}N_2O_2)_2 \cdot H_2SO_4 \cdot 2H_2O$

Molecular Weight: 782.94 gm/mol

Melting point: 233–235°C

Table 6.1: Alkaloid content comparison by *Cinchona* species

Species	Total alkaloids (%)	Quinine content (%)
C calisaya	3–7	0–4
C pubescens	4.5–8.5	1–3
C officinalis	5–8	2–7.5
C ledgeriana	5–14	3–13
C succirubra	6–16	4–14

Extraction of plant constituent is the first step in phytochemical investigations. The air-dried powdered plant material is extracted in soxhlet assembly successively with petroleum ether, benzene, solvent ether, etc. Finally the drug is macerated with chloroform water. Each time before extracting with the next solvent, the powdered material is dried in hot-air oven below 50°C. Each extract is concentrated by distilling off the solvent and then evaporate to dryness on water bath. The extract obtained with each solvent is weighed. Its % yield is calculated in terms of air-dried weight of plant material.

Procedure

1. Mix the powdered bark (50 gm) with sufficient quantity of 20% alcoholic potassium hydroxide, granulate and dry either at room temperature or below 60°C.
2. Powder granulated mass and pack material in soxhlet apparatus are extracted with benzene for 6 hours. Shake benzene extract with three successive portions of 25 ml of sulfuric acid. Decoloris extract with activated charcoal and heat to boiling. Filter solution while hot.
3. Basify the extracts with ammonia solution (pH 8.5) and extract the liberated alkaloids with three successive portions of chloroform. Combine the chloroform extracts.
4. Distill off chloroform to yield total alkaloidal residue. Dry it to constant weight at 80°C and keep in desicator.

5. Recrystallize the quinine sulphate with hot water using activated charcoal. Dry it to constant weight at 60–80 °C. Calculate yield with respect to powdered drug.

Calculation:

$$\% \text{ Yield} = \frac{\text{Practical Yield}}{\text{Theoretical Yield}} \times 100$$

Result: The percentage yield of Quinine sulphate is found to be _____

EXPERIMENT 17

Aim: To carry out isolation of *artemisinin* from *Artemisia annua*.

Theory: *Artemisia annua* L. (Famil: Compositae) is an annual herb native of Asia and has been used for many centuries for the treatment of fever and malaria. Many secondary metabolites of terpene peroxides Linn such as artemisia ketone, artemisinic alcohol, arteannuin B and myrcene hydroperoxide are isolated from artemisinin. Some of them also can be found in essential oil. Leaves of *Artemisia annua* L. contain about 1.2% essential oil. Thirty-two components are identified in the essential oil of *A. annua* L *in which* campher (48.00%), 1,8-cineole (9.39%), camphene (6.98%) and spathulenol (4.89%) are major components. The essential oil shows antibacterial and antifungal activities.

Procedure

1. Coarsely powder the dried leaves of *Artemisia annua* and extract with petroleum ether.
2. Concentrate the petroleum ether extract to dryness and then dissolve in chloroform.
3. Add acetonitrile to the chloroformic solution for the precipitation of waxes and other impurities to filter out.
4. Concentrate the filtrate and fractioned chromatographically on silica gel by eluting with chloroform-ethyl acetate.
5. Collect the fraction containing artemisinin and concentrate where upon crystals of artemisinin get deposite which may be further purified by recrystallization from cyclohexane or ethanol.

Result: The percentage yield of artemisinin is found to be _____.

EXPERIMENT 18

Aim: To carry out isolation of *vincristine* from Vinca.

Procedure

1. Extract dried vinca leaves and herb with aqueous-alcoholic acetic acid solution.
2. Concentrate the aqueous extract then extract the residue further with 2% Hydrochloric acid.
3. After extraction adjust the pH to 4 with sodium hydroxide solution and then extract with toluene.
4. Separated the toluene layer and adjust the pH of aqueous layer to 7 and again extract with toluene.
5. Mix toluene extracts together, concentrate, dry and dissolve in a mixture of toluene: methylene chloride (65:35).
6. Fractionate the mixture chromatographically on neutral alumina column with toluene-methylene chloride as an eluent using gradient elution technique for the separation of vincristine.
7. Evaporate vincristine rich fractions to dryness subsequently crystallized from alcohol.
8. To the alcoholic solution, add aqueous or ethanolic solution of sulphuric acid to convert vincristine into its sulphate salt.

Result: The percentage yield of vincristine sulphate is found to be _____.

EXPERIMENT 19

Aim: To carry out extraction of *strychnine* and *brucine* from Nux Vomica seeds.

Requirement: Powdered nux vomica seeds, slaked lime, chloroform, dilute sulphuric acid, ethanol, oxalic acid, charcoal, acetone, soxhlet apparatus, vacuum distillation unit, desiccators.

Theory: The seeds of nux vomica (*Strychnos nux vomica*, Lin. family Loganiaceae) contain about 1.8–5.2% of indole alkaloids-strychnine and brucine. Nux Vomica yields not less than 1.15% of strychnine. The therapeutic value of nux vomica is due to the two alkaloids, brucine and strychnine, although there are other substances present of some interest. The total alkaloidal content ranges from 2 to 2.7%. The dominating constituent of nux vomica is a complex compound which, in natural form, is an invaluable remedy. By means of chemical reagents it can be split embracing two intensely poisonous alkaloidal products, a glucoside and acids. These alkaloids are strychnine, brucine. The main acid is igasuric Acid, while the glucoside is named loganin. These are all colorless bodies, the alkaloids being very bitter, and energetically poisonous Brucine being a poison similar to Strychnine, acting with less violence and more slowly, than Strychnine. Nux vomica is used as a bitter stomachic, spinal cord stimulant and nerve tonic.

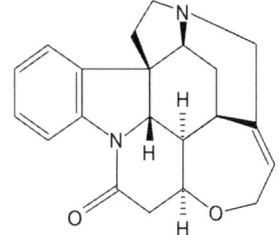

Strychnine

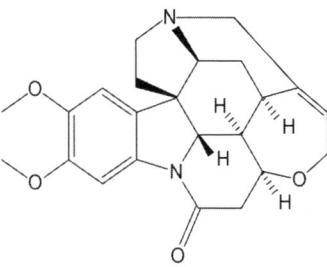

Brucine

Strychnine ($C_{21}H_{22}N_2O_2$): This violently poisonous alkaloid is crystaline, slightly soluble in cold water (1 part in 6700), the solution being alkaline and bitter. It dissolves in 7 parts of chloroform and 150 parts of 90% alcohol. Strychnine is a terrible tetanic poison, affecting the cerebrospinal system, but it kills without producing marked anatomical change, the muscles and nerves being scarcely altered, although the brain and spinal cord may be congested, stomach, four limbs intensely congested, right side of heart gorged (sometimes empty), and the lungs congested, The fatal dose of Strychnine is as low as 4 grain. Indeed, it is recorded that and a grain killed a two-year old child in four hours, while 8 grain killed a man in twenty minutes.

Brucine ($C_{23}H_{26}N_2O_4$): This related alkaloid is also a product of Nux Vomica. It is known as 10,11-Dimethoxystrychnine. Brucine is very bitter, freely soluble in cold alcohol, soluble in 850 parts of cold water. Brucine is crystallizable from aqueous alcohol. The hydrated crystals melt at 105°C, while the anhydrous base melts at 178°C, changing color, and depositing carbon. It forms crystallizable salts with acids. It differs in reaction from Strychnine in that strong sulphuric or nitric acid strikes with it a blood-red color, whereas with Strychnine, no coloration appears. To a hydrochloric acid solution of Brucine and Strychnine, if potassium ferrocyanide solution added Brucine precipitates, while Strychnine remains dissolved. The mixed alkaloids can be quite closely separated by alcohol which freely dissolves Brucine, but scarcely dissolves Strychnine, Brucine is a poison which has the physiological qualities of Strychnine, but in a markedly less degree.

Procedure

1. Mix 50 g powdered nux vomica seeds with 5 g slaked lime paste by addition of water and dry at 100°C.

2. Extract the drug with chloroform in soxhlet apparatus for 6 hours.

3. Separate chloroform extract and shake with successive 3 portions of 25 ml of dilute sulphuric acid. Combine the acid extracts and filter.
4. Add excess of ammonia solution to acid extract to precipitate the alkaloids.
5. Extract the precipitate with 25% ethanol, which dissolves brucine.
6. Filter off undissolved strychnine and purify brucine by repeated crystallization from ethanol.
7. Concentrate the filtrate to one sixth of its volume and precipitate brucine as oxalate by neutralization with sufficient volume of oxalic acid. Wash precipitate with cold ethanol, dissolve in small volume of hot water, decolorize with charcoal, filter and evaporate filtrate to dryness.
8. Extract residue with small volume of acetone, remove the solvent to yield brucine as oxalate.

Chemical Test

For Strychnine: Dissolve strychnine in conc. sulphuric acid and add potassium dichromate solution. Deep violet colour is produced.

For Brucine: Brucine with nitric acid gives orange yellow colour.

EXPERIMENT 20

Aim: To extract *ammonium glycyrrhizinate* from glycyrrhiza powder and to carry out its TLC studies.

Requirements: Glycyrrhiza powder, acetone, conical flask, dilute ammonia solution, dilute nitric acid, water bath, etc.

Theory:

Liquorice
- **Botanical Name :** *Glycyrrhiza glabra*
- **Family Name :** Papilionaceae
- **Common Name :** Calamus, Mulethi, Sweet Liquorice, Sweetwood
- **Part Used :** Root
- **Habitat :** Cultivated in northern and southern india
- **Product offered :** Roots

It is tonic, diuretic, demulcent, expectorant, emmenagogue and laxative. It is used for allaying coughs and catarrhal infections, useful in irritable conditions of mucous membrane of urinary organs. It is useful in sore throat, cough, anorexia and persistent low fever. It is also used in flavoring of tobacco, confectionery, beverages, jams and marmalades. Roots are used in the treatment of Addison's disease, asthma, bronchitis, coughs, peptic ulcer, arthritis and allergic complaints. Externally, the roots are used in the treatment of herpes, eczema and shigles.

Extraction of plant constituent is the very first step in such phytochemical investigations. The air-dried powdered plant material is extracted in soxhlet assembly successively with petroleum ether, benzene, solvent ether, etc. Finally the drug is macerated with chloroform water. Each time before extracting with the next solvent, the powdered material is dried in hot-air oven below 50 °C. Each extract is concentrated by distilling off the solvent and then evaporating to dryness on water bath. The extract obtained with each solvent is weighed. Its percentage is calculated in terms of air-dried weight of plant material.

A. Extraction of ammonium glycyrrhizinate from glycyrrhiza powder

Procedure

1. To about 20 gm of powdered drug add 50 ml acetone and 2 ml of dilute nitric acid. Mix thoroughly, cork the flask and macerate it for two hours.
2. Shaking occasionally, filter the contents. To the marc, add 20 ml of acetone, warm it on water bath and filter. Combine the filtrate and concentrate preferably under vacuum.
3. To combined acetone extracts add sufficient quantity of dilute ammonia solution for precipitation of ammonium glycyrrhizinate.

4. Separate the precipitate by filtration, wash it with 5 ml of acetone twice, dry the product and weigh. Find out the MP and % yield.
5. The yield of ammonium glycyrrhizinate should be approx. 4.5 % w/w.

Calculations:

$$\text{Percentage Yield} = \frac{\text{Practical Yield}}{\text{Theoretical Yield}} \times 100$$

Result: The yield of ammonium glycyrrhizinate is found to be:
   Practical yield = ——— gm.
   % practical yield = ——— % w/w.

B. TLC of ammonium glycerrhyzinate:

Stationary Phase: Silica gel G

Mobile Phase: Toluene: Ethyl acetate:Glacial acetic acid (12.5:7.5:0.5)

Detection: Vanillin sulphuric acid

EXPERIMENT 21

Aim: To carry out isolation of *glycyrrhetinic acid* from Liquorice roots.

Method – I

1. Extract liquorice root powder with boiling water, concentrate the aqueous extract and evaporated to dryness.
2. Dissolve the residue in water and precipitated glycyrrhetinic acid by addition of hydrochloric acid (pH 3–3.5).
3. Filter the precipitate, wash with water and dry to yield crude glycyrrhetinic acid.

Method–II

1. Extract Liquorice root powder with chloroform and discard chloroform layer.
2. Dry the marc and extract with 0.5 M sulphuric acid for the hydrolysis of glycosides.
3. Cool the acidic extract and then extract with chloroform thrice.
4. Concentrate the combined chloroform extract to dryness to yield glycyrrhetinic acid.

Result: The percentage yield of glycyrrhetinic acid is found to be _____

EXPERIMENT 22

Aim: To carry out extraction of *Withania somnifera*.

Requirements: *Withania somnifera,* soxhlet apparatus, petroleum ether, methanol, etc.

Theory:

Withania Somnifera

Botanical Name: *Withania somnifera*

Plant Part Used: Roots

Extraction Method: Water extraction/Alcoholic extraction

Withania somnifera is one of the best known and most researched Ayurvedic herbs and holds a place in the Ayurvedic traditions similar to Ginseng in Chinese therapies. For that reason, *Withania somnifera* has been often referred to as the "Indian Ginseng" and is widely employed as a **pain-killer** and **tranquilizing narcotic**. The extract is derived from the **roots of *Withania somnifera*** belonging to family Solanaceae. It is commonly known as **Ashwagandha**. Its main use, as described in Ayurvedic literature, is as a "rasayana" or rejuvenating drug and hence also traditionally known as Avarada which suggests the application of this plant for enhancing longevity. *Withania somnifera* is used in several indigenous drug preparations for maintaining health as well as treatment of several disease conditions. Its main use is as an immunomodulator and as an antistress. Withania contains number of phytoconstituents, withanolides as the major constituent. It is used to cure anemia, rheumatoid arthritis and is useful in insomnia, tissue-building and nervous breakdown, in fever, constipation and eye diseases.

Withania somnifera Extract

Active Ingredient: Alkaloids 1–2%, Withanolides 1.5–2%

Chemical Constituents and Components: Main chemical components are glycosides, withanolides, withasomnine, hentriacontane, dulcitol, withaniol and withaferin.

The plant material is subjected to preliminary phytochemical screening for the detection of various plant constituents. Extraction of plant constituent is the very first step in such phytochemical investigations. The air-dried powdered plant material is extracted in soxhlet assembly successively with petroleum ether, benzene, solvent ether, etc. Finally the drug is macerated with chloroform water. Each time before extracting with the next solvent, the powdered material is dried in hot-air oven below 50°C. Each extract is concentrated by distilling off the solvent and then evaporating to dryness on water bath. The extract obtained with each solvent is weighed. Its percentage is calculated in terms of air-dried weight of plant material.

Procedure

1. Ashwagandha root is segregated manually to get more than 80% roots of 3-5 mm diameter, as the roots of this dimension contain maximum active principles.
2. It is crushed to a coarse powder (20 mesh) and the powder formed during crushing is removed by sieving.
3. The crushed material is extracted with 55% v/v alcohol in Counter-Current Extractors.
4. The extracted fluid is concentrated at maximum temperature of 55°C and vacuum 650–700 mm to make it free of alcohol.
5. It is further concentrated to 28–30% solids in solution.
6. The solution is homogenized, kept at temperature of 105°C for 10 minutes, filtered through a screen of 80–100 mesh and spray dried at inlet temperature 170°C and outlet temperature of 85°C.
7. The dried powder obtained from the chamber and is uniformly blended, pulverized, and shifted to required mesh. (usually 80–100 mesh) and aseptically packed.

Result:

EXPERIMENT 23

Aim: To carry out extraction of *resins* from jalap roots.

Requirement: Jalap powder, maceration chamber and 90% alcohol.

Theory:

The main constituent of tubers of jalap (*Ipomoea purga,* family-Convolvulaceae) is resin. Jalap resin contains convolvulin, a substance with 18 hydroxyl groups esterified with valeric, exogonic and tiglic acids. *Ipomoea purga* contains 9–18% of resin. Ipomoea means worm-like, referring to the peculiar, twisted nature of the root system. Jalap is used as purgative (powerful cathartic) and vermifuge. Because it is considered a good remedy for kidney problems, the plant is also widely-known as riñona (a Spanish word) for kidneys, *riñones*. The Morning Glory or Jalapa roots are considered to be an effective antispasmodic and are used in syrup to treat epilepsy.

Procedure

1. Macerate about 25 g of powdered jalap root with 100 ml of 90% alcohol for 3 hours with frequent stirring.
2. Filter the alcoholic extract; wash the marc with two 10 ml quantities of 90% alcohol.
3. Combine the alcoholic extracts.
4. Concentrate the combined filtrate on a water bath to about 10 ml and pour it slowly into about 60 ml of hot water with constant stirring.
5. Allow the precipitated resin to subside.
6. Decant the supernatant liquid, wash resin with 10 ml portion of hot water. Collect the resin and dry at room temperature.

EXPERIMENT 24

Aim: To isolate *piperine* from black pepper and carry out its TLC studies.

Requirment:: Soxhlet apparatus, 10% alcoholic potassium hydroxide, ethanol, black pepper, vacuum distillation unit, conical flask, beaker, funnel, measuring cylinder, glass-rod, refrigerator, water bath.

Theory:

Piperine can be isolated in good yield from grounded black pepper, which is made up of 5–9% of alkaloids that also include piperidine, piperettine and piperanine.

Piperine is a piperidine alkaloid which occurs in the unripe fruits of *Piper nigrum, P. longeum* and *P. retrofractum* (Piperaceae). It is responsible for the pungency of pepper. Along with piperine chavicine (an isomer of piperine) also occurs in pepper. It is slightly soluble in water and forms salts with strong acids.

Piperine gives maximum absorption at 245 nm in the UV spectrum. It is tasteless but produces a burning sensation and has a sharp after taste. The initial tastelessness of piperine may be a consequence of its extremely low solubility in water. Pepper is used to cure many illnesses such as cancer, malaria, and cholera; however, today it is most commonly used as a food additive.

A. Alkaloids found in black pepper

Piperine

Piperidine

Piperettine

Piperanine

Principle:

Black pepper fruits are extracted with 95% ethanol. The crude ethanol extract contains piperine, chavicine (its geometric isomer) and some acidic and resinous material. In order to prevent co-precipitation of piperine and the resin acids, dilute ethanolic potassium hydroxide solution is added to the concentrated extract to keep the acidic material in the solution as solid gummy material that is precipitated in the container.

B. Isolation of piperine from black pepper

Procedure

1. Extract 20 gm. of powdered black pepper with 350 ml of 95% alcohol in a soxhlet extractor for 2 hours.
2. Cool and filter the solution.
3. Concentrate the filtrate on water bath at 60°C.
4. Add 20 ml. of 10% alcoholic potassium hydroxide to the filtrate residue and wash with methanol.

5. The filtrate is left over night, where upon yellow needles shape crystals are deposited.
6. Find out the yield, MP and perform TLC.

Recrystalization:

Take crude piperine in test tube, in that add minimum amount of hot Acetone:Haxane (3:2) to dissolve the crude piperine. Keep the test tube aside for 15 minutes at room temperature. Collect rod like yellow crystals by filtration through wattman filter paper. Wash with 2 ml of cold ether. Allow it to dry.

Identification tests:

- Melting Point: 125–126°C
- Piperine when treated with 1,3,5-trinitrobenzene in a 1:1 ratio forms a solid complex in the form of red needles.
- λmax: 245 nm.

C. TLC of piperine

1. Solvent system: Benzene: Ethyl acetate (2:1)
   Detection: Vanillin sulfuric acid.
2. Solvent system: Toluene:diethyl ether: dioxane (62.5:21.5:16).
   Detection: Vanillin sulphuric acid.

EXPERIMENT 25

Aim: To isolate *eugenol* from clove oil.

Requirement: Clove oil, distillation unit, desiccator, solvent ether, potassium hydroxide, sulphuric acid, etc.

Theory:

Isolation of eugenol from cloves

Biological Name: *Caryophyllus aromaticus, Syzygium aromaticum, Eugenia caryophyllus*

Family: Myrtaceae

Other Names: Clove, caryophyllus

Active Compounds: Clove oil contain 60 to 90% eugenol, which has antifungal, anesthetic and antiseptic properties.

Primary Nutrients: Calcium, Magnesium, Phosphorus, Potassium, Sodium, Vitamins A, Vitamin B-complex and Vitamin C.

Preparation: The oil of clove is prepared by steam distillation.

Clove is one of the oldest spices in world, which is the dried, unopened flower bud of a small evergreen tree. Clove used mainly as an ingredient of variety of food specialties, beverages, medicines, cosmetics, perfumery and toiletries. Clove oil can be extracted from the leaves, stem and buds. Clove oil is a natural analgaesic and antiseptic used primarily in dentistry for its main ingredient eugenol. It is a home remedy for dental pain relief, mainly toothache; it is also often found in the aromatherapy. The oil produced by cloves can be used in many things from flavouring medicine to remedies for bronchitis, common cold, cough, fever, sore throat and tending to infections.

There are three types of clove oil:

- **Clove bud oil** is derived from the flower-buds of *S aromaticum*. It consists of 60–90% eugenol, eugenyl acetate, caryophyllene and other minor constituents.
- **Clove leaf oil** is derived from the leaves of *S.aromaticum*. It consists of 82–88% eugenol with little or no eugenyl acetate, and minor constituents.
- **Clove stem oil** is derived from the twigs of *S.aromaticum*. It consists of 90–95% eugenol, with other minor constituents.

Specifications of Clove Bud oil

Description: Oil is obtained by the steam distillation of the dried buds of *Eugenia caryophyllata*

Family: Myrtaceae

Color and Appearance: Violet-or purple-brown colour.

Odour Description: Somewhat harsh, phenolic, slightly sweet.

Refractive Index: 1.525 – 1.545

Specific Gravity: 1.025 – 1.065

Optical Rotation: 0° to –3°

Solubility: Soluble in 70% alcohol.

Main Components: Eugenol (60–90%)

Storage: Store in tight full containers in a cool and dry place protected from light.

Eugenol

Extraction of plant constituent is the first step in phytochemical investigations. The air-dried powdered plant material is extracted in soxhlet assembly successively with petroleum ether, benzene. Finally the drug is macerated with chloroform water. Each time before extracting with the next solvent, the powdered material is dried in hot-air oven below 50°C. Each extract is concentrated by distilling off the solvent and then evaporating to dryness on water bath. The extract obtained with each solvent is weighed. Its percentage is calculated in terms of air-dried weight of plant material.

Procedure

1. Dissolve 10 ml of volatile oil in 100 ml of solvent ether and shake with 3 successive quantities of 100 ml of 10% potassium hydroxide solution.
2. Regenerate eugenol by acidifying the aqueous layer with excess of sulfuric acid and extracting the acidified layer with successive quantities of 50 ml of solvent ethered.
3. Distilled off the solvent with care to ensure minimum loss of eugenol and dry residue in desiccator.

Solvent System:

Tolunc:Ethyl acetate :: 92:7

Detection:

UV-254 nm/Anisaldehyde-Sulphuric acid/Vaniline-Sulphuric acid

Calculation:

$$\text{Percentage Yield} = \frac{\text{Practical Yield}}{\text{Theoretical Yield}} \times 100$$

Result: The percentage yield of eugenol is found to be _____

EXPERIMENT 26

Aim: To carry out isolation of *eugenol* from cinnamon leaf oil.

Requirement: Cinnamon leaf oil, Distillation unit, separating funnel, desiccator, solvent ether, potassium hydroxide, sulphuric acid.

Theory: Cinnamon leaf oil is obtained from the leaves of *Cinnamomum zeylanicum* family *Lauraceae*. It is good source of eugenol.

Botanical Name: *Cinnamomum zeylanicum*

Synonyms: *Cinnamomum*, Laurus cinnamomum, Ceylon Cinnamon, Seychelles Cinnamon, Madagascar Cinnamon, True Cinnamon

Plant Family: Lauraceae

Plant Part: Inner Bark

Extraction Method: Steam Distillation

Colour: Brownish Yellow to Dark Brown

Specific Gravity at 30°C: 1.028 to 1.047

Refractive Index at 30°C: 1.5290 to 1.5370

Optical Rotation at 30°C: +1° to –2°

Major Constituent: The main constituents of the oil are eugenol (76.60%), linalool (8.5%) and piperitone (3.31%).

Odour: Fresh typical Cinnamon Leaf Oil

Cinnamon (*Cinnamomum zeylanicum*) is derived from the scented inner bark of the cinnamon tree. Cinnamon leaf oil produced by the steam distillation of the leaves from the plant Cinamomum verum Presel (Lauraceae). The main constituent of Oil of Cinnamon leaf is Eugenol. The Oil of Cinnamon leaf is used in spice flavours, in perfumery and as a source of Eugenol. Eugenol is a phenylpropene and is a member of the phenylpropanoids class of chemical compounds. It is a clear to pale yellow oily liquid extracted from certain essential oils especially from clove oil, nutmeg, cinnamon, basil and bay leaf. It is slightly soluble in water and soluble in organic solvents. It has a spicy, clove-like aroma. Eugenol exhibits antioxidant and anti-inflammatory activities, eugenol is used in perfumeries, flavorings, essential oils and in medicine as a local antiseptic and anesthetic. It was used in the production of isoeugenol for the manufacture of vanillin, though most vanillin is now produced from phenol or from lignin.

Eugenol

Procedure:

1. Dissove 10 ml volatile oil (cinnamon leaf oil) in 100 ml of solvent ether in a separating funnel and shake with 3 successive quantities of 100 ml of 10% potassium hydroxide solution.
2. Regenerate eugenol by acidifying the aqueous layer with excess of sulphuric acid and extracting the acidified layer with three successive quantities of 50 ml of solvent ether.
3. Distill off the solvent with care to ensure minimum loss of eugenol.
4. Dry residue in a desicator.

Chemical Test:

To 5 ml solution of eugenol, add 2–3 drops of neutral $FeCl_3$ solution. A yellow green colored solution is obtained.

To 5 ml solution of eugenol in chloroform add 1 ml picric acid solution in chloroform. Heat the solution on water for few minutes and cool. Brown red color crystals of picrate are obtained.

Solvent System:

Tolune: Ethyl acetate (93:7)

Detection:

UV-254 nm/Anisaldehyde-Sulphuric acid/Vaniline-Sulphuric acid

Calculations:

$$\text{Percentage Yield} = \frac{\text{Practical Yield}}{\text{Theoretical Yield}} \times 100$$

Result: The percentage yield of eugenol is found to be

EXPERIMENT 27

Aim: To isolate *volatile* oil from fennel.

Requirements: Clavenger apparatus, fennel, water, glycerin.

Principle: Essential oil or volatile oils are odoriferous, volatile principles that are obtained from different plant parts and are characterized by high refractive indexes. Volatile oils are primarily composed of mixture of Monoterpenes ($C_{10}H_{16}$), Sesquiterpenes ($C_{15}H_{24}$) and their oxygenated derivatives. These are generally extracted by steam distillation or hydrodistillation, by solvent extraction or by mechanical expression.

Fennel (*Foeniculum vulgare* Mill., *Apiaceae*) is a well-known aromatic and medicinal plant. Fennel essential oil is extracted from Foeniculum vulgare var. dulce, which is sweet fennel (also known as *F officinale*, *F capillaceum* and *Anethum foeniculum*) of the Umbelliferae (Apiaceae) family and is also known as fennel and Roman fennel.

The main chemical components of fennel oil are α-pinene, myrcene, fenchone, trans-anethole, methyl chavicol, limonene, 1,8-cineole and anisic aldehyde. The principal constituents are anethole and fenchone. Sweet fennel oil is extracted from crushed seeds by steam distillation and yield 1–4% of volatile oil. Estragole is found in the essential oil as the major component; and high levels of *trans*-anethole.

Anethole

Extraction, Isolation, Identification and Estimation of Phytoconstituents

Frenchone

Herbal drugs and essential oil of fennel have antispasmodic, diuretic, anti-inflammatory, analgesic and antioxidant effects. They are active for dyspeptic complaints, flatulence and bloating. The volatile oil showed antioxidant, antimicrobial and hepatoprotective activity. It is also used in cases of obesity. It has a cleansing and toning effect on the skin, helping with bruises, sorting out overly oily skin and to fight wrinkles in more mature complexions (possibly due to the estrogenic properties of the oil). They are also used as flavoring agents in food products.

The apparatus used for the extraction of volatile oil is clavenger apparatus. The volatile oil in fennel is isolated by water distillation.

The volatile oil gets distilled due to the difference in vapour pressure of oil and water. When the drug is allowed to boil in the flask, steam enters into the tissues of the drug and liberates the volatile oil present. The volatile oil by virtue of the difference in the vapour pressure of the distilling liquid travels upward and when reaches the condenser gets cooled, falls and gets collected in the graduated tube.

Procedure

1. Place 150 ml water and 150 ml glycerin and a few pieces of porous porcelain in the flask which is joined to the apparatus and joined with condenser.
2. Introduce water by tube N until it reaches level B and 1 ml of xylene through tube K using a graduated pipette and placing it's tip at the bottom of tube K.
3. Heat the flask until it begins to boil and is continued at a rate that leaves the lower part of the condenser (G).
4. After 30 min heating is discontinued and after at least 5 minutes the volume of xylene in the graduated tube is observed.
5. The drug fennel is then introduced into the flask and distillation is continued for 3 hours. After 3 hours, discontinue heating and after 5 min the volume of oil in the graduated portion of the tube is read. The distillation is then continued further for one hour and read the volume of oil again. The procedure is repeated till the two consecutive readings of the volume of oil occur constant.
6. The volume of xylene is subtracted from the volume of the oily layer and the remainder is taken to be the content of volatile oil in the drugs.

Identification Tests

- *Odour test*: volatile oils have a characteristic odour.
- *Spot test*: volatile oils do not leave a permanent stain on the filter test.
- *Solubility test:* volatile oils are soluble in 90% alcohol whereas fixed oils are not.

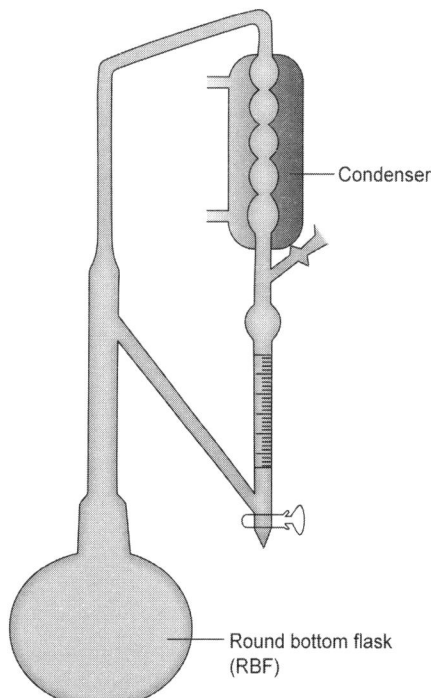

Fig. 6.1: Clavenger apparatus

TLC

Solvent System

Tolune: Ethyl acetate (92:7)

Detection

UV-254 nm/Anisaldehyde-Sulphuric acid/Vaniline-Sulphuric acid

Calculations:

$$\text{Percentage Yield} = \frac{\text{Practical Yield}}{\text{Theoretical Yield}} \times 100$$

Result: The percentage yield of volatile oil is found to be _____

EXPERIMENT 28

Aim: To carry out isolation of *lemon grass oil* from lemon grass.

Requirement: Lemon grass leaves, distilled water.

Theory: Lemon grass oil is a volatile oil or essential oil contains chemical constituents like limonene (terpene) and citral (terpenoid that exhibit aldehyde as functional group), etc. The percentage of citral in lemon grass oil is 3.4–3.6%. Lemon grass oil is used as flavoring agent and carminative. Lemongrass oil has unique therapeutic properties like, analgesic, anti-depressant, antimicrobial, antipyretic, antiseptic, astringent, bactericidal, carminative, deodorant, diuretic, febrifuge, fungicidal, galactagogue, insecticidal, nervine, nervous system sedative and tonic. Lemongrass treats pain arising from indigestion, rheumatism, and nerve conditions. The refreshing fragrance of the oil reduce headache irritability and drowsiness. Moreover, it has proved an antiseptic, suitable for use on various types of skin infections, usually as a wash or compress, and is especially effective on ringworm and infected sores. It is also used in Perfumery Compounds, Soaps and Laundry products, used as a starting material in the production of Vitamin-A or for Isolation of Citral, and in Aromatherapy

Specifications of Lemongrass Oil

Botanical Name: Cymbopogon citratus

Parts Used: Leaves

Extraction: By steam distillation of the leaves of Cymbopogon Citratus

Colour: Yellow coloured liquid

Odour: The odour is strong, sharp, pungent and fresh-grassy Lemon type, herbaceous or tea like odour.

Specific Gravity: 0.894 – 0.904

Refractive Index: 1.4830 – 1.4890

Optical Rotation: – 3° To +1°

Content of total Aldehyde as Citral: 75% – 76 %

Chemical Composition: The main chemical component of Lemongrass oil is Citral. Other constituents are myrcene, citronellal, geranyl acetate, nerol, geraniol, neral and traces of limonene.

Solubility: Soluble in Alcohol and other organic solvents and insoluble in water.

Storage: Store in a cool, dry place in tightly sealed containers, protected from heat and light.

Procedure

1. Take small pieces of lemon grass leaves and distilled water in excess into a round bottom flask of a clavenger apparatus.
2. Heat the contents at less than 100°C.
3. The distillate was collected and allowed to stand aside for 20 min.
4. Separate the volatile oil layer which is immiscible with water phase.

EXPERIMENT 29

Aim: To determine volatile oil content in the given sample of Eucalyptus leaves by hydro-distillation method.

Requirements: Clavenger apparatus, heating mantle, glycerol, plant sample, beaker, water, anhydrous sodium sulphate.

Theory: Oil from the eucalyptus tree (*Eucalyptus globulus*) is used today in many over-the-counter cough and cold products, ointments containing eucalyptus are also applied to the nose and chest to relieve congestion. Eucalyptus oil is also found in creams and ointments used to relieve muscle and joint pain, and in some mouthwashes. Eucalyptus oil is also rich in cineole, an antiseptic that kills bacteria that can cause bad breath. Eucalyptus is used in some antiseptic mouthwashes, along with other oils, and the mouthwashes have been shown to help prevent plaque and gingivitis. On the skin, eucalyptus oil has been used to treat arthritis, boils, sores and wounds. The oil is also used in some insect repellents. *Eucalyptus globulus* leaves contain tannins, which are believed to reduce inflammation; flavonoids, plant-based antioxidants; and volatile oils. *Eucalyptus globulus* leaves also contain 1.5–3.5% volatile oil which contains α-pinene (1.68-26.96%), β-pinene(0.81–28.57%), α-phalendrene (1.19–24.0%), Δ^3 cerene(2.77–27.71%), γ-terpene (5.34–49.24%) and 1,8–cineole (17.46–51.62%).

Procedure

1. Take 100 gm fresh leaves of eucalyptus in 1 litre distillation flask together with 250 ml of water.
2. Add a few pieces of porcelain in order to avoid bumping during distillation.
3. Keep the distillation flask was on heating mantle.
4. Fit graduated receiver of clavenger apparatus filled with water to avoid any air bubbles.
5. Continued distillation for four hours at the rate which keeps lower end of the condenser cool.
6. Allow the distillate to be collected in a graduated receiver in which aqueous portion of distillate automatically separated.
7. Measured the volatile oil volume which separates out as the upper layer in graduated tube and calculated % w/v on a dry weight basis.

Dried leaves of *Eucalyptus globulus* should contain not less than .... % v/w of volatile oil. Characteristics of Eucalyptus oil are:

Color : _____

Odor and Taste : _____

Weight per ml : _____

Solubility : _____

Optical Rotation : _____

Content of Eucalyptus oil: _____

Calculation: _____

Result: _____

EXPERIMENT 30

Aim: To determine volatile oil content in given sample of *Mentha piperita* leaves by hydro-distillation method.

Requirements: Clavenger apparatus, heating mantle, glycerol, plant sample, beaker, water, anhydrous sodium sulphate.

Theory: *Mentha* species [*Mentha piperita*] from the Lamiaceae family contains 1.02% essential oil of twenty nine compounds are identified in leaves oil representing 58.61% of the total oil composition. The major compound in aerial parts are Menthone (29.01%), followed by menthol (5.58%), menthyl acetate (3.34%), menthofuran (3.01%), 1,8-cineole (2.40%), isomenthone (2.12%), limonene (2.10%), α-pinene (1.56%), germacrene-D (1.50%), β-pinene (1.25%), sabinene (1.13%) and pulegone (1.12%).

Procedure

1. Take 50 gm fresh leaves of mentha in 1 litre distillation flask together with 250 ml of water.
2. Add a few pieces of porcelain in order to avoid bumping during distillation.
3. Keep the distillation flask on heating mantle.

4. Fit graduated receiver of Clavenger apparatus filled with water to avoid any air bubbles.
5. Turn heat on and continue distillation for four hours at the rate which keeps lower end of condenser cool.
6. Allow the distillate to be collected in graduated receiver in which aqueous portion of distillate automatically separated.
7. Measured the volatile oil volume which separates out as the upper layer in graduated tube and calculated % w/v on a dry weight basis.

Dried leaves of *Mentha piperita* should contain not less than .... % v/w of volatile oil. Characteristics of Mentha oil are:

Color: _____
Odor and Taste: _____
Weight per ml: _____
Solubility: _____
Optical Rotation: _____
Content of Mentha oil: _____

Calculation: _____

Result: _____

EXPERIMENT 31

Aim: To prepare and submit TLC plate of given crude drug (cinchona bark)

Requirements: Cinchona bark, Chloroform, Methanol, Dragendorff's reagent, Standard quinine, Silica gel G

Aapparatus: Chromatographic chamber (25 × 25 × 10) cm, Glass plate (20 × 20) cm, Oven, UV lamp.

Procedure:

1. Make slurry with about 15 g of silica gel G with 30 ml of distilled water.
2. Clean the chromatographic plates thoroughly with chromic acid mixture followed by washing with distilled water and dry in oven.
3. Spread slurry with the aid of moving hopper spreader on chromatographic plates; the layer of 300 cm width is coated on the cleaned plate. The coating is allowed to dry at room temperature and the plates are activated in an oven at 60°C for 20 minutes.
4. Pour the solvent system chloroform-methanol-ammonia (60:10:1) in the TLC chamber to a depth of 3 cm and allow to saturate for 3 hours. The chamber is lined with filter paper on three sides to maintain equilibrium of mobile phase.
5. Prepared the test solution of total alkaloidal extract and standard solution of quinine in chloroform separately (1mg/ml).
6. Load 10 µl of the solution on activated plates, with the aid of calibrated capillary.
7. Allow the chromatogram to develop for 10 cm.
8. Take out plate, mark the solvent front and dry at room temperature.
9. Observe the plate under UV lamp (254 µm)
10. The alkaloid shows blue fluorescence, spray the plate with dragendorff's reagent and dry by warming.
11. Identify the location of alkaloids which take reddish brown coloration (R_f value = 0.6)

EXPERIMENT 32

Aim: To carry out TLC study of clove oil and Datura.

TLC of Clove oil:

Stationary Phase: Silica gel G.
Mobile Phase: Toluene: Ethyl acetate (93:7).

Detection:

1. Vanillin Sulphuric acid
2. Ethanolic KOH 5%

TLC of Datura:

Stationary Phase: Silica gel G
Mobile Phase: Toluene:Ethyl acetate:Diethyl amine (70:20:10)
Detection: Dragendroff's reagent

EXPERIMENT 33

Aim: To carry out TLC study of Rauwolfia, Cinchona and black pepper.

TLC of Rauwolfia:

Type-1

Stationary Phase: Silica gel G

Mobile Phase: Toluene : Ethyl acetate : Diethyl amine (70:20:10)

Detection: UV at 254 nm.

Type-2

Stationary Phase: Silica gel G

Mobile Phase: n-butanol:Glacial acetic acid:water (40:10:10)

Detection: Dragendroff's reagent

TLC of Cinchona:

Stationary Phase: Silica gel G

Mobile Phase: Chloroform:Diethyle amine (9:1)

Detection: 10% Ethanolic Sulphuric acid

TLC of Black pepper:

Type-1

Stationary Phase: Silica gel G.

Mobile Phase: Toluene : Diethyl ether : Dioxane (62.5 : 21.5 : 16).

Detection: Vanillin sulphuric acid.

Type-2

Stationary Phase: Silica gel G.

Mobile Phase: Toluene:Ethyl acetate (7:3).

Detection: Vanillin sulphuric acid.

EXPERIMENT 34

Aim: To identify constituents of given herbal drug preparation by chromatographic methods.

Requirements: Filter paper, herbal drug preparation, TLC chambers, glass rods, rubber stoppers, solvent system, etc.

Theory: Chromatography comprises a group of methods for separating molecular mixtures that depends on the differential affinities of the solutes between two immiscible phases. One of the phases is a fixed bed of large surface area, whereas the other is a fluid that moves through, or over the surface of the fixed phases. The fixed phase is called the stationary phases, and the other is mobile phases. Thin layer chromatography is an important analytical tool in the separation, identification and estimation of different classes of natural products. The method based on physicochemical phenomenon of adsorption is rapid and permits the use of corrosive spraying reagents.

Procedure

1. Prepare filter paper strips for the purpose of paper chromatography.

2. Prepare the solvent system (chloroform: methanol:ammonia: :60:10:1) and pour it to a depth of 3 cm in the chamber lined from inside with a filter paper to maintain the equilibrium of the mobile phase. Allow the chamber and filter paper strip to saturate for 15 minutes.

3. Apply spots of sample and standard solution on paper strips and allow to dry at room temperature.

4. Develop the chromatogram up to 10 cm. Take out the paper, mark the solvent front and dry at room temperature.

5. Spray the paper with detecting reagent and dry at room temperature for about 5–10 minutes. Identify the components of the herbal preparation by comparing their location and R_f values with that of standard solution.

Calculations:

$$R_f = \frac{\text{Distance travelled by the component}}{\text{Distance travelled by the solvent front}}$$

Result: On comparison of R_f values the given mixtures is found to contain _____

EXPERIMENT 35

Aim: To identify constituents of given herbal drug preparation by circular paper chromatography.

Requirements: Filter paper, herbal drug preparation, petri dishes, solvent system, etc.

Theory: Chromatography comprises a group of methods for separating molecular mixtures that depends on the differential affinities of the solutes between two immiscible phases. One of the phases is a fixed bed of large surface area, whereas the other is a fluid that moves through, or over the surface of, the fixed phases. The fixed phase is called the stationary phases and the other is termed mobile phases. Thin layer chromatography is an import analytical tool in the separation, identification and estimation of different classes of natural products. The method based on physicochemical phenomenon of adsorption is rapid and permits the use of corrosive spraying reagents.

Procedure

1. Prepare filter paper circles for the purpose of paper chromatography.
2. Prepare the solvent system (chloroform: methanol: ammonia : : 60 : 10 : 1) and pour it to a depth of 1 cm in the petri dishes. Allow the petri dishes and filter paper circles to saturate for 15 minutes.
3. Apply spots of sample and standard solution on papers and allow to dry at room temperature.
4. Develop the chromatogram up to 4 cm in all directions. Take out the paper, mark the solvent front and dry at room temperature.
5. Spray the paper with detecting reagent and dry at room temperature for about 5–10 minutes. Identify the components of the herbal preparation by comparing their location and R_f values with that of standard solution.

Calculations

$$R_f = \frac{\text{Distance travelled by the component}}{\text{Distance travelled by the solvent}}$$

Result: On comparison of R_f values the given mixtures is found to contain _____

EXPERIMENT 36

Aim: To identify the amino acids in given mixture by comparing their R_f values with reference standards.

Requirements: TLC plates, Silica gel G, amino acids, Spraying reagents, TLC chamber, etc.

Theory: Chromatography comprises a group of methods for separating molecular mixtures that depends on the differential affinities of the solutes between two immiscible phases. One of the phases is a fixed bed of large surface area, whereas the other is a fluid that moves through, or over the surface of the fixed phases. The fixed phase is called the stationary phases and the other is termed mobile phases. Thin layer chromatography is an important analytical tool in the separation, identification and estimation of different classes of natural products. The method based on physicochemical phenomenon of adsorption is rapid and permits the use of corrosive spraying reagents.

Procedure

1. Prepare slurry of silica gel G by mixing 1 part of the adsorbent with 2.5 parts of water in a glass mortar. Coat the slurry uniformly with the help of an applicator on clean dry glass plates. Allow the plates to dry at room temperature and activate in an oven at 120° C for 30 minutes.
2. Prepare the solvent system (*n*-butanol : glacial acetic acid : water : : 4 : 1 : 5) and pour it to a depth of 3 cm in the chamber lined inside with a filter paper to maintain the equilibrium of the mobile phase.
3. Prepare the standard solutions of amino acids by dissolving about 2 mg of accurately weighed amino acid in 2 ml of distilled water. Prepare the mixture by mixing 1 ml of each amino acid solutions.
4. Apply the spots of individual amino acid solutions with the help of a micropipette

or capillary tube. Apply the spot of mixture of amino acids similarly. Allow the spots to dry at room temperature.

5. Place the glass plate gently inside the chamber. Develop the chromatogram by ascending technique till the solvent front has moved by about 10 cm. Take out the plate, mark the solvent front and dry at room temperature.
6. Spray the plate with ninhydrin reagent and heat the plates at 100°C for about 5-10 minutes. The violet or reddish-violet spots of amino acids would be visible on the plate.

Identify the amino acids of the mixture by comparing their location and R_f values with that of standard solution.

Calculations:

Distance traveled by the component

$$R_f = \frac{\text{Distance travelled by the component}}{\text{Distance travelled by the solvent}}$$

Result: On comparison of R_f values the given mixtures is found to contain _____

EXPERIMENT 37

Aim: To perform paper chromatography of given known sample of protein.

Procedure

Preparation of solvent system and saturation of chamber
- Prepare about 20 ml solvent system water:n-butanol:glacial acetic acid (4:5:1)
- Saturate the chamber with solvent system

Preparation of plate
- Prepare slurry of silica gel and pour on the slide to make a thin layer of silica
- Allow the slide to dry in air and then activate in oven at 80°C for 30 min.
- Apply the sample to the plate using capillary
- Keep the plate in saturated chamber
- Run the solvent to the plate then take it out and dry

- Spray the plate with ninhydrin solution and then air dry
- Calculated the R_f value as follows:

$$R_f = \frac{\text{Distance travelled by sample}}{\text{Distance travelled by the solvent}}$$

Distance of the solvent front

EXPERIMENT 38

Aim: To identify alkaloids in cinchona bark extract by comparing their R_f values with reference standards.

Requirements: TLC plates, Silica gel G, cinchona alkaloids, solvent system, spraying reagents, TLC chamber, etc.

Theory: Chromatography comprises a group of methods for separating molecular mixtures that depends on the differential affinities of the solutes between two immiscible phases. One of the phases is a fixed bed of large surface area, whereas the other is a fluid that moves through, or over the surface of the fixed phases. The fixed phase is called the stationary phases and the other is termed mobile phases. Thin layer chromatography is an important analytical tool in the separation, identification and estimation of different classes of natural products. The method based on physicochemical phenomenon of adsorption is rapid and permits the use of corrosive spraying reagents.

Procedure

1. Prepare slurry of silica gel G by mixing 1 part of the adsorbent with 2.5 parts of water in a glass mortar. Coat the slurry uniformly with the help of an applicator on clean dry glass plates. Allow the plates to dry at room temperature and activate in an oven at 120°C for 30 minutes.
2. Prepare the solvent system (chloroform : methanol : ammonia :: 60 : 10 : 1) and pour it to a depth of 3 cm in the chamber lined inside with a filter paper to maintain the equilibrium of the mobile phase. Allow the chamber to saturate for 15 minutes.

3. Prepare test solution of total alkaloidal extract and standard solution of quinine in chloroform (1 mg/ml). Load the solutions on activated plates with the help of capillary tubes. Allow the chromatogram to develop for 10 cm. Take out the plate, mark the solvent front and dry at room temperature.
4. Spray the plate with Dragendorff's reagent and dry by warming. Identify the location of alkaloids, which take reddish brown color.

Calculations:

Distance traveled by the component

$$R_f = \frac{\text{Distance travelled by the component}}{\text{Distance travelled by the solvent}}$$

Result: On comparison of R_f values the given mixtures is found to contain

EXPERIMENT 39

Aim: Estimation of vasaka alkaloids in *Adhatoda vasica* by titrimetry method and TLC.

Requirements: Conical flask, Beaker, Funnel, Measuring cylinder, Glass rod, Water bath, pH stips

Theory
A. Estimation of vasaka alkaloids:

Procedure

1. Take 10 gm of Vasaka powder in 50 ml of alcohol. Add 2 ml of H_2SO_4. Warm it for 15 min and keep it overnight/reflux it for one and a half hours.
2. Filter it, take the filtrate and concentrate it up to 10 ml by evaporation. Take 10 ml of concentreated extract.
3. Add 30 ml of water and extract it twice with chloroform in separating funnel. Discard chloroform layer and neutralize aqueous layer with Na_2CO_3 and basify it with NH_3 to pH 9–10.
4. Extract the content twice with 10 ml of chloroform. Combine the chloroform extracts and evaporate slowly to dryness.
5. To this add 20 ml of 0.1 N HCl and few drops of methyl red and titrate it against 0.1 N NaOH to end point.

Factor: Each ml of 0.1 N of HCl ≅ 0.0188 gm of vasicine.

B. TLC of Vasaka:

Stationary Phase: Silica gel G

Mobile Phase: Chloroform:Methanol:Ethylacetate:Ammonia (8:2:1:1)

Detection: 1. Dragendroff's reagent.
              2. UV at 254 nm.

EXPERIMENT 40

Aim: Estimation of total tannin in Harad powder.

Requirements: Conical flask, Beaker, Funnel, Measuring cylinder, Glass-rod.

Theory: Tannins are secondary metabolites of plants, non-nitrogenous, phenolic in nature. Tannin is an astringent, polyphenolic compound that binds to and precipitates proteins and various other organic compounds including amino acids and alkaloids. Tannins have molecular weights ranging from 500 to over 3,000 and upto 20,000 (proanthocyanidins). Tannins are incompatible with gelatin, heavy metals, iron, lime water, metallic salts, strong oxidizing agents and zinc sulfate, since they form complexes and precipitate in aqueous solution. Tannins have a property to tan animal skin to convert in to leather. They can be extracted using water-acetone/alcohol mixture. They have a property to precipitate gelatin and heavy metals.

Procedure

1. Add 20 ml of boiling water to about 0.5 gm of accurately weighed Harad powder and heat it on water bath for 15–20 minutes under frequent mixing.

2. Allow the solution to settle for few minutes. Filter it continuously through cotton wool in 100 ml of volumetric flask taking care that no particles of drug should get off cotton wool.
3. Extract drug in flask four times with boiling water as indicated above and filtering the liquid in same volumetric flask.
4. Cool the liquid and make it up to 100 ml.
5. Take 10 ml of extract; add 10 ml of indigo sulphonic acid. Dilute up to 100 ml and titrate it against 0.1 N $KMnO_4$ under constant mixing until a golden yellow colour is obtained.

Factor: Each ml of 0.1 N $KMnO_4 \cong 0.004157$ gm of tannin.

Blank test is carried out simultaneously by titrating only 10 ml of indigo sulphonic acid after made up to 100 ml against 0.1 N $KMnO_4$.

Standardization of $KMnO_4$ Solution

Dissolve 0.8 gm of accurately weighed $KMnO_4$ in water and dilute to produce 250 ml. Titrate this solution against 25 ml of oxalic acid, mixed with 25 ml of water and 5 ml of conc. H_2SO_4. Keeping temp at 70°C during entire titration procedure.

Factor: Each ml of 0.1 N oxalic acid $\cong$ 0.00316 gm of $KMnO_4$.

EXPERIMENT 41

Aim: Estimation of sennoside from Senna powder by colorimetry (IP 1996)

Requirement: Conical flask, Beaker, Funnel, Measuring cylinder, Glass-rod, separating funnel.

Reagent: Powder Senna, Dist. Water, conc. HCL, Chloroform, $FeCl_3$, Solvent ether, 1N KOH, Na_2CO_3.

Procedure:
1. Take 150 mg of accurately weighed Senna powder in 250 ml of conical flask.
2. Add 30 ml distill water. Mix it properly and heat it for 20 minutes on water bath.
3. Filter the solution. Transfer 20 ml of the solution to separating funnel.
4. Add 1 drop of conc. HCl and shake it with two quantity of Chloroform (15 + 15) ml.
5. Allow it to separate and discard the chloroform layer.
6. Transfer 10 ml of liquid to 100 ml capacity container and adjust the pH of solution between 7–8 with 5% solution of Na_2CO_3.
7. Add 20 ml of $FeCl_3$ solution. Mix it and reflux it on water bath continue heating for 20 minutes.
8. Add HCl until the precipitate dissolves.
9. Allow the solution to cool and transfer it to a separating funnel.
10. Extract it with 3 quantities each of 25 ml of ether.
11. Combine the ether extract and dilute up to 100 ml with ether.
12. Take 10 ml of 1 N KOH.
13. Measure the absorbance immediately at 500 nm using KOH as blank.

EXPERIMENT 42

Aim: Estimation of quinine in Cinchona bark powder as per BP 2000.

Requirement: Conical flask, Beaker, Funnel, Measuring cylinder, Glass rod, 1000 ml Glass Beaker.

Reagent: Powder cinchona bark, dil. HCl, Chloroform, Solvent ether, 20% NaOH, Tragacanth.

Procedure

1. Mix 1 gm cinchona powder with 10 ml of distiled water and 7 ml of dil. HCl.
2. Keep it on water bath for 30 minutes, cool and add 25 ml of chloroform, 50 ml of ether and 5 ml of 20% NaOH solution.
3. Shake the mixture repeatedly for 30 minutes.
4. Add 3 gm of Tragacanth.
5. Shake until the mixture becomes clear.

6. Filter it through cotton; rinse the flask and add with 5 quantities each of 20 ml of mixture of chloroform and ether (1:2).
7. Combine the filtrate, evaporate it to dryness.
8. Dissolve residue in 10 ml of ethanol.
9. Evaporate this to dryness, and dissolve again the residue in 0.1 M HCl.
10. Dilute this to 1000 ml with same acid and check the absorbance in UV at 316 nm.

Preparation of standard solution:

Dissolve 30 mg of quinine in 0.1 M HCl and dilute this to 1000 ml and measure the absorbance at 316 nm.

EXPERIMENT 43

Aim: To estimate vitamin C in chyawanprash by colorimetry.

Requirement: China dish, water bath, glass rod, and Whatman filter paper, colorimeter.

Reagent: Chayvanprash, 10% H_2SO_4, 10% Ammonium Molybdate.

Theory: Chyavanprash is a wonderful Ayurvedic heath tonic, which boosts the energy levels and strengthens the immune system of the body. It contains about 25 to 80 herbs and amla (*Emblica officinalis*) or Indian gooseberry is one of them. Chyavanprash is truly an elixir of life, as it helps to prolong the longevity of life. It is known for its nutritional value. It is highly beneficial for the human body and also helps to get rid of various forms of diseases. Chyavanprash has antioxidant properties. Chyavanprash is very high in vitamin C content and helps to strengthen the immune system hence protecting the body from everyday infections like cough, fever and cold. It helps revitalize the mind and body and is the best health supplement to fight stress. It has beneficial qualities for all age groups men and women alike. Chyavanprash is well known as an immunity booster, antioxidant, rejuvenator, a great source of vitamin C and a very good energy provider. It is made from natural herbs, fruits and spices hence it is the preferred antioxidant to fight free radicals in the body.

Procedure

1. Take 5 gm of Chayvanprash in China dish in 10–15 ml of water.
2. Heat on water bath for 15–20 minutes while stirring by glass rod.
3. The solution should be filtered through Whatman filter paper twice.
4. Colouring matter is removed by charcoal (activated) and measure the actual amount of extract.
5. Add 0.5 ml of filtrate and 2 ml of 10 % H_2SO_4 with 4 ml of 10% Ammonium Molybdate and keep for 60 minutes while make the volume up to 10 ml with water.
6. Take λ_{max} at 650 nm and measure the absorbance against standard of absorbance 1 µg – 10 µg/ml solution.

EXPERIMENT 44

Aim: To estimate citral in Lemon oil.

Requirement: Conical flask, Funnel, Measuring cylinder, Glass rod.

Reagent: Lemon oil, hydroxylamine hydrochloride reagent in 60% alcohol, methyl orange, 0.5 N KOH.

Procedure:

1. Weigh 10 gm of lemon oil in a stoppered tube reagent in 60% alcohol and add a drop of methyl orange.
2. Titrate the librated acid with 0.5 N KOH in alcohol (60%) until the red colour change to permanent yellow in the lower layer.
3. Calculate the aldehyde content.

EXPERIMENT 45

Aim: To demonstrate the column chromatography.

Requirement: Glass column, glass rod, filter paper, silica gel, cotton wool, sand, elution solvent.

Theory: Chromatography is a technique employed for the separation of component of mixture by continuous distribution of the components between two phases. One phase moves (mobile) over the other (stationary) in a continuous manner. When the stationary phase is solid (adsorptive nature) and mobile phase is liquid or gaseous phase, it is called adsorptive chromatography, and when the stationary phase is liquid (held on inert support) with mobile phase as liquid or gaseous, it is called as partition chromatography. When the chromatographic operations are carried out using column, it is called as column chromatography.

Types of column chromatography:
1. Adsorption chromatography in which the components of mixture are selectively adsorbed on the surface of packing column material, i.e. adsorbent.
2. Partition chromatography in which component is partitioned between the mobile phase and stationary phase on inert solid support.
3. Ion exchange chromatography in which the constituent of sample is selectively retarded/retained by exchange resin by replacing ions on packing material.
4. Gel chromatography is the method in which column is packed with a permeable gel which bridge out separation by sieving or molecular filtration action.

Principle:
The basic principle underlying in adsorption chromatography is adsorption of component at the solid–liquid interface. For good separation, the component of mixture should have different degree of affinity for the solid support, i.e. adsorbent and the interaction between adsorbent and component should be reversible. The component having strong adsorption for column at faster rate as the elute passes through the column.

Component of mixture is bound to solid surface by specific interaction between polar groups of molecule on adsorbing surface. The atoms, ions, or molecules of adsorbent have properties different at surface than those from the interior. The bonds at the surface layer are perturbed and have higher energy level. This is called surface activity. The attractive force may be ionic (electrostatic), dipole-dipole, dipole-induced dipole or simple London force. Thus, solute from solution when comes into contact gets adsorbed on the surface. Usually the surface loses activity when it is converted by a monolayer of adsorbed species.

Procedure:
Wash the column with acetone and hang it in inverted position overstand and allow drying it. Cut the glass wool of inner diameter of column and place it inside the column with the help of clean and dry glass rod. Now cut the filter paper of the same diameter and place it over the glass wool. Now prepare the slurry of silica gel with your suitable solvent such as *n*-hexane, toluene, etc. and pour it into the column, while pouring care should be taken to avoid the entrapment of air into the column which may lead to chances of breaking of column. Now allow to stand for 5 to 7 minutes for the settlement of silica into the column, now cut the cotton of the inner diameter of the column and place it over the settled silica into the column slowly with help of glass rod without disturbing the column. Now, cut two filter paper of the inner diameter of the column and place your extract between these two filter papers and place it over the cotton. Put some sand over the top most filter paper and pour your solvent in required quantity over it. Run the column and collect the fractions into different cleaned vials and perform the TLC.

Result: _____

EXPERIMENT 46

Aim: Pharmacognostical and phytochemical investigation of tulsi plant.

Theory: The various species of *Ocimum* (Lamiaceae), i.e. *Ocimum gratissimum* Linn., *Ocimum americanum* Linn., *Ocimum sanctum* Linn. and *Ocimum basilicum* Linn. are widely distributed in tribal areas of India. The pharmacognostical examination include the morphological, microscopical characters and physical constants of leaves of various *Ocimum* species including determination of loss on drying, ash values and extractive values. The preliminary phytochemical screening of various leaf extracts and presence of various phytoconstituents like carbohydrates, flavonoids, protein and amino acids, tannins, phytosterols and saponins.

Phytochemical study is also useful to isolate the pharmacologically active principles present in the drug. The other parameters observed are also useful for the future identification of the plant and serve as a standard monograph for identification and evaluation of plant.

1. **Collection and Authentication of Plant:** The leaves of *Ocimum* species (*O. gratissimum* Linn., *O. americanum* Linn., *O. Sanctum* Linn. and *O. basilicum* Linn.) can be collected from the local area. The plant material can be identified and authenticated by Botanical Survey of India. The collected leaves are to be shade dried under normal environmental condition, powdered and store in a closed container for further use.
2. **Macroscopic Examination:** The various leaves of *Ocimum* species can be studied individually for its morphological characters such as colour, odour, taste, shape, size, etc.
3. **Determination of Physical Constants**
    i. **Ash values:** The ash values are useful to determine the quality and purity of the crude drug. Ash contains inorganic radicals like phosphate, carbonates and silicates of sodium, potassium, magnesium, calcium, etc. Such variable are then removed by treating with acid. Different ash values like total ash, water soluble ash, acid insoluble ash and sulphated ash can be determined as per standard procedure mentioned in WHO guidelines.
    ii. **Extractive values:** Extractive values are useful for evaluation of crude drugs. It gives an idea about the nature of the chemical constituents present in the crude drug. Different extractive values like water soluble extractive and alcohol soluble extractive value are to be determined as per standard procedure mentioned in WHO guidelines.
    iii. **Foreign organic matter and moisture montent:** Foreign organic matter can be determined from the weight of the drug taken and moisture content is to be determined by loss on drying method in terms of percent w/w as per standard procedure mentioned in WHO library.
4. **Reaction of Powdered Drug with Different Reagents:** Powdered drug treated with different reagents and colored shown by that treatment is noted down.
5. **Fluorescence Analysis:** Fluorescence characteristic of powdered drug with different reagent can be observed under day light and UV light after drug treatment with different reagents.
6. **Preliminary Phytochemical Screening:** The preliminary phytochemical screening with the various qualitative chemical tests of freshly prepared extracts of leaves revealed the presence of various phytoconstituents like carbohydrate, phenolic compounds, flavonoids, protein and amino acids, tannins, phytosterols and saponins by using reported methods.

EXPERIMENT 47

Aim: Determination of percentage purity of ginger in various samples by Wallis's Lycopodium spore method.

Reagent: Glycerin, Iodine, Ginger powder, Tragacanth, Trikatu churna, Clove, Lycopodium spore.

Introduction: Lycopodium consists of the spores of the club moss, *Lycopodium clavatum* Linn.

Family: Lycopodiaceae and possibly other species.

Lycopodium is a pale yellow, fine powder that floats when thrown on to the surface of water. It has a density of 1.06–1.09. The spores are very resistant to pressure and are unaffected by dilute acids and alkalis. The drug is odourless and tasteless and devoid of grittiness when rubbed between the fingers.

Microscopy: Each spore is tetrahedral and has the shape of the fourth part of a sphere; three faces are flat and triangular while the fourth is rounded-triangular and convex. The length of the straight edges is about 21 microns and the average diameter of the spores is about 25 microns. One mg of the powder contains about 94,000 spores.

The convex surface is entirely covered with a fine network of raised ridges forming meshes which are four to six sided and produce a honey-combed appearance. The three flat faces are similarly covered except towards the apex of the spore where they are nearly smooth; strong ridges mark the lines of union of three flat faces. When firmly crushed, the spores burst and droplets of yellowish fixed oil are liberated. These spores contain about 40–50% of fixed oil, which consists principally of the glycerides of Lycopodium-oleic acid (80%) and myristic acid. Lycopodium-oleic acid resembles ordinary oleic acid but is not identical with it. Sitosterol, hydrocaffeic acid and traces of alkaloids are also present. Pure Lycopodium yields about 1–1.5% of ash; the commercial drug leaves about 3–4% of ash. The moisture present is about 5%.

Uses: Lycopodium is sometimes used as a dusting powder for excoriated surfaces, for preventing the mutual adhesion of pills and for making snuffs (insufflations). It is also used as a standard of reference in quantitative microscopy. The greater part of Lycopodium is used industrially for the manufacture of fireworks.

Foreign organic matter present in the powdered drug can be determined by taking advantage of characteristics particles, i.e. particles which are easily identified and distinguished from the remainder of the powder. They must also be fairly resistant to mechanical forces.

Powdered drug can be evaluated by comparison with Lycopodium spores, if it contains well defined characteristic particles which can be counted (starch grains, pollen grains, etc.) or single layered tissues which can be traced after magnification for actual area calculation (single layer of sclerenchyma, etc.) or characteristics having uniform length and thickness, etc. (trichomes, etc.). In all these cases, the characteristics/area of drug powder is compared with the spores in a fixed quantity.

Procedure

Dry the powdered drug at 105°C and determine its steady weight at room temperature. Weigh accurately powdered material and Lycopodium spores and mix them. Proportion spores of 2:1 powdered drug to Lycopodium has been found to be satisfactory. Mix them on a glass plate with flexible spatula. Make a thin smooth paste by adding a suspending medium (glycerin: tragacanth mucilage: water:: 2:1:2). Transfer the paste into a stopper tube by washing with a more quantity of suspending medium. Adjust the final volume by suspending fluid such that about 10-20 spores may be present in a field of 4 mm objective. Oscillate the tube gently to get a uniform suspension. Place a drop on a slide, spread with a needle, put cover slip and count the characteristics particles of the organic matter as well as the Lycopodium spores in the field. Made one more slide in the same way and count 25 fields. Prepare another suspension as described above, prepared two more slides and count 25 fields each for both preparations as above. Determine the average of 4 sets of counts (4 × 25 = 100 fields in all) and also the percentage of moisture present from the first step. Calculate the number of characteristic particles present in one mg of the powder dried at 105 °C. Determine in a similar way the number of characteristic particles per mg of the pure foreign matter, calculate with reference to the material dried at 105 °C.

Calculated the percentage of foreign organic matter from the formula:

% of foreign organic matter

$$= \frac{n \times w \times 94{,}000 \times 100}{S \times m \times p},$$

where, n = number of characteristics particles in 25 fields

S = number of spores in the same 25 fields

w = weight in mg of Lycopodium taken

m = Weight in mg of the sample

p = number of characteristics particles/mg of the pure foreign matter, i.e. 2, 81,100

94,000 = number spores per mg of Lycopodium

Result:

EXPERIMENT 48

Aim: Determination of Foaming Index of given drug sample (Glycerrhiza and Shatavari).

Requirements: 500 ml Conical Flask, 100 ml Volumetric Flask, Test Tubes, Beaker.

Introduction: Many medicinal plant materials contain saponins that can cause persistent foam when an aqueous decoction is shaken. The foaming ability of an aqueous decoction of plant materials and their extracts is measured in terms of foaming index.

Glycerrhiza

Biological source: It consists of dried, peeled or unpeeled root and stolon of *Glycerrhiza glabra* Linn.

Family: Leguminosae

Chemical constituents: It contains Glycyrrhizin, Glycyrrhizinic acid, Glycyrrhetinic acid, Asparagin, Glucose and Sucrose.

Glycyrrhetinic acid

Uses: Expectorant, Demulcent, Cough Suppresant, Flavouring agent, Antispasmodic, in the treatment of rheumatoid arthritis.

Shatavari

Biological source: It consists of dried roots and leaves of the plant *Asparagus racemosus*.

Family: Liliaceae

Chemical constituents: It contains, Shatavarin I–IV (0.2%), Quercetin, Rutin, Hyperoside, and Diosgenin.

Shatavarin I

Uses: Galactogouge, Tonic, Diuretic, Antioxytoxic, in the treatment of rheumatism and nervine tonic.

Procedure:

Take 1 g of powder in 500 ml conical flask containing 100 ml of boiling water. Maintain the flask at moderate boiling for 30 minutes.

Cool the mixture and filter into 100 ml volumetric flask and add sufficient water to make the volume. Pour the decoction into 10 stoppered test tubes in successive portions of 1 ml, 2 ml, 3 ml, etc. up to 10 ml and adjust the volume of the liquid in each tube with water to 10 ml. Stopper the tubes and shake them in lengthwise motion for 15 seconds, two shakes per second. Allow to stand for 15 minutes and measure the height of the foam. The results are assessed as follows:

1. If the height of the foam in every tube is less than 1 cm and foaming index is less than 100.
2. If a height of foam of 1 cm is measured in any tube, the volume of the plant material decoction in this tube is used to determine the index. If this tube is the 1st or 2nd tube in series, prepare one more intermediate dilution in the similar manner to obtain a more precise result.
3. If the height of the foam is more than 1 cm in every tube the foaming index is over 1000. In this case repeat the determination using a new series of dilution of the decoction in order to obtain a result.

Calculation:

Calculate the foaming index using following formula:

Foaming Index = 1000/A

A = Volume in ml of the decoction used for preparing the dilution in the tube where foaming to a height of 1 cm is observed.

Result:

Foaming index of Glycerrhiza = _____

Foaming index of Shatavari = _____

EXPERIMENT NO: 49

Aim: Determination of Swelling Index of given drug sample (Isapgol and Methi).

Requirements: Measuring cylinder, Seeds

Introduction: Many medicinal plant materials are of specific therapeutic or pharmaceutical utility because of their swelling properties, especially gums and those containing an appreciable amount of mucilage, pectin or hemicellulose. The swelling index is the volume in ml taken up by the swelling of 1 g of plant material under specific conditions. Its determination is based on the addition of water or swelling agent as specified in the test procedure for each individual plant material (either whole, cut or pulverized). Using a glass stoppered measuring cylinder the material is shaken repeatedly for 1 hour and then allowed to stand for required period of time. The volume of the mixture (in ml) is then read. The mixing of whole plant material with the swelling agent is easy to achieve but cut or pulverized material requires vigorous shaking at specified intervals to ensure even distribution of the material in the swelling agent.

Isapgol

Biological source: It consists of dried seeds of the plant known as *Plantago ovata*.

Family: Plantaginaceae

Chemical constituents: Mucilage, pentosan, aldobionic acid, xylose, arabinose, galacturonic acid, rhamnose, fixed oil and proteins.

Uses: Demulcent, laxative, emollient, in the treatment of chronic constipation, in the preparation of tablets, as a stabilizer in ice-cream industry.

Methi

Biological source: It consists of dried seeds of *Trigonella foenum graecum*

Family: Leguminosae

Chemical constituents: Trigonelline

Trigonelline

Uses: Insulin stimulation, as a spice. Potential source of diosgenin, antidiabetic, antiulcer, anticancer.

Procedure

Transfer 1g of the seeds to 25 ml measuring cylinder. Fill up to 20 ml mark on the cylinder with water. Agitate gently and occasionally during 24 hours and allow to stand. Measure the volume occupied by the swollen seeds. The genuine seeds of Isapgol occupy a volume of not less than 10 ml.

Result:

Swelling Index of Isapgol = _____
Swelling index of Methi = _____

EXPERIMENT 50

Aim: To estimate Sennoside B from Senna leaf powder.

Requirements: Conical flask, Separating funnel, Beaker, Pipette, Test-tubes, Filter paper

Reagents: Chloroform, Hydrochloric acid, Ferric chloride, 5% w/v $Na_2CO_3/NaHCO_3$, 1 N Potassium hydroxide, Ether

Principle:

Modified Borntrager test (Oxidative Hydrolysis): The aqueous extract is treated with Ferric chloride solution and HCl. Addition of Ferric chloride converts Dianthrone to Anthrone. Hydrochloric acid will hydrolyze Glycoside into glycone and aglycone moiety. It is then treated with ether and made alkaline using KOH/NH_3. The aqueous layer show pink, red or violet color which is then estimated by colorimetry.

Theory:

Biological source: Sennoside B is Anthrone glycoside obtained from dried leaflets of *Cassia angustifolia*.

Family: Leguminosae

Chemical Constituents: Sennoside A and B which are stereoisomer of each other are dimeric glycoside with rhein dianthrone as aglycone, i.e. 10,10'-bis (9,10 dihydro, 1, 8, dihydroxy, 9-oxanthracene-3-carboxyllic acid)

Structure of Sennoside A or B

Uses: Purgative, Laxative.

Procedure

Weigh accurately about 0.15 g of drug from given fine powder and add 30 ml of water. Place in a water-bath under reflux condenser for 30–40 minutes, allow to cool and filter it and adjust the volume to 30 ml. Take 20 ml of the above filtrate and add 0.1 ml HCl and shake with 3 quantities of 15 ml Chloroform in separating funnel. Discard the Chloroform extract and neutralize the aqueous layer with $NaHCO_3$ and filter it. Take 10 ml of the above filtrate and 20 ml of 10.5% aqueous $FeCl_3$ and heat for 30–40 minutes and add 1 ml concentrated HCl and keep for hydrolysis in a reflux for about 30 minutes till solution becomes clear and cool it completely. Extract the aqueous layer with 15 ml of solvent ether with 3 times in separating funnel and combine the ether layer and make the volume with solvent ether up to 50 ml. Take 10 ml of this solution evaporates it and to the residue add 10 ml of 1M KOH solution. Take the absorbance at 515 nm. Calculate the % content of hydroxyanthracene glycosides expressed as Sennoside B taking 240 as the value of A (1% 1 cm) at the maximum of about 515 nm.

Calculation

Absorbance at 520 nm = 0.07

Now, $A = abc$

$$0.07 = 240 \times C$$

$$C = \frac{0.07}{240}$$

$$C = 0.0002916 \text{ g}/100 \text{ ml}$$

Dilution: 0.15 gm of drug
↓
Add 30 ml of water
↓ reflex (30 – 40 min)
20 ml of above filtrate
↓
10 ml of solution
↓

Make the volume upto 50 ml with ether → 10 ml of above solution

100 ml solution contains = 0.0002916 g Sennoside

50 ml solution contains = 0.0001458 g of Sennoside.

10 ml solution contains = 0.0001458 g Sennoside

20 ml solution contains = 0.0002916 g Sennoside

30 ml solution contains = 0.0004374 g Sennoside

0.15 g powder contains = 0.0004373 g Sennoside

100 g powder contains = 0.29% w/w Sennoside

Result:

The given Senna powder contains Sennoside and it complies with its standard range 0.2% to 0.5% w/w

EXPERIMENT 51

Aim: To determine Barbaloin from Aloe Vera.

Requirement: Soxhlet apparatus, 1000 ml volumetric flask, 10 ml volumetric flask, Beaker, Pipette.

Reagents: Ethanol, $FeCl_3$ solution (60% w/v), HCl, 1 N NaOH, Carbon tetrachloride

Introduction

ALOE

Synonym: Aloe, Musabar, Kumari

Biological Source: Aloe is the dried juice of the leaves of *Aloe barbadensis*.

Family: Liliaceae.

Chemical Constituents: It mainly contains aloin, which is a mixture of glycosides among which barbaloin is chief constituent. It also contains isoberbaloin, β-barbaloin, Aloe-emodin and resin.

Barbaloin

Aloesin

Use: Purgative, Pain and Itching, Slow down the Ulceration and Keratosis, Gel is used in cosmetics as protective due to antiwrinkle properties, inflammation.

Procedure

Moisten 0.2 g of fine powder with 2 ml of ethanol; add 5 ml of water at about 60 °C. Mix, add further 75 ml of water at about 60 °C and shake for 30 minute, filter through filter paper. Wash the flask with 20ml of H_2O and add sufficient H_2O to combine filtrate and washing to produce 1000 ml. Transfer 10 ml of solution to flask containing 1ml of HCl. Heat in water bath under reflux condition for 4 hr so that water level is always above that of liquid in flask. Cool and transfer the solution into separating funnel, rinsing the flask successively with 4 ml of 1 N NaOH and 4ml of H_2O and add the rinsing to the content of separating funnel. Extract with 3 quantities each of 20 ml of CCl_4 and wash to combine the CCl_4 extract with 2 quantities each of 100 ml of H_2O discarding the washings. Dilute the Organic phase to 100 ml CCl_4. Evaporate 20 ml carefully to dryness on water bath and dissolve the resulting residue in 10ml of NaOH. Immediately measure the absorbance at 440 nm and at 500 nm. Calculate the content of anhydrous barbaloin taking 200 as A1% 1cm at 500 nm. The result of assay is not valid unless the ratio of absorbance at 500 nm to that of 440 nm is not less than 1.9.

Calculation:

$$A = abc$$
$$0.065 = 200 \times c$$
$$c = 3.25 \times 10^{-4} \, g/ml$$

0.2 g powder contains = 3.25×10^{-4} g/ml

100 g powder contains = 0.1625 % w/w Barbaloin.

Check point

Ratio of absorbance at 500 nm to 440 nm

$$= 0.065/0.041$$
$$= 1.585$$

Result: The given sample of Aloe Vera contains _____.

EXPERIMENT 52

Aim: To determine volatile oil content of Eucalyptus leaf.

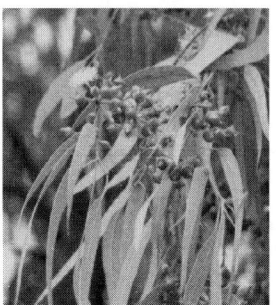

Fig. 6.2: Eucalyptus leaf

Procedure

1. Take about 50 gm of accurately weight of eucalyptus leaf in one liter distillation flask of Clevenger apparatus together with 250 ml of water.

2. Add few pieces of porcelain to it in order to avoid bumping during distillation.

3. Keep the distillation flask/ round bottom flask on the heating mantle and set the distillation assembly (Clevenger apparatus). Fill the graduated receiver with water avoiding any air bubbles. Do not tighten the outlet near the upper end of the receiver. Instead, loosely pack it with cotton.

4. Turn the heat on and continue distillation for four hours at a rate which keeps the lower end of the condenser cool.

5. Allow the distillate to be collected in the graduated receiver in which the aqueous portion of the distillate is automatically separated and returned to the distillation flask.

6. Measure the volume of volatile oil which separates out as the upper layer in the graduated tube.

7. Finally measure the volume of oil in ml.

Chapter 7

Preparation and Standardization of Ayurvedic Formulations

Introduction

Ayurveda: The word ayurveda derived from two sanskrit words, i.e. Ayur and Veda. Means: "the science of life" or "the true knowledge of life". The Charaka, Sushruts, Sharangadhra and many of the persons are having the great working and dedication for ayurveda.

An Ayurvedic medicine (as defined in the Drugs and Cosmetic Act 1940) includes all medicines intended for internal or external use, for the diagnosis, treatment, mitigation or prevention of diseases or disorder in human beings or animals and manufactured exclusively in accordance with the formulae described in the authoritative books of ayurvedic systems of medicine specified in the first schedule of the Act.

The object of Ayurveda is to counteract the imbalance of three essential elements, *vata, pitta and kapha* (air, bile and phlegm respectively), which also called *'Tridosh'* which regularizes the normal working of the human body.

Ayurvedic Dosage Forms:

These are almost similar to the allopathic dosage forms. In this system, the crude drugs, metals, minerals, ghee, oil and stones are used as medicine in various forms.

The basic principles involved in the preparation of these dosage forms are almost similar to those of allopathic processes like distillation, decoction, powders, calcinations, etc. But their technique of preparation is little-bit-different from allopathic drugs.

The various forms are:

1.	Arka	Distillate
2.	Asava and Arishta	Fermented preparations
3.	Avaleha or Leha	Linctus
4.	Kwatha	Decoction
5.	Churna	Fine powders
6.	Ghrita and taila	Medicated ghee and oil
7.	Varti/Anjana	Eye preparations
8.	Pisti	Very fine powders
9.	Bhasma	Calcinated residues
10.	Vati/Gutika	Tablets and pills

Evaluation of Herbal Drug Formulations

Evaluation of a drug means confirmation of its identity and determination of its quality and purity and detection of nature of adulteration. The evaluation of a crude drug is necessary because of three main reasons:

1. Biochemical variation in the drug
2. Deterioration due to treatment and storage
3. Substitution and adulteration, as a result of carelessness, ignorance or fraud.

Over the years the nature and degree of evaluation of drugs has undergone a systematic change. Initially the drugs were identified by comparison only with the standard description available. Due to advancement in the chemical knowledge of various drugs, at present evaluation also includes methods of estimating active constituent present in the formulation. With the advent of separation technique and instrumental analysis, it is possible to perform physical evaluation of crude drugs, which could be both of qualitative and quantitative nature.

Evaluation comprises different chemical test and chemical assay. The isolation, purification and identification of active constituent are chemical methods of evaluation. The purity of crude drug is ascertained by quantitative estimation of active chemical constituent present in them. The method may be useful in determining single active constituent or the group of related constituent present in the same drug. Chemical evaluation also covers phytochemical screening carried out for establishing chemical profile of a crude drug. The commonly employed technique for separation of active substance from crude drug is called Extraction which involves the use of different solvents. The choice of plant material for extraction depends on its nature and the components required being isolated.

The utility of chromatographic techniques and instrumentation in establishing qualitative as well as quantitative profiles of crude drug constituents is well understood and systematically practised in Quality Control and Assurance Laboratories of herbal drugs based industries. The instrumental analysis of the constituents is reliable, quick, reproducible and more convincing.

Thin layer chromatography (TLC)

Presently many chromatographic techniques are available. Thin layer chromatography is widely used for the rapid analysis of drugs and drug preparation. TLC is altogether a new versatile, specialized laboratory technique that evolved in early fifties. It can be employed for both organic and inorganic substances.

Identification can be effected by observation of spots of identical R_f value and about equal magnitude obtained respectively, with an unknown and a reference sample chromatographed on the same plate. A visual comparison of size and intensity of the spots usually serves for semi-qualitative estimation. The major principle involved is either adsorption or partition. The components get separated due to difference in partition coefficient between the mobile phase and stationary phase.

Apparatus

a. A flat glass plate of appropriate dimensions which allow the application at specified points of the necessary quantities of the solution being examined and appropriate reference solution and which allow accommodation of specified migration path length.

b. An aligning tray or a flat surface on which the plates can be aligned and rested when the coating substance is applied.

c. The coating substance consisting of finely divided adsorbent (e.g. Silica gel G, Acetylated Silica gel, Aluminium oxide, etc) materials normally 5 mm–40 mm in diameter suitable for chromatography. It is applied directly to plate with the help of a spreader. Spreader is moved over the glass plate to apply a uniform layer of adsorbent of uniform thickness over the entire surface of plate.

d. A storage rack is to support the plates during drying and transportation.

e. A developing chamber

Preparation of plates

Prepare a suspension of coating substance in accordance with the instructions of the supplier using the spreading device; spread a uniform layer of suspension 0.25–0.30 mm thick on a flat glass plate 20 cm long. Allow the coated plates to dry in air, heat at 100°C– 105°C for at least 1 hr and allow cooling, protected from moisture.

Method

Saturate the development tank for about 1 hour at room temperature. Remove a narrow strip of the coating substance about 5mm wide from the vertical sides of the plates. Apply the solution being examined in the form of circular spots about 2–6 mm in diameter and allowed to air dry. Place the spotted plates in the developing tank close the lid and allow to stand at room temperature, until the mobile phase has ascended to the marked line. Remove the plates dry and visualize as directed in the monograph.

Visualization/ Detections

UV 254 nm and UV 365 nm are mostly used as the detecting agents, e.g. Indoles, Quinoles, Isoquinole, etc.

Spray reagents like anisaldehyde–sulphuric acid reagent, Vanillin–sulphuric acid reagent, Dragon droffs reagent, Iodoplatmate reagent, Van Urks reagent, Ninhydrogen reagent, etc. are used for Alkaloids like Rauwolfia, Cinchona, Berberine, etc.

EXPERIMENT 1

Aim: To perform Phytochemical Screening of Crude Drugs.

Theory: The plant may be considered biosynthetic laboratory not only for the chemical compound such as carbohydrate, protein and lipids that are utilized as food by man but also for multitude of compounds like alkaloids, glycosides, volatile oil, tannins, etc. Those exert a physiological effect. The compounds that are responsible for therapeutic effect are usually secondary metabolites. The plant material may be subjected to preliminary phytochemical screening for the detection of various plant constituents on the following lines. The systemic investigation of plant material for its phytochemical behavior involves the following steps:

1. Authentification (original/real) and extraction of plant materials.
2. Separation and isolation of the constituent of interest.
3. Characterization of isolated compound.
4. Investigation of the biosynthetic pathway to particular compounds.
5. Quantitative evaluation.

Table 7.1: Identification

Plant constituents/Extracts	Test reagent used				
	Petroleum ether	Chloroform	Acetone	Ethanol	Water
Alkaloid					
Carbohydrate					
Phytosterol					
Fixed oil and fats					
Saponins					
Phenols					
Tannins					
Proteins and amino acids					
Gums and mucilage					
Volatile oil					

Methods for extraction
1. Maceration
2. Percolation
3. Decoction

Procedure
Successive solvent extraction
1. Extract about 50g of air dry powdered plant material successively with following solvent in Soxhlet extractor
   a. Petroleum ether (60–80°)
   b. Benzene
   c. Chloroform
   d. Acetone
   e. Ethanol (95%)
2. Finally macerate the marc with chloroform water for 24 hours to obtain the aqueous extract
3. Concentrate each extract by distilling off the solvent and then evaporating to dryness on water bath
4. Weigh the extract obtained with solvent and calculate its % in terms of air-dry weight of plant material and also note the consistency of extract.

Qualitative chemical identification:
The extracts are subjected to various qualitative chemical tests to determine the presence of various phytoconstituents like alkaloids, glycosides, carbohydrates, phenolics and tannins, phytosterols, fixed oils and fats, proteins and amino acids, flavonoids, saponins, etc. using reported methods.

1. **Alkaloids:** Dissolve extracts individually in dilute hydrochloric acid and filter. The filtrates are tested carefully and treated with alkaloid reagents.

   Mayer's test: Filtrates are treated with Mayer's reagent (potassium mercuric iodide). The formation of a yellow cream precipitate indicates presence of alkaloids.

   Wagner's test: Treat filtrates with Wagner's reagent (iodine in potassium iodide) and observe. Formation of brown or reddish brown precipitate indicates presence of alkaloids.

   Dragendorff's test: Treat filtrates with Dragendorff's reagent (solution of potassium bismuth iodide). Formation of red precipitate indicates presence of alkaloids.

   Hager's **test:** Treat filtrates with Hager's reagent (saturated picric acid solution). Formation of yellow colored precipitate indicates the presence of alkaloids.

   TLC
   Solvent system: Ethyl acetate: Methanol: Water (100:13.5:10)
   Spraying reagent: Dragendorff's reagent
   Colour: Orange

2. **Proteins and Amino acids:**

   Millons test: Treat filtrates with 2 ml of Millons reagent. The formation of white precipitate, which turned to red upon heating indicates presence of proteins and amino acids.

   Biuret test: Treat filtrates with 1ml of 10% sodium hydroxide solution and heat. Add a drop of 0.7% copper sulphate solution to the above mixtures. The formation of purplish violet colour indicates presence of proteins.

   Ninhydrin test: Add 0.25% Ninhydrin reagent to the extracts and boil for few minutes. Formation of blue colour indicates presence of amino acid.

3. **Carbohydrates:** Dissolve extracts individually in 5ml of distilled water and filter. The filtrate is used to test the presence of carbohydrates.

   Benedict's test: Treat filtrates with Benedict's reagent and heat on water bath. Formation of an orange red precipitate indicates presence of reducing sugars.

   Molisch's test: Treat filtrates with 2 drops of alcoholic α-naphthol solution in a test tube and add 2 ml concentrated sulphuric acid carefully along the sides of the test tube. Formation of violet ring at the junction indicates presence of carbohydrates.

Fehling's test: Hydrolyse filtrates with dilute hydrochloric acid, neutralize with alkali and heat with Fehling's A and B solutions. A red precipitate is formed which indicates presence of carbohydrates.

Barfoed's test: Treated filtrates with Barfoed's reagent and heat on water bath. Formation of an orange red precipitate indicates presence of reducing sugars.

4. **Flavonoids:** To a 2–3 ml of ethanolic extract, a piece of magnesium ribbon and 1 ml of concentrated hydrochloric acid is added. Pink red or red coloration of the solution indicates presence of flavonoids in the drug.

TLC

Solvent system: Ethyl acetate: Methanol: Water (100:13.5:10)

Ethyl acetate: Formic acid: Glacial acetic acid: Water (100:11:11:26)

Spraying reagent: NP/PEG reagent/ UV

Colour: Orange/yellow/green (UV–365 nm)

5. **Phenols:** A drop of ethanolic extract is spotted on a filter paper and a drop of phosphomolybdic acid reagent is added on it. The spot is then exposed to ammonia vapor. Blue coloration of the spot indicates presence of phenols.

6. **Glycosides:** Extracts are hydrolysed with dilute hydrochloric acid and the hydrolysate is subjected to glycosides tests.

Modified Borntrager's test: Treat the extracts with ferric chloride solution and heat on boiling water bath for about 5 minutes. Cool the mixture and shake with equal volume of benzene. Separate the benzene layer and treat with half of its volume of ammonia solution. The formation of rose pink or cherry red colour in the ammoniacal layer indicates presence of anthranol glycoside.

Legal's test: Treat the extracts with sodium nitroprusside in pyridine and methanolic alkali. The formation of pink to red colour indicates presence of cardiac glycosides.

Baljet test: Treat the extracts with sodium picrate and the formation of a yellowish orange colour confirmed the presence of cardiac glycosides.

Killer–Killiani test: Dissolve 0.5 g of dried extract in 2 ml of glacial acetic acid containing one drop of ferric chloride solutions. Add 1 ml of concentrated H_2SO_4. A brown ring obtained at the presence of a cardenolides.

TLC

Solvent system: Ethyl acetate: Methanol: Water (100:13.5:10)

Spraying reagent: Kedde reagent (cardiac glycoside)

Colour: pink/violet

Spraying reagent: KOH reagent (anthraquinone glycoside)

Colour: red

7. **Saponins:**

   Froth's test: Dilute the extracts (alcoholic and aqueous) with 20 ml of distilled water separately and shake for 15 minutes in a graduated cylinder. A layer of foam measuring about 1 cm is formed which indicates presence of saponins.

TLC

Solvent system: Ethyl acetate: Methanol: Water (100:13.5:10)

Chloroform: Glacial acetic acid: Methanol: Water (64:32:12:8)

Spraying reagent: Anisaldehyde sulphuric acid/Vanillin sulphuric acid

Colour: Blue

8. **Tannins (Phenolic compounds):**

   Ferric chloride test: Treat the extracts with few drops of neutral ferric chloride solution (5%). The formation of bluish black colour indicates presence of phenolic nucleus.

Lead acetate test: Treat the extracts with few drops of 10% lead acetate solution. The formation of yellow precipitate confirmed the presence of flavonoids.

Alkaline reagent test: Treat the extracts with few drops of sodium hydroxide separately. Formation of intense yellow colour, which turned colourless on addition of few drops of dilute acid, indicates presence of flavonoids.

Shinoda test: Treat the extracts with few fragments of magnesium metal separately, followed by drop wise addition of concentrated hydrochloric acid. The formation of magenta colour indicates presence of flavonoid.

Vanillin hydrochloric test: Treat the extracts with few drops of vanillin hydrochloride reagent. The formation of pinkish red colour indicates presence of tannins.

9. **Steroids and Triterpenoids:**

   Libermann–Burchard test: To one ml of ethanolic extract of drug add one ml of chloroform and 2 to 3 ml of acetic anhydride. To the above mixture, 1 to 2 drops of concentrated Sulphuric acid is added. Dark green coloration of the solution indicates the presence of steroids and dark pink or red coloration of the solution indicates presence of triterpenoids.

   Salkowski's test: Treat the extracts with in chloroform with few drops of concentrated sulphuric acid, shake well and allow standing for some time, red colour appears in the lower layer indicates presence of sterols and formation of yellow colored lower layer indicates presence of Triterpenoids.

TLC

Solvent system: Hexane: Diethyl ether (7:3)

Benzene: Diethyl ether (9:1)

Spraying reagent: 50% H_2SO_4 in ethanol

80% potassium dichromate in H_2SO_4

Colour: Orange

10. **Fixed Oils and Fats:**

    Stain test: Press small quantity of extracts between two filter papers separately. An oily stain on filter paper indicates presence of fixed oil.

    Saponification test: Heat the extracts on water bath with 0.5 N alcoholic potassium hydroxide solution. Formation of soap indicates presence of fixed oils and fats.

11. **Gums and mucilage:** Add about 10 ml aqueous extract slowly to 25 ml of absolute alcoholic extract with constant stirring. Filter the precipitates and dry in air. Examine the precipitates for its swelling.

12. **Volatile oil:** Take 50 g of powdered material. Subject it to hydrodistillation. Collect the distillate in the graduated tube of assembly in which the aqueous portion is automatically separated from the volatile oil, if it is present in the drug and return back to distillation flask.

Table 7.2: Observation table for qualitative chemical tests

Plant constituents/Extracts	Test reagent used					
	Petroleum ether	Benzene	Chloroform	Acetone	Ethanol	Water
Alkaloid						
Mayer's test Wagner's test Dragendorff's test Hager's test						

Contd.

Table 7.2: Observation table for qualitative chemical tests (Contd.)

Plant constituents/Extracts	Test reagent used					
	Petroleum ether	Benzene	Chloroform	Acetone	Ethanol	Water
Carbohydrate						
Benedict's test						
Molisch's test						
Fehling's test						
Barfoed's test						
Phytosterol						
Libermann-Burchard test						
Salkowski's test						
Fixed oil and fats						
Stain test						
Saponification						
Saponins						
Froth's test						
Haemolysis test						
Phenolic compounds and tannins						
Alkaline reagent test						
Lead acetate test						
Ferric chloride test						
Proteins and amino acids						
Millon's test						
Biuret test						
Ninhydrin test						
Gums and mucilage						
Alcoholic precipitation						
Volatile oil						

Table 7.3: Observation table for TLC

Plant constituents/Extracts	Test reagent used				
	Petroleum ether	Chloroform	Toluene	Ethanol	Ether
Alkaloid					
Carbohydrate					
Fixed oil and Fat					
Saponin					
Phenol					
Tannin					
Protein and amino acid					
Gum and Mucilage					
Volatile oil					
Phytosterol					

EXPERIMENT 2

Aim: To prepare and evaluate marketed formulation of *Churna* (Hingastak *churna* and Trikatu *churna*).

Theory

Definition: *Churna* is a fine powder of drug or drugs.

General method of preparation: Drugs mentioned in the Yoga are cleaned and dried properly. They are finely powdered and sieved. Where there are a number of drugs in yoga, the drugs are separately powdered and sieved. Each one of them (powder) is weighed separately, and well mixed together. In industry, however, all the drugs are cleaned, dried and powdered together by disintegrators. Mechanical sifters are also used. Salt, sugar, camphor, etc. when mentioned are separately powdered and mixed with the rest at the end. Asafoetida (Heeng) and salt may also be roasted, powdered and then added. Drugs like satavari, Guduci, etc. which are to be taken fresh, is made into a paste, dried, and then added.

Characteristics and preservation: The powder is fine of at least 80 mesh sieves. It should not adhere together or become moist. The finer the powder, the better is its therapeutic value. They retain potency for one year and should be kept in air tight containers.

1. Hingastak churna

Table 7.4: Formulation composition of Hingastak Churna

Common name	Botanical name	Quantity
Sunthi	*Zingiber officinalis*	3 g
Marica	*Piper nigrum*	3 g
Pippali	*Piper longum*	3 g
Ajmoda	*Apium leptophyllum*	3 g
Saindhava lavana	Rock salt	3 g
Sveta jiraka	*Cuminum cyminum*	3 g
Krsna jiraka	*Carum carvi*	3 g
Hingu	*Ferula foetida*	3 g

Procedure

Grind the entire ingredients separately. Mix all the ingredients to heeng and make kappad chan *churna*.

Storage conditions: Store in well closed container.

Dose: 1 to 2 g churna with water/ Ghee.

Important Therapeutic Uses

Agnimandya (digestive impairment), Sula (colic Pain), Gulma (Abdominal lump), Vataroga (disease due to vata dosa), Gastric disorder.

2. Trikatu Churna

Table 7.5: Formulation composition of Trikatu Churna

Common name	Botanical name	Quantity
Pippali	*Piper longum*	1 Part
Marica	*Piper nigrum*	1 Part
Sunthi	*Zingiber officinalis*	1 Part

Procedure: Grind the entire ingredients separately. Mix all the three ingredients and make kappad chan churna.

Storage conditions: Store in well closed container.

Dose: 1 to 3 g churna with equal quantity of honey/with ghee or it may be taken with warm water.

Important Therapeutic Uses

Cough, Sneezing, Fever, Arocaka (Tastelessness), Agnimandya (Digestive impairment), Amadosa (Products of impaired digestion and metabolism/consequences of Ama), Gala Roga (Diseases of throat), Pinasa (Chronic rhinitis/sinusitis), Kustha (Diseases of skin), svasa (Dyspnoea/Asthma), Kasa (Cough), Gulma (Abdominal lump), Meha (Excessive flow of urine), Sthaulya (Obesity), Slipada (Filariasis).

Evaluation Procedure

For the evaluation of marketed formulation of curna following tests to be performed:

1. Loss on drying
2. Total ash
3. Acid insoluble ash
4. Alcohol soluble extractive
5. Water soluble extractive
6. pH (1% aqueous solution)
7. Powder microscopy of curna
8. TLC Study.

1. **Loss on drying:** Procedure set forth here determines the amount of volatile matter (i.e., water drying off from the drug). For substances appearing to contain water as the only volatile constituent, the procedure given below is appropriately used. Place about 10 g of drug (without preliminary drying) after accurately weighing (accurately weighed to within 0.01 g) it in a tared evaporating dish. For example, for unground or unpowderd drug, prepare about 10 g of the sample by cutting shredding so that the parts are about 3 mm in thickness. Seeds and fruits smaller than 3 mm should be cracked. Avoid the use of high speed mills in preparing the samples and exercise care that no appreciable amount of moisture is lost during preparation and that the portion taken is representative of the official sample. After placing the above said amount of the drug in the tared evaporating dish, dry at 105 °C for 5 hours, and weigh. Continue the drying and weighing at one hour interval until difference between two successive weighing corresponds to not more than 0.25%. Constant weight is reached when two consecutive weighing after drying for 30 minutes and cooling for 30 minutes in a desiccator show not more than 0.01 g difference.

2. **Total ash:** Incinerate about 2 to 3 g accurately weighed ground drug in a tared platinum or silica dish at a temperature not exceeding 450°C until free from carbon, cool and weigh. If a carbon free ash cannot be obtained in this way, exhaust the charred mass with hot water, collect the residue on an ashless filter paper, incinerate the residue and filter paper, add the filtrate, evaporate to dryness, and ignite at a temperature not exceeding 450°C. Calculate the percentage of ash with reference to the air-dried drug.

3. **Determination of acid-insoluble ash:** To the crucible containing total ash, add 25 ml of *dilute hydrochloric acid*. Collect the insoluble matter on an ashless filter paper (Whatman 41) and wash with hot water until the filtrate is neutral. Transfer the filter paper containing the insoluble matter to the original crucible, dry on a hot-plate and ignite to constant weight. Allow the residue to cool in a suitable desiccator for 30 minutes and weigh without delay. Calculate the content of acid insoluble ash with reference to the air-dried drug.

4. **Determination of alcohol soluble extractive:** Macerate 5 g of the air dried drug, coarsely powdered, with 100 ml of alcohol the specified strength in a closed flask for twenty-four hours, shaking frequently during six hours and allowing to stand for eighteen hours. Filter rapidly, taking precautions against loss of solvent, evaporate 25 ml of the filtrate to dryness in a tared flat bottomed shallow dish and dry at 105°C, to constant weight and weigh. Calculate the percentage of extractive with reference to the air-dried drug.

5. **Determination of water soluble extractive**: Macerate 5 g of the air dried drug, coarsely powdered with 100 ml of water the specified strength in a closed flask for twenty-four hours, shaking frequently during six hours and allowing to stand for eighteen hours. Filter rapidly, taking precautions against loss of solvent, evaporate 25 ml of the filtrate to dryness in a tared flat bottomed shallow dish, and dry at 105°C, to constant weight and weigh. Calculate the percentage of alcohol soluble extractive with reference to the air-dried drug.

6. **Determination of pH values:** The pH value of an aqueous liquid may be defined as the common logarithm of the reciprocal of the hydrogen ion concentration expressed in g per litre. Although this definition provides a useful practical means for the quantitative indication of the acidity or alkalinity of a solution, it is less satisfactory from a strictly theoretical point of view. No definition of pH as a measurable quantity can have a simple meaning, which is also fundamental and exact. The pH value of a liquid can be determined potentiometrically by means of the glass electrode, a reference electrode and a pH meter either of the digital or analogue type.

7. **Powder microscopy churna:**

   For Hingvastak churna:

   Ginger: starch grain, septate fibre with attached vessel, yellow colored oleo resin cells.

   Black pepper: Stone cells, oleo resin cells.

   Long pepper: Stone cells, oil gland, starch.

   Carum carvi: Lignified piited sclerides, vittae, endosperm with oil globule and crystal of calcium oxalate.

   Cumin: Covering trichome, vittae, endosperm.

   For Trikatu churna:

   Ginger: Starch grain, septate fibre with attached vessel, yellow colored oleo resin cells.

   Black pepper: Stone cells, oleo resin cells.

   Long pepper: Stone cells, oil gland, starch.

8. **TLC Study: (Alcoholic extract)**
   - **For Hingvastak churna**

     Mobile phase: Ethyl acetate: Methanol: Water (100:13.5:10)

     Toluene: Ethyl acetate (93:7)

     Spray reagent: Dragendorff's reagent, vanillin sulfuric acid reagent

   - **For Trikatu churna**

     Mobile phase: Ethyl acetate: Methanol: Water (100:13.5:10)

     Toluene: Ethyl acetate (93:7)

     Spray reagent: Dragendorff's reagent

Table 7.6: Results of evaluation parameters

Sl. No	Evaluation parameter	Hingastak churna	Trikatu churna
1	Loss on drying		
2	Total ash		
3	Acid insoluble ash		
4	Alcohol soluble extractive value		
5	Water soluble extractive value		
6	TLC study		

EXPERIMENT 3

Aim: Estimation of total tannin from amla, baheda, harde by titrimetric method.

Requirement: Burette, Conical flask, Volumetric flask, Beaker, Pipette, Thermometer, Measuring cylinder.

Drugs: Amla powder, Baheda powder, Harde powder.

Reagents: 0.1 N $KMnO_4$ solution, 0.1 N Sodium Thiosulphate, Indigo carmine solution, Distilled water, Concentrated H_2SO_4, Starch solution.

Principle: This method is based on redox titration; $KMnO_4$ oxidized tannic acid, Gallic acid, ellagic acid after completion of all tannins. It will oxidize reagent indigo carmine. It is oxidized product give first to green and lastly garden yellow color.

Theory: Tannins constitute a large group of complex organic, non nitrogenous, phenolic compound of high molecular weight and widely distributed in plant kingdom.

Properties of tannin:
- Precipitate protein
- Produce acidic reaction with which are due to polyphenones or carboxylic group

- Solubility: Soluble in water, dilute alkali, glycerin and alcohol.
- Taste: Astringent.

Classification of tannin:

There are mainly three classes of tannins:

1. **Hydrolysable tannins:** For example, Chebulic acid, Gallic acid in myrrobalan
   - Hydrolyzed by acids or enzyme quickly.
   - The products of hydrolysis are Gallic acid or ellagic acid.
   - These tannins show the following tests with $FeCl_3$ gives blue or black color.
   - On heating with HCl, Gallic acid is produced.

2. **Condensed tannins:** For example, catechu, Ketasteral in ashoka bark, Aeaeatechin, Qurcetin in black catechu, Catechin in pale catechu, Kinatannic acid, Kinared in pteraearpus
   - These formed by condensation of many catechu units also known as catechal tannins or phlobatannins.
   - These tannin shows following reaction with $FeCl_3$ they produce green color with dilute hydrochloric acid. Tannins produce phloroglucinol.
   - With vannilin: Alcohol: Hydrochloric acid (1:10:110) shows red color.

3. **Pseudo tannins:** For example, Chlorogenic acid in coffee and nux vomica, Ipecacuanhic acid in ipecacuanha, Catechin in cocoa. They do not obey to gold beater's skin test and low molecular weight compounds.

Chemical tests:

1. With ferric salts gives blue color green, blank or violet color of precipitate this is true tannins.
2. Produce deep red color with $K_4Fe(CN)_6$ and ammonia.
3. **Gold beater's skin test:** It is proto type of untanned fresh skin of an animal and is obtained as a membrane from treated intestine of ox. This membrane is treated with HCl. Rinse with distilled water and then placed in tannin solution for 5 minutes. It is followed by washing with distilled water and putting in $FeSO_4$ solution. A brown or black color is developed, on the skin due to tannins.

Amla

Synonyms: Embelica, Indian goose berry, Amla

Biological Source: It consists of dried as well as fresh fruits of the plant *Embelica officinalis*.

Family: Euphorbiaceae

Chemical Constituents: Rich source of Vitamin C, also contain 0.5% fat, phyllembin and 5% tannins-rich in mineral source like phosphorus, iron and calcium.

Uses

- As an acrid, diuretic, refrigerant.
- Dried fruit given in diarrhea and dysentery also used in jaundice and anemia along with iron compound.
- Alcoholic extract of the fruits is antiviral
- Seed gives asthma and bronchitis.

Harad

Synonyms: Chebulic, Myrrobalan, Haritaki.

Biological Source: It consists of dried ripe and fully matured fruits of *Terminalia chebula*.

Family: Combretaceae.

Chemical Constituents: It is important source of tannin. Tannins are pyrogallol type (hydrolysable) which on hydrolysis yield chebulic acid and α-gallolyl glucose. It also contains Chebulic acid, Ellagic acid and Gallic acid.

Uses

- As an astringent, laxative, stomachic and tonic.
- As an antihelmintic.
- Fruits pulp to treat bleeding
- In treatment of piles and external ulcers.

Bahera

Synonym: Belaric Myrrobalan, Bibhitak.

Biological Source: It consists of dried ripe fruits of the plant *Terminalia belerica*.

Family: Combretaceae

Chemical Constituents: It contains about 20–30% tannins and 40–45% water soluble extractive also contains colouring matter. It contains gallic, ellagic acid, phyllembin, ethyl gallate and gallolyl glucose-seed contain non edible oil.

Uses:
- Use as an astringent in treatment of dyspepsia and diarrhea.
- Gum is used as a demulcent and purgative
- Oil is used for the manufacture of soap.

Procedure

Preparation of drug extract: Weigh accurately 1 gm of each powdered drug and extract in 100 hour distilled water by heating at 70–80°C for 1 hr. Filter the solution and make the volume up to 100 ml.

Estimation of tannins: Take 10 ml prepared extract from stock solution, add 10 ml indigo carmine solution as an indicator, then dilute the solution to 300 ml with distilled water. Heat the solution for 20 minute at 70–80°C. Ttitrate the solution against 0.1N $KMnO_4$ solution till blue to parrot green colour changes to golden yellow. Determine a blank reading also.

Standardization of 0.1 N $KMnO_4$ solution: To 25 ml of $KMnO_4$ solution in a glass stopper flask, add 2 gm of KI followed by 10 ml of 1M H_2SO_4. Titrate the liberated iodine with 0.1M sodium thiosulphate using 3 ml of starch solution added toward the end of the titration as indicator. Perform blank determination and make any necessary correction.

Reagent Preparation

1. **Potassium permanganate:** 0.1N may be prepared by dissolving 31.8 gm of $KMnO_4$ in 900 ml of water heating on water bath for 1 hour cool, filter through sintered glass filter and add sufficient water to produce 1000ml.

2. **Sodium thiosulphate:** 0.1 M may be prepared by dissolving 24.8 gm of sodium thiosulphate in sufficient carbon dioxide free water to produce 1000ml.

3. **CO_2 free water:** water which has been boiled vigorously for few min. and protected from environment during cooling and storage.

4. **Indigo carmine:** 10 ml of HCl and 990 ml 20% W/V nitrogen free sulfuric acid in water and 0.2 gm indigo carmine.

5. **Nitrogen free Sulphuric acid:** A grade of commerce containing not less than 96.0% w/w of H_2SO_4.

6. **Sulphuric acid:** 0.1 M may be prepared by adding 5.4 ml to an equal quantity of water and diluting to 1000 ml with water.

7. **Starch solution:** Triturate 1 gm starch with 5ml of water and add to 100 ml boiling water containing 10 mg of mercuric iodide.

Result: In given powder total amount of tannin found to be:

Amla =

Bahera =

Harad =

Standard Value:

Amla:

Bahera:

Harad:

EXPERIMENT 4

Aim: To prepare and evalute swarna bhasma.

Theory

Bhasmas (Calcinated residue)

It is ashes which are obtained by calcinations of metals, tanin, vegetable and mineral substances by a special process inclosed crucibles or in pits covered with cow dung cakes (puta) is known as Bhasma.

Preparation

The method of preparation of bhasma consists of two steps, the first being sodhana and the second marana. Both the processes are time consuming and need special attention all the white.

Stage I-Shodhan

Purification of mineral, metal or other material used for preparaion of bhasma is called shodhen (Purification). This is two tupes:

1. **Rasaynic (chemical) purification:** Involves removal of the extrageneous contaminating materials.
2. **Aushedhiya purification:** This is performed for following objects.
   a. To removal contaminating substance away from drugs.
   b. To bring/activate the rest medicinal properties of drugs.
   c. To treat drug to achieve some specific/special effects.
   d. To increase the potency of drug.

   Shoden is carried out in two ways depending on the drugs.

1. **Simple Shodhan:** This is applied to most of metals and minerals. Fine parts of metal are heated and are then applied in oil or drug.
2. **Special Shodhan:** Used for certain liquid drugs. This involves the process of:
   1. Bhavano
   2. Swaden
   3. Marden

Stage II- Marana

This is the stage where bhasma is prepared. Here the material obtained from shodhen (stage-I) is mixed with other ingradients for special period of time. Then the mass is converted to small tablets. The shape and size of tablet is determined by the density of material, higher the density of material, thinner should be the tablet. The tablets are dried in sun thoroughly. Dried tablet are placed as single layer in earthen bowel. Its mouth is converted by another bowel, here upside down onces it. The junction between the two is sealed with cloth coated with wet clays by forming 7-layers of such cloth.

Now a pit is prepared in open even which is half filled with dry clay. In the pit, earthen sealed bowels are placed and the remaining part of pit is again filled with clay. Where clay has burned and the pit has cooled. The earthen bowel is removed and tablet permit are recovered which are then finely powdered to fineness, generally ball mill is used for this purpose.

Properties of Bhasma

1. It should be very fine so that it can fill the tiny marks of finger.
2. The bhasma should flat on surface of water where sprinkled over it float.
3. It should not revert back to material as waste stage-1
4. Colour varies form black, gray brown, blooded or red.

Evaluation or Standardisation

1. **Morphological or organoleptic standardization:**

Colour	: Black, gray, brown, blooded or red
Odour	: Odourless
Taste	: No specific
Solubility	: Bhasma float on surface of water
Size and shape	: Very fine powder

2. **Physical evaluation:** Various physical contents are employed:

   Solubility (No. of ml solvent in ml required to dissolve 1 gm of drug)

   Specific gravity:

   Optical rotation:

Refractive index (to establish ientity and purity):

Melting point (Identification of solid substance):

Moisture Content (By loss on drying):

3. **Microscopical standardization:**

   Stomatal index:

   Palisade ratio:

   Vein-islet number:

   Vein-termination number:

4. **Chemical evaluation:**

   Various chemical tests are employed to identify certain drug or their purity.

5. **Biological standardisation:**
   1. **Biological assay:** Biological activity of different drug on different tissue or estimation of poteney of crude drug is done by its effect on living organism like bacteria, virus, fungi, etc.
   2. **Toxicological studies:** Necessary for safe use of drug and its proper dosage.
   3. **Microbial content and potential impurities:** A limit should be deined for microbial content such as total count should 10^3, 10^4 etc or pathogen should be totally absent.
   4. **Metabolic studies:** Drugs are also important to control of the dose to be administered.

6. **Analytical method:**
   a. **Quantitative analysis:**
      i. **Extractive value:** Drug is extracted with solvent such as $CHCl_3$, alcohol, water.
      ii. **Ash value:** Determine inorganic content and amount of salt present in drug.
      iii. **Bitter value:** Evaluated by different bitter taste.
      iv. **Fluorescence analysis:** The fluorescence of drug extract is obtained in UV light.
   b. **Qualitative analysis:**
      i. **Isolation of active principle:** Drug extracted by using different solvent, e.g. H_2O, alcohol, etc. but they don't alter the active principle.
      ii. **Stability of active principle:** The extract should show maximum physical and chemical stability.
      iii. **Identification of active principle:**
          Example of Bhasma:
          1. Tamra
          2. Godanti
          3. Pravala
          4. Mukta
          5. Lauha
          6. Survarna
          7. Shankha
      iv. Colour varies from black, gray, brown, blooded or red.

Storage

- They are stored in air tight, glass or earthen container.
- Bhasmas are quite stable products and maintain their potency for a long time.
- Taste: No specific taste.

Surna Bhasma

Mercury	2 Part
Gold Leaf	1 Part
Lemon juice	q.s.
Sulphur	3 Part

Procedure: Rub the 2 parts of mercury and 1 parts of leaf gold into a mass with lemon juice. Place the mass in crucible with 3-parts of sulphur. The crucible is then covered and expressed to heat. This is repeated for 10-times. When the gold completely losses its metallic character and becomes reduced to dark brown impalable powder.

Storage conditions: Store in well closed container.

Dose: Take the Bhasma with equal quantity of honey/ with ghee/cream.

EXPERIMENT 5

Aim: To prepare and evalute sitoplodi churna.

Theory

Churna (fine powder): These are solid dosage form of medicament for internal use.

Types of Churna: These may be simple or compound.

Simple churna: These contain only one medicament.

Compound churna: These contain two or more than two medicament and prepared by mixing dry mineral, animal or vegetable substances in a pestle mortar.

The dose is 2–3 gm which may be incrased or decreased according to age and seerity of disease. It is administered with water, milk, fruit juices or ether suitable liquid depending on the nature of disease. It may be given by mixing with gur or honey in equal quantity, with sugar twice the quantity and with milk four times the quantities as that of drug.

Preparation of Churna

The drugs are cleaned property, dried throughly and pulverized in a pestle mortar to obtain a better fineness. The powder mixture is then passed through cloth, linen or fine sieve. In case aggery is to be mixed with powder, it should be equal to the quantity of churna and in case of sugar, it should be double the quantity of churna.

Precautions

1. Throughly cleaned and dried drugs should be used for the preparation of churans.
2. They hould be finely sifted.
3. Each substance should be powdered separately and then mixed.
4. Pestle and Mortar used for reducing the particle size and mixing the substances should be clesn and dry.
5. They must be stored in a dry container.
6. They should not be prepared in rainy season.
7. They should dissolve in the stomach contents.

Standardisation

A. Physical standardisation-Techniques used for physical stand of the drugs includes:
- Macroscopic examination.
- Microscopic examination
- Determination of physical constants.

Physical standards are also determined:
1. Foreign matter
2. Moisture content
3. Extractive value
4. Volatile content
5. Ash value
6. Refractive index
7. Optical rotation
8. R_f value

B. Chemical standardization- These are:
1. Extractive value
2. Bitter value
3. Ash value
4. Fluorescence analysis.
5. Volatile content
6. Specroscopy

   1. **Extractive value:** Extracted with different solvent such as ether, chloroform, alcohol, water and their constant extractive value with different solvent are established.
   2. **Ash value:** By finding ash value we can know inorganic content or excessive soil contamination.
   3. **Bitter value:** Bitter drug are used as stomachic and are evaporated by their bitter value evaluation.
   4. **Fluroscence analysis:** Flurosence is obtained under UV light, e.g. Sudarshan churna, Triphala churna, Trikuta churna.

Storage

They are stored in air light, glass or plastic containers.

The churna is free flowing and retains potency for one year.

Examples:

Triphala churna, Trikatu churna, Drakshadi churna and Sudarshan churna.

Sitoplodi Churna

1. Mishri		160 gm
2. Banch lochan		80 gm
3. Piper Badi		40 gm
4. Choti Elaychi (cardnamom) dana		20 gm
5. Dal Chini (*Cassia cinnamon*)		10 gm

Procedure

Grind the entire ingredients separately. Mix all the five ingredients starting from below to upward and make kappad chan churna.

Storage conditions: Store in well closed container.

Dose: Take the churna with equal quantity of honey with ghee or it may be taken with water.

Use: Used in TB, Cough, etc.

EXPERIMENT 6

Aim: To prepare and evaluate Triphala Churna.

Theory: Triphala is a combination of the dried fruits of *Terminalia chebula, Terminalia belerica, and Embelica officinalis* in equal proportions. These are popularly known in India as Harde, Baheda and Amla. Harde and Baheda have a warm energy, while Amla is cool. Triphala, being useful as an internal cleansing, detoxifying formula for everyone including more sensitive type individuals and vegetarians.

Triphala Churna:

Harad chhal ⎫
Baheda chhal ⎬ Equal part
Amla chhal ⎭

Procedure: Grind the entire ingredients separately. Mix all the three ingredients and make kappad chan churna.

Uses: Traditionally Triphala ("three fruits") is a highly esteemed and widely utilized Ayurvedic formula for **gastrointestinal health**. It is traditionally used for digestion and purification and also to maintain a healthy colon, improve digestion and rejuvenate and strengthen tissues. It is taken as a general health tonic, useful for all body types and a variety of conditions. It is commonly prescribed to tone and strengthen the digestive system, particularly in cases of weak digestion and constipation. It is a gentle laxative that can be used daily and is not habit-forming, and has no adverse effects on the intestinal flora (the microorganisms that aid digestion). It is said to improve the function of the stomach and intestines, and is also prescribed for cases of excess stomach acid. It regulates and detoxifies the bowels, improves overall health by increasing the efficiency and absorption of digestion, and reduces gas. It has a balancing effect on the body's metabolism, and is prescribed to restore appetite. It helps the body to eliminate excess fat, by improving metabolism. It also has anticholesterol and antimucus properties in the body. Because of its gentle properties, it is recommended as a digestive aid for the elderly and for those with sensitive stomach. In addition to restoring the balance of the digestive tract, it is used as a blood builder and purifier, and may increase red blood cell count and hemoglobin levels. It is also prescribed for diabetes, for its balancing effect on blood sugar levels. It is believed to strengthen the kidneys and liver, and is prescribed for hepatitis sufferers. It is a source of vitamin C and is believed to improve the function of the immune system. The herbs in Triphala have antiinflammatory properties. The remedy is prescribed for gout (a form of arthritis caused by excess uric acid in the body, and other inflammatory conditions). It also having a calming and tonic effect on the nervous system, and is recommended for

Alzheimer's disease and other degenerative disorders of the nervous system. Another use is to strengthen the eyes, particularly in cases of cataracts, glaucoma, and conjunctivitis. It can be used as eyewash and may reduce soreness and redness in the eyes. It can also be applied topically to the skin to speed the healing of bruises and sunburn.

Modern Pharmacology

Triphala chemically contains compounds known as Anthraquinone, which stimulate intestinal contractions to speed the digestive process. It combines both nutritional as well as blood and liver cleansing (detoxifying) actions. The nutritional aspect is partly in the form of its bioflavonoid, high vitamin C content and the presence of linoleic oil, phospholipids and other important nutrients which it makes more of a tonic. It has little function as a local demulcent but is more of a lubricating source of nourishment and also possesses some bitter anthraquinone which help stimulate bile flow and peristalsis. It is an effective blood purifier that stimulates bile secretion as it detoxifies the liver, helps digestion and assimilation, and significantly reduces serum cholesterol and lipid levels throughout body. It shows cleansing effect by promoting bowel movement. It exerts following actions:

Improves digestion, Antioxidant action, Improves circulation (cardiotonic and capillary strengthening flavonoids), Potentiates adrenergic function (helps the body recover from stress), Lowers blood pressure, Exerts a marked heart-protective and cardio-tonic effect, Reduces serum cholesterol, Improves liver function and is liver protective, Anti-inflammatory action (constituents include Vit C and quercetin), Expectorant action, Anti-viral (HIV, AIDS, herpes, CMV) properties, Anti-bacterial properties, Anti-cancer properties, Anti-allergy properties.

Dose and Dosage Formulations

There are two ways to take Triphala, as a powder or tablet. Traditionally Triphala is taken as a Churna or powder. Stir 2 or 3 g of the powder with warm water and consume the entire amount each evening or divided into three doses throughout the day, between meals if possible or take two to six tablets one to three times daily. Tablets and capsules can be swallowed, while the powder can be mixed thoroughly in a small amount of cold or warm water. The powder can also be simmered in water and drunk as a medicinal tea. Children may only require one or two tablets in the evening. The larger dose is more laxative while the smaller dose tends to be more gradually blood purifying. Triphala can be taken daily as a digestive tonic and laxative; it is best taken in the evening, about two hr. after eating, and at least 30 minutes before bedtime. No food should be eaten for one and a half hours after ingestion. It is not addictive; it can be taken over long periods of time. As eyewash, one teaspoon of Triphala powder can be added to one cup of boiled and cooled water. The solids should be removed by straining through a dense cloth. The eyewash can be applied to the eyes three times per day. For topical application to the skin, the powder can be mixed with a small amount of water to make an easily applied paste.

Precautions:

Triphala is not recommended during pregnancy or nursing. It's 'downward flowing' energy is believed to favor miscarriage and should not be used with cases of diarrhea and dysentery. The most common problem is constipation and bowel irregularity. This can lead to poorer general digestion and liver function, less vitality and perhaps even less optimism and an overall poorer outlook and quality of life.

Side Effects

The use of Triphala may increase intestinal gas at first, as a possible by-product of the cleansing and detoxification effects in the digestive tract. Loose stools or diarrhea may indicate too high dosage, and the amount ingested should be reduced.

Storage conditions: Store in well closed container

Dose: Take the churna with water.

Use: Purgative, Liver tonic, Preserving eyesight, fever.

Standardization

Methodology: A laboratory sample of Triphala churna is evaluated for following parameters to gather the information regarding the quality. The procedures mentioned by WHO guidelines were followed to evaluate these parameters for the standardization. The parameters are:

A. **Physical Standardisation:** Techniques used for physical stand of the drugs includes:
- Macroscopic examination
- Microscopic examination
- Determination of physical constants.

Physical standards are also determined:
1. Foreign matter
2. Moisture content
3. Extractive value
4. Volatile content
5. Ash value
6. Refractive index
7. Optical rotation
8. R_f value

B. **Chemical standardization-** These are:
1. Extractive value
2. Bitter value
3. Ash value
4. Fluorescence analysis
5. Volatile's content
6. Specroscopy
1. **Extractive value;** Extracted with different solvent such as ether, chloroform, alcohol, water and their constant extractive value with different solvent are established.
2. **Ash value:** By finding ash value we can know inorganic content or excessive soil contamination.
3. **Bitter value:** Bitter drug are used as stomachic and are evaporated by their bitter value evaluation.
4. **Fluroscence analysis-** Flurosence is obtained under UV light, e.g. Sudarshan churna, Triphala churna, Trikatu churna.

A. **Description:** Laboratory formulation of Churna was more or less free flowing powder having color dull yellow to olive brown, with a characteristic odour and an astringent as well as a bitter taste.

B. **Powder microscopy of Triphala Churna:** All the three added ingredients of the laboratory samples could be microscopically identified.

Crystals and stone cells were common to all the three ingredients, and therefore did not serve to distinguish between them. Certain epidermal characteristics were, however, useful for the evaluation purpose.

Evaluation parameters of Triphala churna

Loss on drying: A very useful form of dish for the determination of moisture and ash is a thin flat porcelain dish. If a platinum dish is available it may be used. The burning of the powder should proceed slowly and the material must not be allowed to catch fire or to give off smoke as dense fumes.

The most common method for the determination of moisture is to heat the drug till one gets constant weight at 100°C as is done for digitalis however many substances loose other volatile constituents or some of their constituents undergo change with consequent loss of weight at a temperature of 100°C.

Procedure: Weigh about 2 g of the powdered drug into a weighed flat and thin porcelain dish. Dry in oven at 100°C or 105°C. Cool in desiccator and watch the loss in weight which would be recorded as moisture.

Ash Value:

Total ash:

Incinerate about 5 g of drug accurately weighed drug in tared silica crucible at a temperature not exceeding 450°C until free from Carbon (i.e. the residue inside the crucible should become white/Ash colored in appearance) Cool it and weigh. Calculate the percentage of ash with reference to the air-dried drug.

$$\% \text{ Total ash} = \frac{100(W_2 - W)}{(W_1 - W)},$$

where, W = weight of Empty Crucible.

W_1 = Weight of Crucible + Sample before ignition

W_2 = Weight of Crucible + Sample after ignition

Acid insoluble Ash: Boil the ash obtained from total ash content for 5 minutes with 25 ml of dilute HCL. Collect the insoluble matter in Gooch crucible or on the ash less filter paper. Wash with hot water and ignite to constant weight. Calculate the percentage of acid insoluble ash with reference to the air dried drug.

Water soluble Ash: Boil the ash for 5 minutes with 25 ml of water and collect the insoluble matter in Gooch Crucible or ashless filter paper. Wash with hot water and ignite for 15 minutes at a temperature not exceeding 450° Subtract the weight of insoluble matter from the weight of the ash, the difference in the weight represents the water soluble ash. Calculate the percentage of water soluble ash with reference to air dried drug.

$$\% \text{ Total ash} = \frac{100(W_2 - W)}{(W_1 - W)},$$

where, W = Weight of Empty Crucible.

W_1 = Weight of Crucible + Sample before ignition

W_2 = Weight of Crucible + Sample after ignition

Table 7.7: Results of evaluation parameters

S. No.	Evaluation parameter	For laboratory formulation
1.	R_f value	
2.	LOD	
3.	Ash value	
	Total ash value	
	Acid insoluble ash	
	Water soluble ash	

EXPERIMENT 7

Aim: Comparative TLC study of Ellagic acid, Gallic acid, Curcumin in given marketed Pathayadi Kwatha (Sadanga) Churna.

Reagent: Toluene, Ethyl acetate, Formic acid

Theory:

KWATHA CHURNA

Certain drugs or combination of drugs are made into coarse powder (Yavakuta) and kept for preparation of Kasaya. Such powders are called Kwatha *Churna*.

Method of preparation: Drugs are cleaned and dried. They are coarsely powdered weighed as per formula, and then mixed well.

Characteristics and preservation: Kwatha churna as retain potency for one year and should be kept in an air tight container.

Table 7.8: Composition of kwatha churna

Sl. No.	Drug	Quantity
1	Pathya (Haritaki)	1 part
2	Aksa (Bibhitaka)	1 part
3	Dhatri (Amalaki)	1 part
4	Bhunimba (Kiratatikta)	1 part
5	Nisa (Haridra)	1 part
6	Nimba	1 part
7	Amrata (Guduci)	1 part

Dose: 48 g in divided doses

Anupana: Guda

Important Therapeutic Uses: Siroroga (Disease of head), Bhru-sankha-karnasula (Trigeminal neuralgia), Ardhavabhedaka (Migraine), Suryavarta (Sinusitis), Dantapida (Pain in Teeth), Naktandhya (Night blindness)

TLC

Solvent System: Toluene: Ethyal acetate: Formic acid :: 4.5 : 3 : 0.4

Spraying agent: $FeCl_3$ solution

EXPERIMENT 8

Aim: To determine the particle size of the given sample (Nagod) by Sieving method and Optical microscopy.

Theory:

1. Sieving method:

- Particles having size range between 50–1500 μm are estimated by the sieving method. Here the size is expressed as d_{sieve}, which describes the diameter of a sphere that passes through the sieve aperture as the asymmetric particle. This method directly gives weight distribution.

- The sieving method finds application in dosage form development of tablets and capsules. Normally 15% of fine powder of (pass through mesh 100) should be present in granulated material to get a proper flow of material and achieve good compaction in tableting. Therefore % of coarse or fine powder can be quickly estimated.

- Sieves for pharmaceutical testing are constructed from wire cloth with square meshes, woven from wire of brass, bronze, stainless steel or any other suitable material. Sieves should not be coated or plated. There must be no reaction between the material of the sieve and the substance to be sieved.

Table 7.9: Designations and dimensions of IP specification sieves

Sieve no.	Aperture size (μm)	Sieve no.	Aperture size (μm)
10	1700	44	325
12	1400	60	250
16	1000	85	35
22	710	100	36
25	600	120	34
30	500	150	36
36	425	170	35

2. Optical microscopy: Particle size in the range of 0.2–100 μm can be measured by optical microscopy. In this method size is expressed as d_p (projected diameter), which describes diameters of a sphere having the same area as asymmetric particle when observed under microscope. This method directly gives number distribution, which can be further converted to weight distribution. The optical microscope has a limited resolving power (of the lens). The lower limit can be brought down using ultra microscope and electron microscope. Optical microscopy method is used to determine

a. Particle size analysis in suspensions.
b. Globule size distribution in emulsions.
c. Particle size analysis in aerosols.

3. Nagod: Drug consisting of dried leaves of *Vitex nergundo* Linn. Family: Verbenaceae. It is a large shrub of 3–5 m high, distributed throughout the country ascending to an altitude of 1500 m in hills.

Description

Fresh leaf: Lathery, palmatyl trifoliate to pentafoliate, the middle leaflet largest in size, 6–12 cm long, 1.5–3 cm wide with 1–3 cm long petiolate at the base, two lowest lateral leaflet of the pentafoliate leaves are very small and almost sessile, rachis long.

Leaflets lanceolate, acute, entire or rarely crenate, pubescent and dark green on upper surface, tomentose and whitish on lower surface; venation, unicostate reticulate, lateral veins arising at an angle of 45°, almost running parallel to each other.

Characteristic aromatic odour: Bitter in taste

Procedure:

1. Sieving method:
- Arrange the sieves in a net with the coarsest at the top.
- A sample of 50 g of the powder is placed on the top sieve.

- Sieves set is fixed to the mechanical shaker apparatus and shaken for a certain period of time (10 min).
- Powder retained on each sieve is weighed.
- Frequently the powder is assigned the mesh number of screen through which it passes or on which it is retained. It is expressed in terms of arithmetic or geometric mean of two sieves.
- Calculations are done.

2. Optical microscopy:

- Eye piece of microscope is fitted with a micrometer.
- This eye piece micrometer is calibrated using a standard stage micrometer.
- Take powder sample and prepare a suspension with a suitable vehicle such as paraffin oil.
- When water is used as a vehicle, verify the aspects of hydration (swelling) of the particles.
- The sample of suspension is mounted on a slide or a ruled cell and is placed on the mechanical stage.
- Size of the particle is estimated with the help of eye piece micrometer.
- Around 625 particles must be counted in order to estimate the true mean.

Table 7.10: Optical microscopy

Sl.No.	Sieve size (μm)	Sieve size (μm)	Sieve size range	Size range	Mean size (d)	Log mean size	Weight retain in sieve (n)	% frequency
1.	10	1700	10 – 16	1700 – 1000	1350	3.130	0.350	0.350
2.	16	1000	16 – 36	1000 – 425	712.5	2.852	0.140	0.140
3.	36	425	36 – 60	425 – 250	337.5	2.528	85	85
4.	60	250	60 – 100	250 – 150	200	2.3010	3.690	3.690
5.	100	150	> 100	> 150	75	1.875	0.320	0.320
	% cumulative frequency			nd		nd^2		nd^3
	0.350			472.5		223256.25		105488578.1
	0.49			99.75		9950.0625		9925149938
	85.140			2868.75		822972656.3		$2.581090578 \times 10^{12}$
	88.690			738		544644		401947272
	4.01			24		576		13824

$\Sigma nd = 4203$ $\Sigma nd^2 = 823751082.6$

$\Sigma nd^3 = 2.591523164 \times 10^{12}$

1. Average particle size: $\Sigma nd / \Sigma n$

    $= 4203 / 89.5 = 46.93089385$

2. Volume surface mean: $\Sigma nd^3 / \Sigma nd^2$

    $= (2.591523164 \times 10^{12}) / 823751082.6$

    $= 3146.002745$

3. Surface length mean: $\Sigma nd^2 / \Sigma nd$

    $= 823751082.6 / 4203$

    $= 195991.2164$

4. Surface no mean: $\sqrt{\Sigma nd^2 / \Sigma nd}$

    $= 6.82870905$

5. Volume no mean: $\sqrt{\Sigma nd^3 / \Sigma nd}$

    $= 38.30170946$

Particle Size

100 division of eye piece = 94 division of stage micrometer

$$1 \text{ division of eye piece} = 94/100 = 0.94 \text{ μm}$$

8	4	3	6	2	5	7	3	10	4
5	3	8	2	3	5	7	5	4	2
1	3	7	2	6	8	5	6	3	2
1	3	2	6	1	2	8	5	4	3
2	1	1	3	5	8	3	3	2	5
4	3	8	12	5	3	4	15	10	2
2	3	3	4	5	3	4	6	5	3
7	3	5	4	8	5	5	4	3	1
3	5	12	4	4	5	2	1	3	7
8	4	5	5	5	6	5	4	6	2

Table 7.11: Particle size calculation

Class (d)	No of particles (f)	fd
1	7	7
2	13	26
3	21	63
4	14	56
5	20	100
6	7	42
7	5	35
8	8	64
10	2	20
12	2	24
15	1	15
		$\Sigma fd = 452$

$$\text{Average} = 452/100$$
$$= 4.52 \times 0.94$$
$$= 4.25 \text{ μm}$$

Result: The average particle size of the give powder by optical microscopic method is **4.25 μm.**

EXPERIMENT 9

Aim: To prepare and evaluate Chyawanprash Avaleha.

Theory:

Avaleha or leha and Paka–"Linctus"

Avaleha or leha is a semisolid preparation of drugs prepared by addition of sugar, jaggery (gur) or sugar candy and boiled with prescribed drug-juice or decoction. These drugs carry fruit pulp and active ingredient produced in decoction and having natural flavouring agent.

Avaleha having following ingredients:

1. Rshya or other liquid
2. Sugar or jaggery
3. Powdered drug
4. Oil or ghee
5. Honey

Preparation: Sugar candy or jaggery/gur are first dissolved in liquid or Rshya, then filtered to remove foreign particles from it. The solution is then boiled on medium flame till the sugar solution such a consistency where a drop of water added to it sinks rather then dissolves. To such solution the powdered drug is then added slowly with homogenous mixing to form the paste.

When still hot, oil/ghee is added and mixed property. If honey is also required to incorporate as per formula, it must be added when the paste becomes cool. Then mix homogeneously to form final homogenous mass.

Precaution:

1. The Avaleha should neither hard nor a thick fluid.
2. When pulp of the drugs is added and ghee or oil is present, this can be rolled between the fingers.
3. Growth of fungus indicates deterioration.
4. The colour and smell of the preparation depends upon the drugs used.

Storage

1. Avaleha should be kept in glass or porcelain jars.
2. Metal containers which have no reaction with Avaleha may be used.
3. Should be used within one year.

Uses

1. It has antioxidant properties and strengths body's internal defence mechanism.
2. Proetecting infections, cough and cold, stress, etc.

Example:

1. Chayavanaprash
2. Kutajavaleha
3. Draksavaleha
4. Vasavaleha
5. Bilvadileha
6. Surnavaleha
7. Amla ka Avaleha

1. Chyawanprash Avaleha:

These have following ingradients:
 a. Amla Pitthi (roasted in oil or ghee) 8 kg
 b. Prakshep Draviya–have following ingredient:
  1. Bansh lochan- 16 parts.
  2. Piper Badi-8 parts.
  3. Tej Pat
  4. Nagkesar
  5. Dalchini (cinnamom)
  6. Choti ilaychi (cardamom)
 c. **Kwath (Liquid Preparation)** have following ingredients:
  1. Dashmool (10 drugs)
  2. Austawerga (8 drugs)
  3. Punarnava
  4. Agarkashta
  5. Bhumiamlaki
  6. Meda
  7. Mahameda
  8. Ashwagandha
  9. Satavari
  10. Vidarikand
  11. Mulathi (Liquorice)
  12. Draksha
  13. Pushkarmool
  14. Gajpiper
  15. Neel kamal
  16. White chandan
  17. Kateri
  18. Guruchi
  19. Karkatshring
  20. Sugar   20 kg
  21. Honey   2.5 kg

Procedure

1. **Preparation of Amla Pitthi:** Take fresh amla fruit and tied in a muslin cloth and hang up into boiling water and boil the fruits untill they are as soft as broken to touch. Then the fruits are taken out and rubbed on a jute cloth by which a soft mass without fibrous matter is obtained. Then this soft mass of fruits is rosted with oil or ghee or both (According to Charakh both ghee and oil in 1:1 ratio or according to sharangdhar only ghee is used in steel container.
Then this Amla Pitthi is store in steel container or plastic container.

2. **Preparation of Prakshep Draviya:** Grind all the ingredients separately and mixed properly and then make kappad chan churna.

3. **Preparation of Kwath:** Take equal parts of all ingradients of kwath and mixed with 10-time of water (water is used for boiling amla). The mixture is boiled until the concentration of mixture remaining 8-times. Now filter the mixture.

4. **Preparation of final products:** Take filtrate kwath (1/2 or 1/4 volume of kwath obtained by heating). Add sugar and mixed until sugar completely mixed and heat the mixture till the sugar solution such a consistency where a drop of water when added to it sinks rather then dis-

solves. To such solution the Amla Pitthi is then added slowly with homogeneously mixing to form the paste. Honey is added when the paste becomes cool. Now finally prakshel dravya is added and mixed homogeneously to form final homogeneous mass.

Uses:

1. Antioxidant, strengths body internal defence mechanism.
2. Protecting infections, cough and cold, stress, etc.

Estimation of Vitamin-C in Chyawanprash by colorimetry:

Procedure

1. Take 5 gm of Chayvanprash in china dish in 10–15 ml of water.
2. Heat of water bath for 15–20 minutes while stirring by glass rod.
3. The solution should filter through wattman filter paper twice.
4. Colouring matter removed by charcoal (activated) and measures the actual amount of extract.
5. Add 0.5 ml of filtrate and 2 ml of 10 % H_2SO_4 with 4 ml of 10 % Ammonium Molybdate and keep for 60 minutes while make the volume up to 10 ml with water.
6. Take max at 650 nm and measure the constant against standard of 1µg – 10µg ml.

EXPERIMENT 10

Aim: To prepare and evaluate Dhatryaristha.

Theory:

Aristas: "Fermented Preparation"

Definitions: Arisths are medicinal preparations made by soaking the drugs either in powder or in the form of decoction (kasaya) in a solution of sugar or jaggery for a specified period of time. During this process, fermentation takes place and alcohol generated which facilitates the extraction of active principles contained in the drugs.

Arisths having following ingradients:
1. Volatile oil
2. Glycosides and alkaloids
3. Alcohols

Preparation of Arisths: Absolute cleanliness is maintained during the preparation of Aristhas. The wooden pots (vessels) are fumigated with Pippali churna and also smeared with ghee before the fermentation liquids are poured into them. In the processing of aristhas [the crude drugs mentioned in the formula (Patha)] are coarsely powdered and decoction (ahaya) is prepared, fitered and transferred to wooden pots. Sugar, honey or jaggery is added to it, dissolved and boiled. Dravyas, other finely powdered ingradients and Dhataki Pushpa (wood fordia fruticosa) are added to it. The vessel is closed with lid and edges are sealed with clay smeared cloth wrapped in seven consecutive layers. Normally the vessels used for processing of arishta are placed in cellar (basement) for a specific period in order to facilitate Sandhana process (fermentation). The contents are examined for completion of sandhana process and the arishta is filtered and bottled.

Standardization of Arisths

In ayurvedic literatures preparations of different Aristh have been described but no standard have been mentioned regarding the quality of their product and difference in their pharmaceutical preparation.

Generally Arisths contains Volatile oils, gycosides, alkaloids and alcohols. So for determination of these products, standeradization of these compounds are required.

a. Standardization of percentage of volatile oil or evalution of its composition:

By chromatographic method: Volatile oil is removed by treating the arishtas with equal amount of saturated solution of sodium chloride. This is treated with petroleum ether and equal volume of Aristas. Salt solution replaces volatile oil and it is dissolved in light petrol and is removed by distillation. Percentage of volatile oil is determined by TLC or GLC.

b. Isolation and determination of other chemical composion by:
   1. Specific gravity of Arishta's
   2. Total residue drying
   3. Total ash, acid insoluble ash
   4. Clarity, colour, odour, etc.
   5. Microbial examinations, etc.

Determination of alcoholic Contents: This is done by distillation procedure. Following steps are involved:
1. Removal of volatile substances.
2. Distillation of all ethyl alcohol, some ether or water.
3. Dilute the disilllate to four-times, the original volume determining the specific gravity of resulting solution.

Alcohol contents calculated from sp. gravity using table in B.P.C.

Storage Conditions:
1. Solution stored in clear, dried bottles and without any forth (foam) at the top.
2. It should not become sour on tanding.
3. It has characteristic, aromatic and alcoholic odour.
4. Bottles are never filled fully becose of over fermentation in these bottle may burst.

Examples

Kumariasava, Kutarista, Draksharista, Dashmulaista, Vidangarista, Ashokarista, Khadirarista, Dhatryaristha

Dhatryaristha:

Fresh Amla fruits (*Phylanthis amblica*)	2000 pieces
Honey	1/8 of the juice
Powder of Peeper	1/2 Tola
Sugar	1/2 Tola

Procedure

Extract the juice from 2000 fresh Amla fruits and mixes it with 1/8 of its quantity of honey, then peeper churna and sugar. Keep the mixture in an earthen pot soaked with ghee for 15 days. After 15-days, filter the mixture.

Storage: Store in bottles.

Uses: Used for fever, anorexia, respiratory disorder, heart, etc.

EXPERIMENT 11

Aim: To prepare and evalute dashmularishtha.

Theory:

Arista

The medicinal preparations made by soaking the drugs, either in powder form or in the form of decoction (Kasaya), in a solution of sugar or jaggery, as the case may be, for a specified period of time, during which it undergoes a process of fermentation generating alcohol, thus facilitating the extraction of the active principles contained in the drugs. The alcohol so generated, also serves as a preservative.

Method of Preparation

The drugs mentioned in the composition are coarsely (Yavakuta) powdered and Kasaya is prepared. The Kasaya is strained and kept in the fermentation vessel. Sugar, jaggery or honey, according to the formula, is dissolved, boiled, filtered and added. Drugs mentioned as Praksepa Dravyas are finely powdered and added. At the end, Dhataki Puspa, if included in the formula, should be properly cleaned and added. The mouth of the vessel is sealed. The container is kept either in a special room (Alternatively, in an underground cellar or in a heap of paddy, so as to ensure that for the duration of fermentation, as far as possible, a constant temperatures may impede or accelerate the fermentation). After the specified period, the lid is removed, and the contents examined to ascertain whether the process of fermentation (Sandhana) has been completed. The fluid is first decanted and then strained after two or three days. When the fine suspended particles settle down, it is strained again and bottled.

Dashmularishtha

Dasamularishtha is a fermented liquid preparation, made with the ingredients in the formulation composition given below. It contains not more than 10% and not less than 5% of alcohol that is self generated in the preparation over a period of time.

Standardization of Aristh:

Protocol for Standardization:

Standardization of Aristh included the parameter listed below:

1. Description
2. Determination of pH
3. Determination of specific gravity
4. Determination of total solid
5. Determination of alcohol content
6. Determination of total sugar and Reducing sugar
7. Phytochemical analysis
8. Chromatographic fingerprinting
9. Spectroscopic analysis

1. **Description:** It involves organoleptic characteristic like Type, Clarity, Odour, Taste, etc.
2. **Determination of pH:** The pH value of an aqueous liquid may be defined as the common logarithm of the reciprocal of the hydrogen ion concentration expressed in g per liter. The pH value of a liquid can be determined potentiometrically by means of the glass electrode, a reference electrode and a pH meter either of the digital or analogue type.
3. **Determination of specific gravity:** The specific gravity of a liquid is the weight of a given volume of the liquid at 25°C (unless otherwise specified) compared with the weight of an equal volume of water at the same temperature, all weighing being taken in air.

Method: Proceed as described under weight per ml. Obtain the specific gravity of the liquid by dividing the weight of the liquid contained in the pycnometer by the weight of water contained, both determined at 25°C unless otherwise directed in the individual monograph.

4. **Determination of Total solid:** Determination of total solids in Asava/Arista is generally required. Asava/Arista containing sugar or honey should be examined by method-1, sugar or honey free Asava/Aristha and other material should be examined by method 2.

Method 1: Transfer accurately 50 ml of the clear Asava/ Aristha an evaporable dish and evaporate to a thick extract on a water bath. Unless specified otherwise, extract the residue with 4 quantities, each of 10 ml, of dehydrated ethanol with stirring and filter. Combine the filtrates to another evaporating dish which have been dried to a constant weight and evaporate nearly to dryness on a water bath, add accurately 1 g of diatomite (dry at 105 °C for 3 hours and cooled in a desiccator for 30 min), stir thoroughly, dry at 105 °C for 3 hours, cool the dish in a desiccator for 30 min, and weigh immediately. Deduct the weight of diatomite added; the weight of residue should comply with the requirements stated under the individual monograph.

Method 2: Transfer accurately 50 ml of the clear Asava/Aristha to an evaporable dish, which has been dried to a constant weight and evaporate to dryness on a water bath, then dry at 105°C for 3 hours. After cooling the dish containing the residue in a desiccator for 30 min, weigh it immediately. The weight of residue should comply with the requirements stated under the individual monograph.

5. **Determination of total sugar:**

Procedure

1. Pipette out 10 ml Benedict's quantitative reagent solution in a 100 ml conical flask.

2. Add 20 ml of water, 5 g of anhydrous sodium carbonate and a few piece of porcelain to prevent bumping. Heat the flask on a flame to boiling. Keeping the mixture just boling, add this sample (diluted if necessary) in the flask rapidly, until white precipitate begins to form.
3. After this add sample drop by drop at the intervals of 10 seconds until the blue color just disappear. The solution must be kept vigorously boling and be stirred continuously throughout the entire titration.

Dilution: The sample is diluted in such a way that the burette reading is between 5-15 ml, for 10 ml of reagent. For this taken 5 ml of Benedict's Quantitative reagent, add 8 drop of sample, boil and cool.

Green precipitate dilute sample 1 in 2 or 3.

Yellow precipitate dilute sample 1 in 5 or 8.

Brick red precipitate dilute sample 1 in 10 or more.

End point: Complete disappearance of blue color.

Reagent:

1. Benedicts' Quantitative reagent:
 a. Dissolve with aid of heat, 100 g of anhydrous sodium carbonate, 200 g of sodium or potassium citrate and 125 g of dry potassium in 800 ml water and filter if necessary.
 b. Dissolve the 18 g of copper sulphate in 100 ml of water, cool the solution.
    - Add (b) to (a) with constant stirring. Add 5 ml of 5% potassium ferricyanid solution. Add water to make 1000ml.
    - 25 ml of reagent is reduced by 50 ml of glucose.
    - Check the strength by titrating with standard solution of glucose.
    - 1 ml of reagent = 2 mg of glucose.

Principle:
- Benedict's quantitative reagent consist of copper sulphate, potassium thiocynate and other chemicals in alkaline media, copper sulphate is reduced to cuprous oxide by glucose.
- Potassium thiocynate react with cuprous oxide and forms white precipitate of cuprous thiocynate instead of usual precipitate of cuprous oxide.
- Disappearances of blue tint from solution indicate complete reduction of copper sulphate.

Note: In Benedict's quantitative reagent small amount of potassium ferricyanide assist in maintaining the cuprous oxide in solution. The use of sodium carbonate as alkaline instead of sodium hydroxide prevents the destruction of small amounts of sugar.

6. Determination of Alcohol Content:
- The ethanol content of a liquid is expressed as the number of volumes of ethanol contained in 100 volumes of the liquid, the volumes being measured at 24.9 °C to 25.1 °C. This is known as the *percentage of ethanol by volume*. The content may also be expressed in g of ethanol per 100 g of the liquid. This is known as the *percentage of ethanol by weigh*.
- **Apparatus:** The apparatus consist of round bottom flask fitted with distillation head with a steam traps and attached to a vertical condenser. A tube is fitted to the lower part of the condenser and carry distillate into the lower part of 100 ml or 250 ml volumetric flask. The volumetric flask is immersed in a beaker containing a mixture of ice and water during the distillation. A disc with circular aperture, 6 cm in diameter is placed under the distillation flask to reduce the risk of charring of any dissolved substances.
- Transfer 25 ml of the preparation being examined, accurately measured at 24.9°C to 25.1°C, to the distillation flask. Dilute with 150 ml of water and

add a little pumice powder. Attach the distillation head and condenser. Distil and collect not less than 90 ml of the distillate into a 100 ml volumetric flask. Adjust the temperature to 24.9°C to 25.1°C and dilute to volume with distilled water at 24.9°C to 25.1°C. Determine the relative density at 24.9°C to 25.1°C from the Table (in I.P). The value indicated in column II of Table I are multiplied by four in orders to obtain the percentage of ethanol by volume contained in the preparation. The values of Alcohol content is read from table given in Ayurvedic Pharmacopoeia/Indian Pharmacopoeia. If the specific gravity is found to be between two values, the percentage of ethanol should be obtained by interpolation. After calculation of the ethanol content, report the result to one decimal place. If excessive frothing is encountered during distillation render the solution strongly acid with phosphoric acid or treat with a small amount of liquid paraffin or silicon oil. The distillate should be clear or not more than slightly cloudy. When steam volatile acids are present, make the solution just alkaline with one molar sodium hydroxide using solid phenolphthalein as indicator before distillation.

Table 7.12: Observation parameters of Dashmularistha

S. No.	Standard parameter	Standard	Test	Inference
1.	pH			
2.	Specific gravity			
3.	Total solid content			
4.	Alcohol content			
5.	Sugar content: 1. Reducing 2. Nonreducing			

EXPERIMENT 12

Aim: To prepare and evaluate Mahavasava.

Theory

Asava-(fermented alcohol)

These are medicated alcoholic liquors prepared by the fermentation of raw vegetable juices with honey or jaggery or treacle.

Asava having following ingradients:
1. Volatile oil.
2. Glycoside and alkaloids
3. Alcohols

Preparation of Asava

Absolute cleanliness is maintained during the preparation of asava. The wooden pots (vessels) fumigated with pippali churn and also smeared with ghee before the fermentation liquids are poured into them. In the preparation of asava, required quantity of water and jaggery or sugar is taken, boiled, cooled and transferred to fermentation vessel or barrel. Finely powdered crude drugs and other ingredients as mentioned in the formula (Patha) are added to it. The container is covered with the lid and edges are sealed with clay smeared cloth, wrapped in seven consecutive layers. Normally the vessels used for processing of asava are placed in cellar (basement) for a specific period in order to facilitate sadhana process (fermentation). The contents are examined for completion of sandhana process and the asava is filtered and bottled.

Storage Conditions

1. Solution stored in clear, drued bottles and without any forth (foam) at the top.
2. It should not become sour on tanding.
3. It has characteristic, aromatic and alcoholic odour.
4. Bottles are never filled fully because of over fermentation in these bottle may burst.

Examples

Madhukasava, Purnavasava, Arvindasava, Chandanasava, Kanakasava, Lohasava, Mahavasava.

Mahavasava

Ingredients:

1. Khadir (*Aceasia katechu*)	8-parts
2. Devdaru	8-parts
3. Honey	1-parts
4. Loha Bhasma	8-parts
5. Amla, Harad, Bheda, Badi Elychi, Dalchini, Marich, Tejpat, Nagkesar	1- parts
6. Sugar	1-parts

Procedure: Make a kwath (decoction) of khadir and devdaru and filter it. Then powder of all the other ingredient except sugar are mixed in stated quantity with the prepared quath and add sugar and honey. Keep the mixture in a covered iron pot for one month (pot may be kept underground). The Asava is filter and bottled.

Storage Conditions

1. Solution stored in clear, drued bottles and without any forth (foam) at the top.
2. It should not become sour on standing.
3. It has characteristic, aromatic and alcoholic odour.
4. Bottles are never filled fully becose of over fermentation in these bottle may burst.

EXPERIMENT 13

Aim: To find out the Antioxidant activity of kwath.

Reagents: Diphenyl picryl hydrazyl, Ethylene diamine tetrachloro acetic acid, Nitro blue tetrazolium, Riboflavin, Potassium ferricyanide.

Principle:

Mechanism of DPPH method

Free radical scavenging potentials of the extracts are tested against a methanolic solution of 1, 1-diphenyl-2-picryl hydrazyl (DPPH). Antioxidants react with DPPH and convert it to 1-1-diphenyl -2-picryl hydrazine. The degree of discoloration indicates the scavenging potential of the antioxidant extract. The change in the absorbance produced at 517 nm can be used as a measure of antioxidant activity.

Super oxide free radical scavenging activity: Super oxide dismutase enzyme prevents oxidation. EDTA is a best antioxidant. EDTA chelates Riboflavin to prevent degradation of Riboflavin.

Reducing power assay:

Theory: Antioxidants help organisms deal with oxidative stress, caused by free radical damage. Free radicals are chemical species, which contains one or more unpaired electrons due to which they are highly unstable and cause damage to other molecules by extracting electrons from them in order to attain stability. Reactive oxygen species (ROS) formed *in-vivo*, such as superoxide anion, hydroxyl radical and hydrogen peroxide, are highly reactive and potentially damaging transient chemical species. These are continuously produced in the human body, as they are essential for energy supply, detoxification, chemical signaling and immune function. ROS are regulated by endogenous superoxide dismutase, glutathione peroxidase and catalase but due to overproduction of reactive species, induced by exposure to external oxidant substances or a failure in the defense mechanisms, damage to cell structures, DNA, lipids and proteins occur which increases risk of more than 30 different disease processes.

The hydroxyl radical is known to react with all components of the DNA molecule, damaging both the purine and pyrimidine bases and also the deoxyribose backbone. Besides DNA, ROS also attack other cellular components involving polyunsaturated fatty acid residues of phospholipids side chains of all amino acid residues of proteins, in particular cysteine and methionine residues. Interestingly the body possesses defence mechanisms against free radical-induced oxidative stress, which involve preventative mechanisms, repair mechanisms, physical defenses and antioxidant defenses.

Enzymatic antioxidant defenses include superoxide dismutase (SOD), glutathione

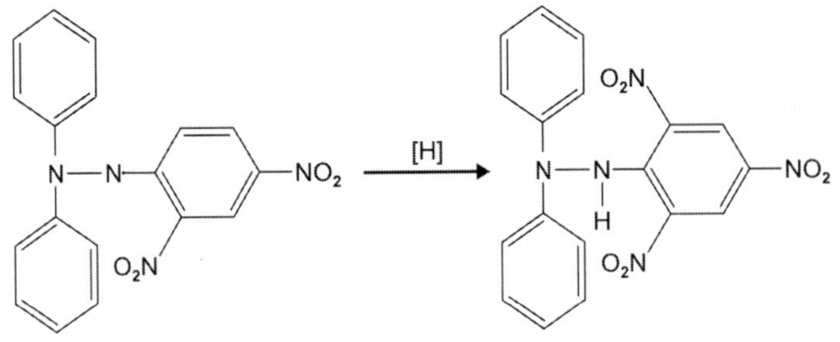

1, 1-diphenyl-2-picryl hydrazyl (DPPH) → [H] → 1, 1-diphenyl-2-picryl hydrazine

Diphenyl picryl hydrazyl

(Purple in color)

↓

(H_2)
Forms nitroxide radicals

↓

As reduction occurs, decrease in colour

peroxidase (GPx), catalase (CAT), etc. Non-enzymatic antioxidants are ascorbic acid (vitamin C), α-tocopherol (vitamin E), glutathione (GSH), carotenoids, flavonoids, etc. All these act by one or more of the mechanisms like reducing activity, free radical-scavenging, potential complexing of pro-oxidant metals and quenching of singlet oxygen. It is possible to reduce the risks of chronic diseases and prevent disease progression by either enhancing the body's natural antioxidant defense or by supplementing with proven dietary antioxidants.

A compound might exert antioxidant actions *in-vivo* or in food by inhibiting generation of ROS, or by directly scavenging free radicals. Additionally, *in-vivo* an antioxidant might act by raising the levels of endogenous antioxidant defences (e.g. by up regulation of gene expression of the genes encoding SOD, catalase or glutathione peroxidase).

Procedure

DPPH method: Dissolve 4.3 mg of DPPH (1, 1-Diphenyl-2-Picryl Hydrazyl) in 3.3 ml methanol and protect from light by covering the test-tube with aluminum foil. Add 150 µl DPPH solutions to 3 ml methanol and take absorbance immediately at 516 nm for control sample. Take different concentration of Kwath and make the volume uniformly to 150 µl using methanol. Dilute each of the samples with methanol up to 3 ml and add 150 µl DPPH to each. Take absorbance after 15 minutes at 516 nm using methanol as blank on UV-visible spectrophotometer. Calculate IC_{50} value for kwath.

Super oxide radical scavenging activity: Mix 100 µl Riboflavin solution, 200 µl EDTA solution, 200 µl methanol and 100 µl NBT (nitro blue tetrazolium) solution in test tube and dilute reaction mixture up to 3 ml with phosphate buffer. Measure the absorbance of solution at 590 nm using phosphate buffer as blank after illumination for 5 minutes. Consider this as control. Take different concentrations of kwath and dilute up to 100 µl with methanol to each of this, mix 100 µl Riboflavin, 200 µl EDTA, 200 µl methanol and 100 µl NBT in test tube and further dilute up to 3 ml with phosphate buffer. Measure absorbance (after illumination for 5 minutes) at 590 nm on UV-visible spectrophotometer. Calculate IC_{50} value for kwath.

Reducing power assay: Dissolve different concentrations of kwath in 1ml methanol and mix with 2.5 ml of phosphate buffer (0.2M, pH 6.6) and 2.5 ml of 1% potassium ferricyanide. Add 2.5 ml of 10% trichloroacetic acid to the mixtures after incubation for 20 minutes at 50 °C. After centrifugation, dilute 2.5 ml of the upper layer with distilled water and add 0.5 ml of 0.1% Ferric chloride. Measure the absorbance at 700 nm. Increase in absorbance of the reaction indicates the reducing power of polyphenol test samples.

In-vitro antioxidant activity of kwath

1. **DPPH (1, 1Diphenyl-2 Picryl Hydrazyl) scavenging activity:** Kwath possessed significant antioxidant activity in a dose dependent manner in DPPH assay with IC_{50} value 89.58 µg/ml.

Table 7.13: Effect of kwath on DPPH free radical scavenging activity

Concentration (µg/ml)	Absorbance ± SD (n = 3)	% inhibition	IC_{50}
Control	0.9		
20	0.650 ± 0.020	27.7 ± 2.2	
40	0.590 ± 0.023	34.4 ± 2.6	
60	0.530 ± 0.027	41.1 ± 3	89.58 µg/ml
80	0.480 ± 0.018	46.6 ± 2	
100	0.420 ± 0.025	53.3 ± 2.8	

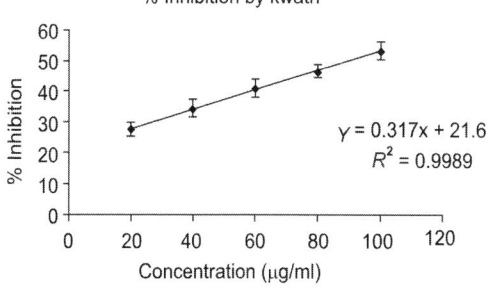

Fig. 7.1: Effect of kwath on DPPH free radical scavenging activity

2. **Superoxide free radical scavenging activity:** Kwath shows dose dependent superoxide free radical scavenging activity with IC_{50} value 91 µg/ml.

Table 7.14: Effect of kwath on super oxide free radical scavenging activity

Concentration (µg/ml)	Absorbance ± SD (n = 3)	% inhibition	IC_{50}
Control	0.834		
20	0.592 ± 0.016	29.01 ± 2	
40	0.550 ± 0.020	34.05 ± 2.4	
60	0.500 ± 0.016	40.04 ± 2	91 µg/ml
80	0.454 ± 0.032	45.56 ± 3	
100	0.385 ± 0.024	53.83 ± 2.6	

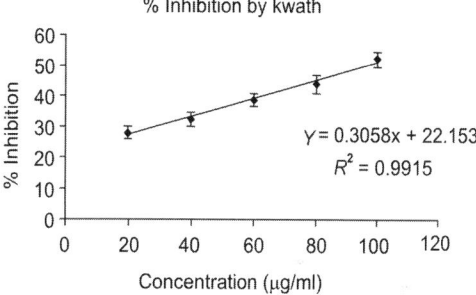

Fig. 7.2: Effect of kwath on superoxide free radical scavenging activity

3. **Reducing power assay:** In this assay absorbance is increased at 700nm with increasing concentration of kwath (20 µg/ml 100 µg/ml) shows reducing power of kwath. The reducing capacity of kwath may serve as a significant indicator of its potential antioxidant activity.

Table 7.15: Reducing power assay of kwath

Concentration (µg/ml)	Absorbance ± SD (n = 3)
20	0.271 ± 0.02
40	0.399 ± 0.1
60	0.554 ± 0.03
80	0.632 ± 0.02
100	0.781 ± 0.01

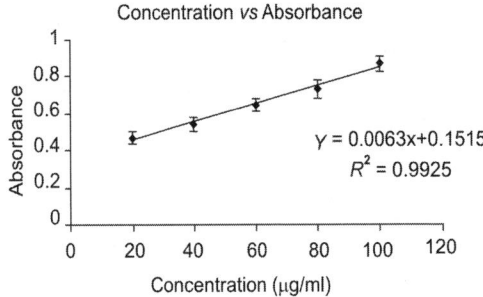

Fig. 7.3: Reducing power assay of kwath

Result: _____

EXPERIMENT 14

Aim: Estimation of total flavonoids content of Kwath.

Requirement: Test tube, Measuring cylinder, Distilled water, Tissue paper, Beaker.

Principle: Aluminium chloride colorimetric method was used for flavanoid determination. The method is based on the quantification of yellow color produced by interaction of flavonoids with $AlCl_3$ reagent.

Procedure:

Preparation of stock solution for quantification of flavonoids: Stock solution of kwath methanolic fraction 1mg/ml was prepared in methanol and used for the estimation of flavonoids.

Preparation of test solution for quantification of flavonoids: 1 ml of sample from stock solution was mixed with 3 ml methanol, 0.2 ml of 10% $AlCl_3$, 0.2 ml of 1 M Potassium acetate and 5.6 ml distilled water. The solution was maintained at room temperature for 30 min; the absorbance of the reaction mixture was measured at 415 nm with UV- Visible spectrophotometer. The % of total flavanoid was calculated from calibration curve of standard flavanoid (rutin) plotted under similar procedure.

Table 7.16: Calibration curve data for rutin

Concentration of rutin (µg/ml)	Absorbance ± SD (n = 3)
10	0.05 ± 0.03
20	0.09 ± 0.01
30	0.13 ± 0.01
40	0.18 ± 0.01
60	0.27 ± 0.02

Fig 7.4: Calibration curve data for Rutin

Table 7.17: Quantification of Flavonoids in kwath

Concentration of Kwath (µg/ml)	Absorbance ± SD (n = 3)	Rutin (µg/ml)	Total flavanoid calculated as rutin per gm dry wt. of kwath Curna
1000	0.231	52.60	3.55 ± 0.25 mg

EXPERIMENT 15

Aim: Estimation of Total Phenolic content of given compound.

Requirement: Test tube, Measuring cylinder, Distilled water, Tissue paper, Beaker

Reagents:

1. *Folin Ciocalteu reagent (1 N):* Dilute commercially available Folin-Ciocalteu reagent (2 N) with an equal volume of distilled water. Transfer it in a brown bottle and store in refrigerator (4°C). It should be golden in colour. Do not use it if it turns olive green.
Laboratory preparation: Dissolve 100 g of sodium tungstate and 25 g of sodium molybdate in 800 ml of water in a 1500 ml flask, add 50 ml phosphoric acid and

100 ml of hydrochloric acid and reflux for 10 hours, cool, add 150 g of lithium sulphate, 50 ml of water. Add 4 to 6 drops of bromine and allow standing for 2 hours. Boil for 15 min cool filter. The reagent should have no greenish tint. Protect from dust. Dilute a portion with an equal volume of water before use.

Principle: The entire phenolic compound is oxidized by folon ciocalteu reagent. This reagent consists of mixture of phosphotungstic acid and phosphomolybdic acid. This is reduced, during the oxidation of phenolic of substance into a mixture of blue molybledenum and tungsten oxide. The blue coloring product produced has a maximum Absorbance at about 750–760 nm. It is proportional to the quantity of oxidized phenolic compound.

2. *Sodium carbonate* (20%): Weigh 40 g sodium carbonate (x $10H_2O$), dissolve it in about 150 ml distilled water and make up to 200 ml with distilled water.

3. *Standard tannic acid solution* (0.1 mg/ml): Dissolve 1 mg in 10 ml of distilled water (always use a freshly prepared solution). Use standard tannic acid sample which is found to be the best. Total phenol content in plant extract is generally determined according to Folin Ciocalteu method.

Principle: This colorimetric method is based on the reduction of a Phoshotunstate phosphomolybdate complex by phenolic to blue color product in alkaline condition. The entire phenolic compound is oxidized by Folin ciocalteu reagent. This reagent consists of mixture of phosphotungstic acid and phosphomolybdic acid which is reduced, during the oxidation of phenolic substance, into a mixture of blue molybledenum and tungsten oxide. The blue color product produced has a max.absorbance at about 750–760 nm. It is proportional to the quantity of oxidized phenolic compound.

Procedure

Preparation of stock solution for quantification of polyphenol: Stock solution of kwath methanolic fraction 1 mg/ml is prepared in methanol and used for the estimation of polyphenol.

Preparation of test solution for quantification of polyphenol: Each of 100 µl of sample is taken in 25 ml volumetric flask, to which 10 ml of water and 1.5 ml of Folin Ciocalteu reagent is added. The mixture is then kept for 5 minutes and 4 ml of 20% w/v sodium carbonate solution is added. The volume is made up to 25 ml with double distill water. The mixture is kept for 30 minutes until blue color developed. The samples are then observed at 765 nm in UV-visible spectrophotometer. The % total phenolic content is calculated from calibration curve of Gallic acid plotted under similar procedure.

Table 7.18A: Calibration curve data for gallic acid

Concentration of gallic acid (µg/ml)	Absorbance ± SD (n = 3)
20	0.05 ± 0.03
40	0.17 ± 0.02
60	0.24 ± 0.03
80	0.39 ± 0.03
100	0.48 ± 0.02

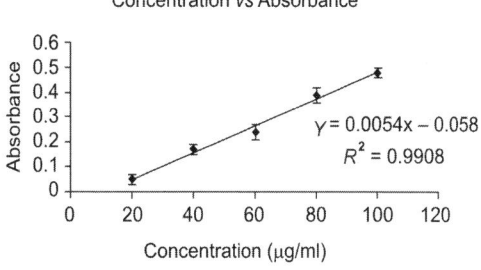

Fig. 7.5: Calibration curve for gallic acid

Table 7.18B: Quantification of polyphenol in kwath

Concentration of Kwath (µg/ml)	Absorbance ± SD (n=3)	Gallic acid (µg/ml)	Total Phenol calculatedas as Gallic acid per gm dry wt. of kwath Curna
100	0.267 ± 0.005	60.18	40.5 ± 0.13 mg

Result: _____

EXPERIMENT 16

Aim: Determination of various Leaf Surface Data (leaf constant of stomatal number and stomatal index).

Requirements: Compound microscope, Stage micrometer, Camera Lucida, Drawing board with black sheet, Chloral hydrate, Glycerin, White pencil

Theory: Microsomal measurement can be made using a stage micrometer in conjunction with eyepiece micrometer camera Lucida or micro projector.

This size of an object or part of it can be measured with the help of two type of micrometer.

1. Stage micrometer
2. Eyepiece micrometer

Stage micrometer:

It is a glass slide (7.6 × 2.5) cm × (3 × 1) inch with a scale engraved on it. The scale is usually 1 or 1.1 mm long and is divided into 0.1 and 0.01 parts of an nm means 1 mm divided into 100 divisions.

$$1 \text{ division} = 1/100 \text{ mm} = 0.01 \text{ nm}$$
$$\text{Or}$$
$$1000/100 = 10 \text{ micron}$$

Eye piece micrometer:

It is a circle of glass with scale attached on the surface. It is small base of glass with a linear scale of 10 mm divided into 1mm and 0.1 mm parts. The value of division varies of with the combination of eye piece of objective lenses.

Camera Lucida:

Magnified image of the object under microscope may be traced on paper. With proper adjusted camera Lucida and illumination it is possible to see simultaneously the drawing paper, the object under microscope, the pencil point and it is easy to trace the required outline. This is much quicker and more accurate than the most skilled freehand drawing but it required. Subsequent addition of details by freehand. Commonly used instruments are:

1. Swift Ives camera Lucida
2. Abbe drawing apparatus.

1. **Swift Ives camera Lucida:** It consists of two prisms. The former fits over the eyepiece and when in use, light to the observer's eye through an opening in the silvered surface of the left hand prism. At the same time light from drawing paper and pencil is reflected by the right hand prism by the silvered surface so that the pencil appear superimposed on the object which may thus be handed.

2. **Abbe drawing apparatus:** It consists of prism fitted over the eyepiece of the microscope and slide draw carrying a mirror which is supported vertically over the tracing a paper. Swift Ives camera Lucida is preferred over the abbe model because; it is small sized and corresponding smaller weight and put strain upon the microscope.

Easy to handle: It does not required adjustment at every reading which abbe model requires adjustment of mirror for each reading

Use of micrometer: It is used to measure microscope object. It is useful for the measurement of starch grains, calcium oxalate, fibers, and oil cells content in the powdered or ignored crude drugs. Mainly for quantitative microscopy it includes:

1. Measurement of length of fibre
2. Determination of umber of fibre
3. Determination of palisade ratio

4. Determination of palisade cells.
5. Determination of stomatal index
6. Determination of vein islet number.
7. Determination of veinlet termination
8. Determination vein termination number

Introduction: Leaves are appendages to the stem which shows a great variety of external form and this makes it difficult to formulate a definition which is to all leaves. There are however two features which are constant, viz Leaves posses neither nodes nor internodes. Branches arise in their axis in the great majority of plants leaves may recognize. In addition by four well-marked character, their flattened form, their thinness, the presence of chlorophyll, the presence of supporting and conducting strands the veins. Leaves are characterized by certain diagnostic structures. Most of the diagnostic characters are microscopic one such as stomata and trichomes, stomatal Index, palisade ratio, vein islet number, etc. All the characteristics shall be referred in detail under microscope character of the leaves.

Stomata: It is made up of two identical guard cells forming a core in centre (stoma means porous or opening). During the formation of stoma the surrounded cells, cut off from the mother Epidermal cells and gets slightly different shape and sizes and these cells are called as subsidiary cells. The primary and secondary function is transportation.

Dicotyledons stomata: Classified into following type depending on number, nature and arrangement of subsidiary cells:

Paracytic stomata (rubiaceous/parellal glands): It comprises two glands cells covered by two subsidiary cells, the long axes of which are parallel to that of stoma, e.g. coca and senna leaves.

Diacytic stomata (caryophyllaceous/cross cells): It comprises two subsidiary cells covered by two subsidiary cells as in case of paracytic stoma but the arrangement of subsidiary cells on guard cells is at right angle to that of stoma, e.g. peppermint, vasaka.

Anisocytic stomata (cruciferous/unequal cells): Number of guard cells are two as in all other cases, but the guard cells covered by the 3 subsidiary cells of which one is markly smaller than the other two, e.g. belladonna, datura.

Anomocytic stomata (ranunculaceous/irregular cells): This type of stomata is surrounded by varying number of subsidiary cells resembling other epidermal cells.

Aclinocytic (radiate cells): The two guard cells are surrounded by a circle of radiating subsidiary cells.

Stomatal number: It is the coverage number of stomata per square mm of the epidermis of the leaf. Stomatal number is affected by various factors like age of plant, size of leaf, environmental conditions, etc. Stomatal index is not affected by these factors. It is relatively constant hence it is more significant in the evaluation of leaf drug.

Stomatal index: It is the % which the numbers of stomata from to the total no. of epidermal cells each stomata being counted as one cell stomatal index can be calculated by using following equation:

$I = S/(E + S)\ 100$

E = Stomatal index

S = number of stomata per unit area

E = number of the epidermal cells in the same unit area.

Procedure:

Determination of stomatal number: Clear the piece of the leaf (midrib part) by boiling with chloral hydrate solution alternatively with chlorinated soda. Peel out upper part and lower part of epidermis separately by means of forceps. Keep it on slide and mount in glycerin water. Arrange a camera Lucida and drawing board (black sheet) for making the drawing to scale. Draw a square of 1 mm by means of stage micrometer. Place the slide with cleared leaf (epidermis) on the stage. Trace the epidermis and stomata. Count the number of stomata present in the area of

1 mm². Include the cell of if at least half of its area lies within the square. Record the result for each of the ten fields and calculate the number of stomata per sq.mm.

Determination of stomatal index: Preparation is same as mentioned above. Count the number of stomata also the number of epidermis cells in each field. Calculate the stomatal index using the formula. Determine the values for upper and lower (epidermis) separately.

Result:

Table 7.19: Determination of various leaf surface data

Sl.No	Stomatal number	Number of epidermal cell	Stomatal index
1			
2			
3			
4			

Average

EXPERIMENT 17

Aim: To determine the total ash and acid insoluble ash of given drug. (*Withania Somnifera*/Black pepper*)*.

Requirements: Silica crucibles, Desiccator, Ashless filter paper, dilute hydrocholic acid, powdered drug

Theory: Ash value are helpful in the determining the quality and purity of crude drug, especially in powdered form.

Procedure

a. Determination of total ash
1. Weigh accurately 3 gm of powdered drug in silica silica crucible.
2. Incinerate the powdered drug by gradually increasing the heat until free from carbon and cool. Keep it in desiccator.
3. Weigh the ash and calculate the percentage of total ash with reference to the air dried drug sample.

b. Determination of acid- insoluble ash
1. Boil the total ash obtained as above for 5 minutes with 25 mL of dilute HCl.
2. Filter and collect the insoluble matter on ashless filter paper, wash the filter paper with hot water, ignite in silica crucible, cool and keep in desiccator.
3. Weigh the residue and calculate acid-insoluble ash of drug with reference to air dried drug.

Result:
1. Total ash of given powdered drug is found _____ %.
2. Acid–insoluble ash of given powdered drug is found_____

EXPERIMENT 18

Aim: To determine ash value of a given powdered crude drug (Liquorice).

Procedure

Determination of total ash value:
1. Weigh and ignite flat, thin, porcelain dish or a tared silica crucible.
2. Weigh about 2 g of the powdered drug into the dish/crucible.
3. Support the dish on a pipe-clay triangle placed on a ring of retort stand.
4. Heat on a burner, using a flame about 2 cm high and supporting the dish about 7 cm above the flame, heat till vapors almost cease to be evolved; then lower the dish and heat more strongly until all the carbon is burnt off.
5. Cooled in a dessicator.
6. Weighed the ash and calculated the percentage of total ash with reference to the air dried sample of the crude drug.

If a carbon free ash cannot be obtained in this way then any one of the following method can be used:
1. Exhaust the charred mass with hot water, collect the residue on an ash less filter paper incinerate the residue and filter paper, add the filtrate, evaporate

to dryness and ignite at a temperature not exceeding 450°C.

2. Cooled the crucible; add 15 ml of alcohol, break up the ash with glass rod burn off the alcohol and again heat the whole to a dull red heat. Cool and weighed the ash.

Calculation:

weight of the empty dish = X

weight of the drug taken = Y

weight of the dish + ash (after complete incineration) = Z

weight of the ash = $(Z - X)$ gm

'Y' g of the crude drug gives $(Z - X)$ gm of the ash

Hence, 100 g of the crude drug gives $100/Y \times (Z - X)$ gm of the ash.

Total ash value of the sample
$$= 100 (Z - X)/Y \%$$

Determination of Acid – Insoluble Ash Value:

1. Using 25 ml of dil. HCl acid, washed the ash from the dish used for total ash into a 100 ml beaker.
2. Placed a wire gauze over a Bunsen burner and boil for five minutes.
3. Filtered through an ash less filter paper, washed the residue twice with hot water.
4. Ignite a crucible in the flame, cool and weigh.
5. Put the filter paper and residue together into the crucible; heated gently until vapors cease to be evolved and then more strongly until all carbon has been removed.
6. Cool in a dessicator.
7. Weigh the residue and calculated acid – insoluble ash of the crude drug with reference to the air-dried sample of the crude drug.

Calculation:

Weight of the residue = 'A' gm
(acid insoluble ash)

'Y' gm of the air-dried drug gives = 'A' g of acid insoluble ash.

Hence, 100 g of the air-dried drug gives $100 \times A/Y$ gm of acid insoluble ash

Acid – insoluble ash value of the sample = $100 \times A/Y \%$

Acid-insoluble ash value of a crude drug is always less than total ash value of the same drug.

Determination of Water soluble ash:

This is determined in a similar way to acid insoluble ash, using 25 ml. of water, in place of dil. HCl acid.

Result: _____

EXPERIMENT 19

Aim: To determine extractive value of a given powdered crude drug (Liquorice).

Procedure

Determination of Alcohol-soluble extractive values:

1. Weighed about 4 gm of the powdered drug in a weighing bottle and transfer it to a dry 250 ml. conical flask.
2. Filled a 100 ml. graduated flask to the delivery mark with the solvent (90% alcohol).
3. Washed out the weighing bottle and pour the washings, together with the remainder of the solvent into the conical flask.
4. Cork the flask and set aside for 24 hrs, shaking frequently (maceration).
5. Filtered into a 50 ml cylinder. When sufficient filtrate has collected, transfer 25 ml. of the filtrate to a weighed, thin porcelain dish, as used for the ash values determinations.
6. Evaporated to dryness on a water bath and complete the drying in an oven at 100°C.
7. Cooled in a dessicator and weighed.
8. Calculated the percentage w/w of extractive with reference to the air-dried drug.

Calculation

25 ml. of alcoholic extract gives 'x' gm of residue.

100 ml. of alcoholic extract gives = '$4x$' gm of residue.

Since 4 gm of air dried drug gives $4x$ gm of alcohol (90%) soluble residue.

Hence 100 gm of air dried drug gives $75x$ gm of alcohol (90%) soluble residue.

Alcohol (90%) soluble extractive value of the sample = $75x$ %

Determination of Water-soluble extractive values:

Steps are similar. Use Chloroform water instead of alcohol (90%).

Chloroform acts as a preservative.

Result: _____

EXPERIMENT 20

Aim: To determine the amount of ethanol present in the given sample of Asava or Arista.

Apparatus

The apparatus consist of round bottom flask fitted with distillation head with a steam traps and attached to a vertical condenser. A tube is fitted to the lower part of the condenser and carry distillate into the lower part of 100 ml or 250 ml volumetric flask. The volumetric flask is immersed in a beaker containing a mixture of ice and water during the distillation. A disc with circular aperture, 6 cm in diameter is placed under the distillation flask to reduce the risk of charring of any dissolved substances.

Method

Transfer 25 ml of preparation being examined accurately measured at 24.9 °C to 25.1 °C to the distillation flask. Dilute with 150 ml of water and add a little pumice powder. Attach the distillation head and condenser. Distill and collect not less than 90 ml of distillate into 100 ml volumetric flask. Adjust the temperature to 24.9°C to 25.1°C and dilute to volume with distilled water with at 24.9 °C to 25.1 °C. Determine the relative density at 24.9 °C to 25.1 °C from the Table (in I.P). The value indicated in column II of table I are multiplied by four in orders to obtain the percentage of ethanol by volume contained in the preparation. If the specific gravity is found to be between two values, the percentage of ethanol should be obtained by interpolation. After calculation of the ethanol content, report the result to one decimal place.

Note

1. If excessive frothing is encountered during distillation render the solution strongly acid with phosphoric acid or treat with a small amount of liquid paraffin or silicon oil.

2. The distillate should be clear or not more than slightly cloudy. When steam volatile acids are present, make the solution just alkaline with one molar sodium hydroxide using solid phenolphthalein as indicator before distillation.

EXPERIMENT 21

Aim: Estimation of total alkaloids.

Reagents: H_2SO_4, NH_3, $CHCl_3$

Theory: The general method for extraction of alkaloid can be summarized as following:

Principle: The moistened drug is treated with alkali so as to set free the base as it exist in salt in salt form and then to separate free base with organic solvent. Then treat with acid for complete excretion. After complete extraction, the aqueous phase is made alkaline with ammonia. The basic aqueous solution is then extracted with convenient organic solvent followed by drying of alkaloid containing solution, normally with sodium sulphate.

Procedure: Take accurately weighed quantity of 10 gms of the drug, then moistened with 10% alcoholic potassium hydroxide and then extract three times with 50, 30, 20 ml benzene.

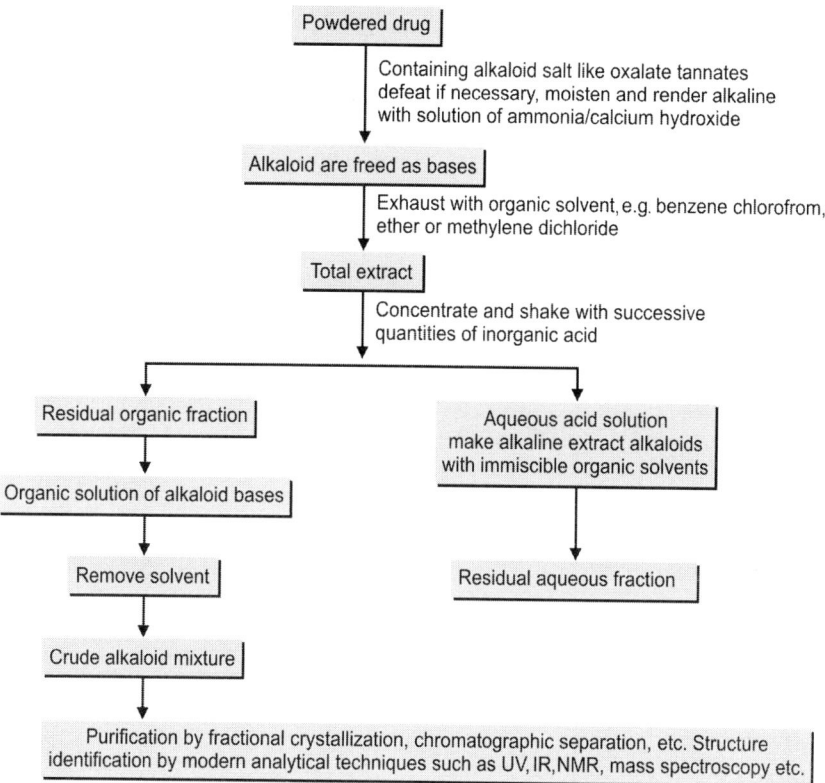

Fig. 7.6: Flow diagram for estimation of total alkaloids

Pour out all extract and shake with 20, 15, 10 ml of 0.5 N H_2SO_4 for complete extraction. Filter all the combined extract in to a separating funnel, make alkaline to litmus with dilute NH_3 solution. Extract the liberated alkaloids with successive portions of 20, 15, 10 ml of chloroform to bring complete extraction and wash the combined organic extract with 10 ml portion of H_2O. Again extract two 10 ml portion of chloroform. Add the chloroform washing to the main chloroform extract and filter the whole in a 100 ml conical flask. Evaporate $CHCl_3$ on a water bath until a few ml are left and remove the solvent completely by using a vaccum dessicator. Add 5 ml of alcohol (90%) of the residue and again evaporate the solvent. Repeat the evaporation with alcohol, dry the residue to a constant weight in the vaccum dessicator and weigh as total alkaloids and perform TLC.

Solvent system: Ethyl acetate: Methanol: Water

Spraying reagent: Dragendorff 's reagent

Result: _____

EXPERIMENT 22

Aim: Preparation and evaluation of prepared herbal cream.

Introduction

Cold cream: The term 'cold' is possibly due to the cooling sensation caused by evaporation of the water in the cream after it is applied to the skin. Creams (cold creams, cleansing creams) may be divided into oil in water (beeswax borax types) and water in oil creams (beeswax without additional alkali). Absorption bases are to be recommended for the preparation of water in oil emulsions that are stable, white and fine textured and has emollient value, these products consist of special grade of petrolatum containing concentrated derived from lanolin which has a great water holding power. These bases can hold almost five times their weight of water and when properly used lead to fine products. Water in oil creams is generally made by melting together the oily components of the mixture and then allowing the mixture to cool about 40°C or to incipient solidification.

Table 7.20: Formula of beeswax borax type cold cream (Tulsi and Neem leaf extracts)

Ingredients	Quantity prescribed	Quantity taken
A Beeswax	2.0 gm	1.0 gm
Almond oil	50.0 gm	25 gm
Lanolin	0.5 gm	0.25 gm
B Borax Tulsi and Neem leaf extract	2.0 gm 35.5 gm	1.0 gm 17.75 gm
Preservatives	q.s	q.s
C Perfume	q.s	q.s
Total weight	**100 gm**	**50 gm**

General procedure for manufacturing

As these preparations are emulsion type, the total ingredient can be classified into oil phase and aqueous phase. Ingredients of oil phase should be taken in increasing melting point. The materials of least melting point should be taken and melt it. Add the other oil or wax gradually in increasing melting point and melt them with continuous stirring. Take separately the ingredients of aqueous phase and mix them and heat to same temperature as oil phase. Emulsifying agents should be added to specific phase. Mix the two phases with continuous stirring until a smooth cream is formed. Finally the product can be milled by triple roller mill. Preservatives should be dissolved in the water before making cream. Perfume should be added after the primary cream is formed and cooled but before final milling.

Table 7.21: Formula of emulsified cleansing cream (Turmeric extract)

Ingredients	Quantity prescribed	Quantity taken
Bees wax	4.0 gm	2.0 gm
Paraffin	10.0 gm	5.0 gm
White petrolatum	10.8 gm	5.4 gm
Mineral oil	55.0 gm	27.5 gm
Turmeric extract (5%)	18.0 gm	9.0 gm
Borax	1.2 gm	0.6 gm
Glycerin	1.0 gm	0.5 gm
Total weight	**100 gm**	**50 gm**

Procedure for cream: Heat the oily phase in a jacketed vessel at about 70°C. Pour the aqueous phase into the oily phase. Stir continuously for a period till a smooth, white emulsion is produced. Add perfume at about 40°C and mix well. Pour into jars or fill into tubes.

Table 7.22: Formula of soft cold cream (Turmeric cream)

Ingredients	Quantity prescribed	Quantity taken
Bees wax	6.0 gm	3.0 gm
Paraffin	12.5.0 gm	6.25 gm
White petrolatum	8.0 gm	4.0 gm
Mineral oil	58.0 gm	29.0 gm
Turmeric extract (5%)	15.6 gm	7.8 gm
Borax	0.2 gm	0.1 gm
Total weight	**100 gm**	**50 gm**

Procedure for cream: The waxes, petrolatum and mineral oil are melted together and brought to 65 °C–70 °C. The water containing the potassium carbonate and borax in solution is run in at the same temperature. Stirring is continued until cool. After adding perfume, the cream is allowed to stand overnight and filled by warming slightly until just liquid.

Evaluation Parameter of Preparaed Herbal Creams

A. Physical Evaluation: It include following parameters:
- pH
- Hardness
- Viscosity
- Turbidity
- Emulsion type
- Softening point
- Water evaporation

B. Rheology: It is very important as these creams are marketed in tubes or containers. The rheology or viscosity should remain constant. As these products are normally nonnewtonian in nature, the viscosity can be measured using viscometer used for such liquids. It include following parameter:
- Spreadibility
- Pourability

Sensitivity test: As various types of ingredients are used with occasional use of antiseptics, hormones, etc. there is a possibility of sensitization of the skin. This should be tested before hand. This test is normally done by patch test on skin and can be either open or occlusive. The test sample is applied along with a standard marker product at different places and effect is compared after period of time.

C. Accelerated stability test studies: This method of evaluation not only indicates stability of functional ingredient. Following are test included in that,

Cyclical temperature tests: These tests are not carried out at fixed temperature and humidity. In these tests, temperature is changed cyclically every day e.g. low- high-low-high, to stimulate changes in temperature daily.

Stress test: This test has been designed taking into consideration the overall stress and time period of actual usage. This test indicates the stable life span of the product from the physical changes that may be monitored include changes in separability and emulsion particles. It is commonly applied to liquid emulsion.

    I. Centrifugal separation method: In this method, the cosmetics product in its container is subjected to centrifugal force. Speed of centrifugation is kept constant. After spinning, separation is measured. These results can be compared with stability testing in static condition.

    II. Vibration test: This method is used to assess effect of vibrations. This will required study of the amplitude. After assessing these, vibration machine can be set for carrying out experiments.

Result: _____

EXPERIMENT 23

Aim: To determine saponification value of the given sample of oil.

Appratus: 200 ml flask with a reflex condenser, water bath.

Method:

Introduce about 2 gm of the substance being examined, accurately weighed into a 200 ml flask of borosilicate glass fitted with a reflex condenser. Add 25 ml of 0.05M ethanolic potassium hydroxide and a little pumice powder and boil under reflex on a water bath for 30 minutes. Add 1 ml of Phenolphthalein solution and titrate immediately with 0.5M hydrochloric acid (a ml). Repeat the operation omitting the substance being examined (b ml). Calculate the saponification value from the expression:

$$\text{Saponification value} = \frac{28.05\,(a-b)}{W}$$

where, W = Weight of the substance.

Note: If the oil has been saturated with carbon dioxide for the purpose of preservation, gently reflex the solution of the oil in ethanol

(95%) and either for 10 minutes, before titration. The oil may be freed from the carbon dioxide by exposing it in a shallow dish in a vacuum desicator for 24 hr before weighing the same.

EXPERIMENT 24

Aim: Determination of Leaf Constant Data (leaf constant of vein islet and veinlet termination number).

Requirement: Leaf sample, Microscope, Camera Lucida, Stage micrometer, Drawing sheet, White pencil

Reagents: Chloral hydrate solution.

Determination of vein-islet number

Theory

Definition: A vein-islet is the small area of green tissue surrounded by the veinlets. The vein-islet number is the average number of vein-islets per square millimeter of a leaf surface. It is determined by counting the number of vein-islets in an area of 4 sq.mm. of the central part of the leaf between the midrib and the margin.

The drugs and its vein-islet number are given below:

Cassia angustifolia:	19 to 23
Cassia acutifolia:	25 to 30
Digitalis purpurea:	2 to 5.5
Digitalis thapsi:	8.5 to 16

Procedure: Clear a piece of the leaf by boiling in chloral hydrate solution for about 30 minutes. Arrange camera lucida and drawing sheet for making drawings to scale. Place stage micrometer on the microscope and using 16 mm objective, draw a line equivalent to 1 mm as seen through the microscope. Construct a square on this line. Move the paper so that the square is seen in the eye piece in the centre of the field. Place the slide with the cleared leaf (epidermis on the stage). Trace off the veins which are included within the square completing the outlines of those islets which overlap two adjacent sides of the square. Count the number of vein islets in the square millimeter. Where the islets are intersected by the sides of the square include those on two adjacent sides and exclude those islets on the other sides. (To obtain a critical result for a leaf, 4 mm should be used, preferably in one large area of 4 mm^2). Find the average number of vein number of vein islets from the four adjoining squares to get the value for one sq.mm.

Determination of veinlets termination number:

Theory

Definition-Vein termination number is defined as the number of vein termination per sq. mm of the leaf surface, midway between midrib of the leaf and its margin. A vein termination is the ultimate free termination of veinlet.

Vein termination number of *Cassia acutifolia* is between 25–29.5

Procedure: Same as for 'Determination of Vein-islet number'. Count the number of veinlet termination present within the square. Find the average number of veinlet termination number from the four adjoining squares to get the value for one mm^2.

Result: _____

EXPERIMENT 25

Aim: To identify constituents of given herbal drug preparation by chromatographic method.

Requirements: Filter paper, herbal drug preparation, TLC chambers, glass rods, rubber stoppers, solvent system, etc.

Theory: Chromatography comprises a group of methods for separating molecular mixtures that depends on the differential affinities of the solutes between two immiscible phases. One of the phases is a fixed bed of large surface area, whereas the other is a fluid that moves through, or over the surface of the fixed phases. The fixed phase is called the stationary phase, and the other is termed the mobile phase. Thin layer chromatography is an important analytical tool in the separation, identification and estimation of different classes of natural products. The method based on physico-chemical phenomenon of adsorption is rapid and permits the use of corrosive spraying reagents.

Procedure

1. Prepare filter paper strips for the purpose of paper chromatography.
2. Prepare the solvent system (chloroform: methanol: ammonia: : 60 : 10 : 1) and pour it to a depth of 3 cm in the chamber lined from inside with a filter paper to maintain the equilibrium of the mobile phase. Allow the chamber and filter paper strip to saturate for 2–3 hours.
3. Apply spots of sample and standard solution on paper strips and allow to dry at room temperature.
4. Develop the chromatogram up to 10 cm. Take out the paper, mark the solvent front and dry at room temperature.
5. Spray the paper with detecting reagent and dry at room temperature for about 5–10 minutes. Identify the components of the herbal preparation by comparing their location and R_f values with that of standard solution.

Calculations:

$$R_f = \frac{\text{Distance travelled by the component}}{\text{Distance travelled by the solvent front}}$$

Result: On comparison of R_f values the given mixtures is found to contain

EXPERIMENT 26

Aim: To separate active principles of plant materials by Column Chromatography and High Pressure Liquid Chromatography (HPLC).

Theory: Natural products are those chemical compounds derived from living organisms, plants, animals, insects and the study of natural products is the investigation of their structure, formation, use and purpose in the organism. Drugs derived from natural products are usually secondary metabolites and their derivatives and today those must be pure and highly characterized compounds. A plant cell produces two types of metabolites:

Primary metabolites involved directly in growth and metabolism, viz., carbohydrates, lipids and proteins.

Secondary metabolites considered as end products of primary metabolism and are in general not involved in metabolic activity, viz. alkaloids, phenolics, essential oils, steroids, lignins, tannins, etc. Primary metabolites are produced as a result of photosynthesis and these products are further involved in the cell component synthesis.

In general, primary metabolites obtained from higher plants for commercial use are high-volume low-value bulk chemicals. They are primarily used as industrial raw materials, foods or food additives; for examples- vegetable oils, fatty acids (used for making soaps and detergents) and carbohydrates (sucrose, starch, pectin and cellulose). However, some primary metabolites like myo-inositol and β-carotene are expensive because their extraction, isolation and purification are difficult.

Secondary metabolites are compounds biosynthetically derived from primary metabolites but more limited in occurrence in the plant kingdom, may be restricted to a particular taxonomic group (genus, species or family). As mentioned above, secondary metabolites are mostly accumulated by plant cells in smaller quantities than primary metabolites. These secondary metabolites are synthesized in specialized cells at particular developmental stages, making their extraction and purification difficult (compared to the primary product produced by the whole plant or organ).

Since the medicinal plants are those rich in secondary plant products their compounds are termed as 'medicinal' or 'officinal'. These secondary metabolites or products exert in general, a profound physiological effect on the mammalian system and thus known as the active principle of that plant. The physiological effect of these active principles is used for curing ailments and therefore these are drugs of plant origin or natural drugs. The use of crude drugs of plant origin (unpurified preparations of active principles, plant extract or some times powdered plant material) is used in the Indian system of medicine or 'Ayurveda'.

Extraction procedure: The following procedure is used for preparation of extracts and column chromatography.

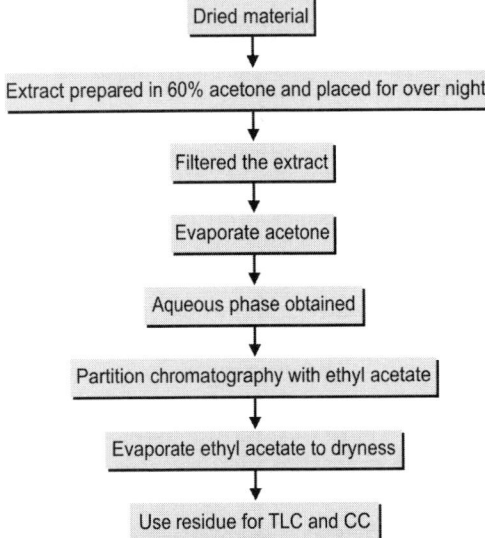

Fig. 7.7: Flow diagram of extraction

Thin Layer Chromatography (TLC)

Thin layer chromatography of crude extract, fractions obtained by column chromatography and other solvent fractions are performed using pre-coated silica gel G60 plates with/without fluorescent indicator using following solvent systems. The R_f is calculated as follows:

$$R_f = \frac{\text{Distance travelled by substance}}{\text{Distance travelled by solvent}}$$

Solvent used in TLC analysis of the crude extract are listed below:

1. Chloroform : Methanol : Acetic Acid :: 85 : 15 : 3
2. Chloroform : Methanol : Acetic Acid :: 90 : 10 : 0
3. Chloroform : Methanol : Acetic Acid :: 90 : 7 : 3
4. Chloroform : Methanol : Acetic Acid :: 90 : 10 : 3

Out of four solvents used, the solvent system at No. 3 is observed best for the separation.

Column Chromatography

The drug extract is used for column. Separation of compounds by column chromatography is one of the most widely used techniques in biochemical work and is the only technique for the separation of secondary metabolites in large quantities.

Preparation of the material: A wide range of materials is used in chromatographic separations (silica, alumina, sephadex, resin) and all need to be equilibrated with the solvent before preparing the column. In addition, some form of pretreatment is often required; for example some gel filtration materials need to be swollen, adsorbents need to be activated by heating or acid treatment, and ion exchange resins have to be obtained in the required ionized form by washing.

During the equilibration with solvent the material is allowed to settle and the fine particles remaining in suspension are removed by decantation. If this is not carried out, the flow rate of solvent down the column will be considerably reduced due to clogging by these fine particles.

a. **Pouring of the column:** The chromatography column is packed with silica by filling it about one-third full with solvent and slowly adding slurry of the material in the solvent. This is carefully poured down a glass rod, as shown to stop air bubbles being trapped in the column. The suspension is allowed to settle and excess solvent run off. This process is repeated until the column is the required height. The column is then washed thoroughly with solvent and the level of the liquid kept just above the surface of the material.

A filter paper disc may be placed carefully to pour mixture without disturbing the column.

b. **Application of the sample:** Weighed quantity of the sample is first dissolved in the solvent before loading it on to the column. In most class experiments the concentrated sample is carefully pipetted on to the surface and the tap opened until the top of the column is just below the level of the meniscus. The solvent reservoir is connected, and a constant head of liquid maintained at the top of the column from a pressure reservoir.

c. **Elution:** The next stage is to remove the materials from the column in order by eluting with an appropriate solvent. In displacement development, the solvent interacts more strongly with the chromatographic material than the compound on the column, than displacing the bound molecules. Large quantities of material can be separated in this way since about 50% of the total column capacity is used. The separation is adequate but for better resolution of peaks elution development is preferred. In this case, no more than 10% of the total capacity is loaded on to the column. The solvent interacts with the column weaker than the solute molecules and overrides the bound molecules gradually eluting them from the column. This is probably the most commonly used means of elution and

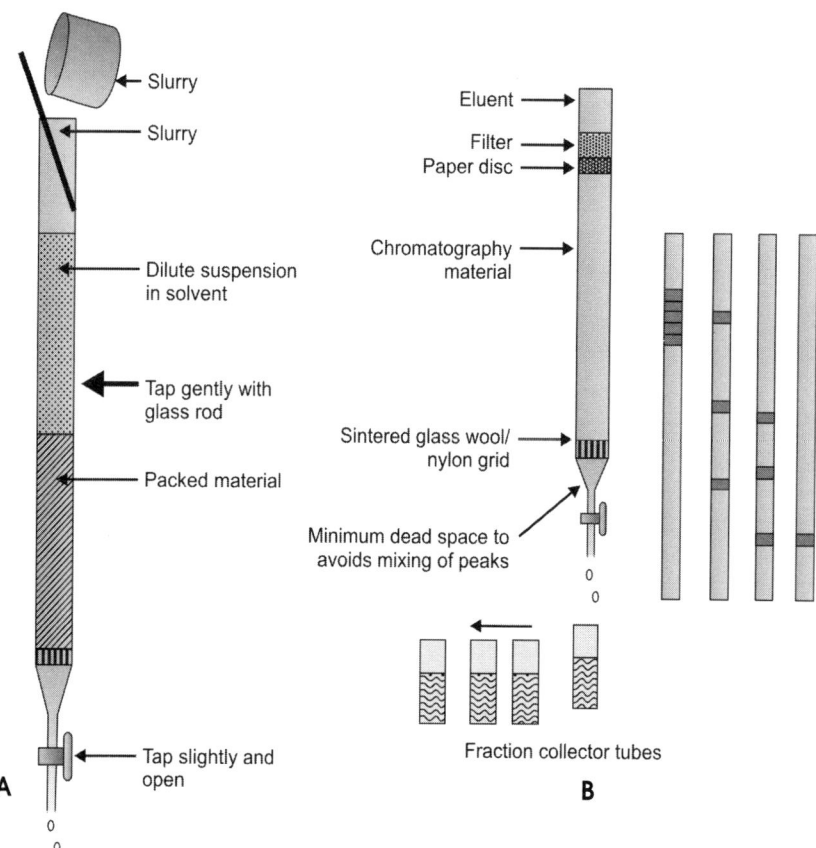

Fig. 7.8: (A) Preparation of a column; (B) separation of compounds in a mixture which are collected as different fractions

different molecules are removed from the column by changing the strength of solvent in a stepwise fashion or by means of a gradient which can be linear concave or convex. The following solvent gradient was used for elution:

Table 7.23: Solvents used for elution

S. No.	Solvent System	Solvent ratio	Amount taken (ml)	No. of fraction
1.	Chloroform	100 %	150	6
2.	Chloroform: Methanol	99.5:5	150	6
3.	Chloroform: Methanol	99:1	150	6
4.	Chloroform: Methanol	95:5	150	6
5.	Chloroform: Methanol	92.5:7.5	150	6
6.	Chloroform: Methanol	90:10	150	6
7.	Chloroform: Methanol	85:15	150	6
8.	Chloroform: Methanol	75:25	150	6
9.	Chloroform: Methanol	50:50	150	6
10.	Methanol	100%	150	6

LC of each fraction is carried out and similar fractions were pooled.

Table 7.24: Liquid chromatography and pooled fractions

Pooled fraction	Sample ID	Wt. of extract (mg)
1–6	01	92.5
7–16	02	54.5
17–23	03	92.0
25	04	176.4
26–29	05	484.8
30–33	06	352.2
34–37	06-A	149.2
38–42	07-A	289.7
43–46	08-A	12.5
47–50	09	1.2475
51–55	10	3.8533
56–60	11	1.0065

Sub Column A: ID No. 05 and 09 are selected fraction for further separation by small column.

The summary of fraction A

Size of column A: 30 × 1.5 cm ID = Internal diameter
Weight of silica gel: 12.73 gm
Type of silica gel: 60–120 mesh
Sample type: Drug fraction ID No. 5 of column
Sample ID: 05(26–29)
Weight of sample: 0.4848 gm

Table 7.25: Solvents system used

S. No.	Solvent system	Ratio	Volume (ml)	No. of fractions
1.	Chloroform: Methanol	95:5	25	1
2.	Chloroform: Methanol	95:5	25	1
3.	Chloroform: Methanol	92.5 :7.5	25	1
4.	Chloroform: Methanol	92.5 :7.5	25	1
5.	Chloroform: Methanol	90:10	25	1
6.	Chloroform: Methanol	90:10	25	1
7.	Chloroform: Methanol	87.5:12.5	25	1
8.	Chloroform: Methanol	87.5:12.5	25	1
9.	Chloroform: Methanol	85:15	25	1
10.	Chloroform: Methanol	85:15	25	1
11.	Chloroform: Methanol	50:50	125	5
12.	Chloroform: Methanol	40:60	100	4
13.	Chloroform: Methanol	20:80	100	4
14.	Methanol		225	9

TLC analysis of each fraction of sub column is carried out with solvent system **(Chloroform: Methanol :: 93: 7)**. After comparison of their TLC profile the similar fractions are taken in vials and weighed.

Table 7.26: Pooled fractions

S.No.	Sample ID	Pooled fraction	Wt. of extract (gm)
1	001 (X)	3–5	0.0584
2	002 (Y)	6–8	0.0832
3	003 (Z)	16–32	0.0275

Sub column (B): (Fraction ID No 9)
The summary of column B: 47–50 fractions
The summary of fraction B is:
Size of column B: 40 × 2 cm ID.
Weight of silica gel: 32.28 gm
Type of silica gel: 60–120 mesh
Sample ID: 09 (47–50)
Weight of sample: 1.2475 gm

Table 7.27: TLC analysis of different fractions

S. No	No. of fraction	Solvent system (Chloroform: Methanol)	Volume (ml)	No. of fractions
1.	1	70:30	50	2
2.	3	60:40	50	2
3.	5	50:50	100	4
4.	9	40:60	50	2
5.	11	30:70	50	2
6.	13	20:80	50	2
7.	15	10:90	400	16

TLC analysis of each fraction of sub column is carried out with solvent system (chloroform: methanol). After comparison of their TLC profile the similar fractions can be taken in tubes and weighed.

Thin layer chromatography (TLC)

The TLC is carried out by **(Chloroform: Methanol: Acetic acid:: 85:15:1)** solvent system.

The pooling of fractions are as below:

Table 7.28: Pooling of fractions

Sample ID	Pooled fraction
001 (II)	1 – 2
002 (II)	3
003 (II)	4
004 (II)	5 – 8
005 (II)	9 – 14
006 (II)	15 – 20
007 (II)	21 – 30

The preparatory TLC was done of pooled fraction 003 (II) in Chloroform: Methanol: Acetic acid (85:15:1) solvent system. 30 μl sample was taken for this purpose. Two bands were detected in UV light. The bands were named as A and B.

The R_f values of both bands are:

$$R_f \text{ value of A} = \frac{3.3}{8} = 0.41 \text{ cm}$$

$$R_f \text{ value of B} = \frac{3.3}{8} = 0.56 \text{ cm}$$

Both the bands are scrapped and taken in separate vials. The both scrapped sample are dissolved in methanol and centrifuged at 1000 rpm for 15 minutes. The both supernatant are taken in separate vials and concentrated with the help of vacuum rotary evaporator.

Spectrophotometry

Spectroscopic measurements are taken in a double beam spectrophotometer. The pure samples taken from TLC/CC are dissolved in methanol and λ_{max} is determined by scanning mode and graphs are printed through an attached printer.

Table 7.29: Spectrophotometric analysis

S. No	Sample ID	Dissolve	λ_{max}	O.D.	R_f value
1.	Sample A	800 ml ↓ 20 μl	260.2 206.2	0.146 0.258	0.4125
2.	Sample B	800 ml ↓ 20 μl	207.2 258.4	0.229 0.107	0.5625

High Pressure Liquid Chromatography (HPLC)

Samples obtained from chromatography are injected in HPLC. The mobile phase is composed of two solvents: A. [water with 0.0025% (v/v) Tri fluoro acetic acid] and B. 80% acetonitrile and 20% solvent A. Each sample is dissolved in 50% aqueous methanol and filtered through a 0.05 mm filter and 200 ml is injected in the injector. Analysis is performed with a C_{18} column (250 mm × 4 mm ID, 5 nm particle size) at 280 nm.

HPLC Results:

HPLC profile of the column fraction shows three major and three minor compounds. The initial attempts is made to separate these compounds resulted in impure compounds hence identification could not be achieved.

Table 7.30: Gradient analysis

Time	Solvent A	Solvent B
0	41.0	59.0
1	40.0	60.0
11	40.0	60.0
18	34.0	66.0
35	10.0	90.0
38	12.0	88.0
45	0.0	100.0
46	41.0	59.0
55	41.0	59.0
60	41.0	59.0

Flow rate: 1.500 ml/min

Discussion:

During this work isolation of active principle from drug sample has been attempted. It is evident from the group testing that the plant contains terpenoids, alkaloids, phenols, steroids and several other compounds. Partial success has been achieved in separating several functional groups. These groups are being evaluated for their antimicrobial and other biological properties. Activity based isolation would be useful in isolation and identification of bioactive molecules.

EXPERIMENT 27

Aim: To develop method in HPTLC and estimate Sennoside B and Glycerrhizin from Capsule and simultaneous estimation of Sennoside and Glycerrhizin.

Theory:

High performance thin layer chromatography (HPTLC) is a sophisticated and automated form of TLC. Evaluation of conventional TLC into a modern instrumental technique started in 1975 with the introduction of so called high performance material. Modern TLC is a powerful, reliable and cost efficient method for qualitative and quantitative analysis. High performance thin layer chromatography refers to the layer, which has a smaller particle size (6 µm), which are slightly thinner (100 or 200 µm) and particularly whose particle size distribution is significantly closer than that of

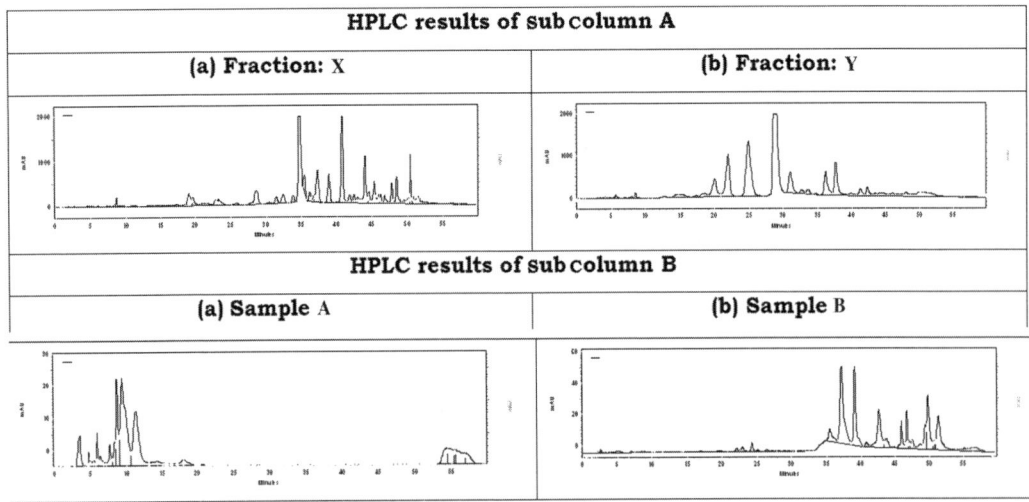

Fig. 7.9: HPLC spectras of different fractions

conventional TLC sorbets. Because of these specifications the optimum separation distance of a HPTLC layer is around 50mm instead of 100–120 mm on a conventional TLC plate.

HPTLC can almost assess the quality of a drug without elaborate laboratory facilities. Simultaneous multi-sample analysis on a single plate that allows a real in-system calibration in contrast to other on-line Chromatographic procedure leads to precise and accurate result with low uncertainty have made HPTLC a versatile, powerful but basically a simple separation technique. Of many chromatography method presently available, HPTLC provide the rapid and positive analysis of plant drugs leading to semi quantitative/quantitative information on chief constituent of the formulation. It can provide fingerprinting for monitoring the identity and purity of drugs and detection of adulteration/substitution. The various steps involved in HPTLC study are shown below:

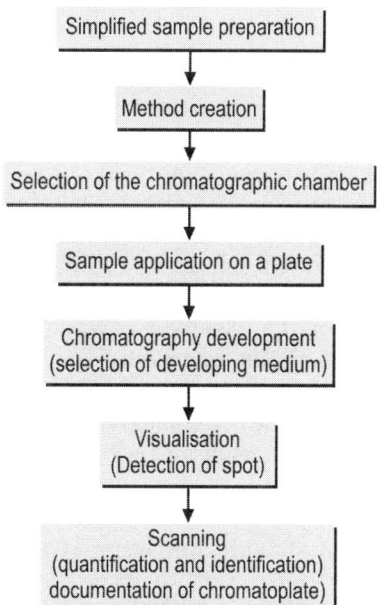

Fig. 7.10: Flow diagram of HPTLC study

Methodology for HPTLC Analysis

Carried out the analysis of the extract and the Capsule formulation using the Standard compound Sennoside B and Glycerrhizic acid by using the highly sophisticated HPTLC instrument

Sample Preparation

The sample preparation procedure is to dissolve the sample in a suitable solvent with complete recovery of intact compounds of interest with a suitable concentration of analytes for direct application on the HPTLC plate. 50 mg of Hydro-alcoholic extract of Senna leaves and dried rhizome extract of Liquorice were refluxed in 40 ml of methanol for a half hour. Filtered while hot and washed the residue with 10ml of methanol. Final volume was made to 50 ml with methanol to get a concentration 1 mg/ml.

20 capsules are weighed and then total weigh is determined. The capsule granules are subjected to fine powder with the help of mortal and pestle. 5 gm powders are refluxed with methanol and final volume is made to 25 ml to get concentration 200 mg/ml and used. Standard solution are prepared by dissolving 10mg of Standard Sennoside and 20 mg Standard Glycerrhizinic acid in 10 ml methanol and sonicate for 15 min and used as a stock solution.

Selection of HPTLC Plates

HPTLC separation material is available in the form of precoated layers supported by glass, plastic sheets or aluminum foil. Although precoated layers of aluminum oxide, cellulose polyamide, ion exchange materials, reversed phase silica (alkyl bonded) have been commercially available for quite sometime, the vast majority of separation is carried out on normal phase silica gel. Pre-coated HPTLC plate in size of 20 × 20 cm with aluminum or polyester support is usually procured mainly for economic reason. These plates can be cut to size and shape to suit particularly analysis by using general-purpose scissors. Silica gel pre-coated plates with aluminum support can be used for the present study.

Application of Sample

The suitable sample volume may be applied either spot wise with a device with controlled delivery speed or they are sprayed on in the form of narrow bands. Sample application in the form of narrow bands provides the highest resolution. The Linomate 5 allows sample application in narrow bands by a spray on technique under an inert gas (Nitrogen) blanket. All the sample solution were applied as a thin band of 8mm width containing a sample volume 7 µl for the Senna (1mg/ml) and Glycerrhiza (1mg/ml) extract, 15 µl and 7 µl of capsule formulation and the std Sennoside (1mg/ml) ranges from 0.5 µl to 2.5 µl, std Glycerrhiza (2mg/ml) 1µl to 5µl on five different tracks in duplicate on the plate by using Camag Linomat 5, which is a microprocessor controlled and programmable applicator.

Development of optimum mobile phase

The qualitative/quantitative analysis can be done only if an ideal mobile phase or developing medium, that can resolve the maximum number of compound present is made available. A number of different individual solvents as well as combination of solvents may be tried to obtain a well separated, resolved and stable peak. The present mobile phase used for simultaneous separation of two or more active component of formulation.

Mobile Phase:

2-Propanol : Ethyl acetate : Water : Ammonia
    50   :   35   : 25 :   2

Chromatographic Development

Ascending, descending, two dimensional, horizontal, multimodal, forced flow planar chromatography are the most common modes of chromatographic development. Rectangular glass chamber, twin-trough chambers, sandwitch chambers, etc. are commonly used for carrying out different types of TLC/HPTLC development. All the plate after drying were developed in previously saturated Camag Twin trough chamber using the above mentioned mobile phase. After proper development, the plate can be removed from the chamber and air dried with the help of dryer to effect faster removal of the mobile phase.

Densitometric Chromatogram Evaluation (Scanning)

For densitometric measurements of a thin layer chromatogram, its separation tracks are scanned with a light beam in the form of slit selectable in length and width. Diffusely reflected light is measured by photo sensor. Densitometric measurement can be made by absorbance or fluorescence; the substances are excited by UV light, most often at 254 and 366 nm. The photo sensor measures the emitted light, which is always of longer wavelength. and the measured light intensity is directly proportional to the amount of the flouroscencing substance. In order to avoid systemic error, scanning should always be done in or against the direction of chromatography. The decrease in the light reflectance due to adsorbed compounds gives rise to a signal in the detectors. The light thus generated is amplified and transmitted to a recorder where the spot by absorbing some of the light cause a signal to lessen and a resultant peak or dip is printed by the detector. The areas included in those peaks measured and related to amount of material in the spot. The scanner is linked to the personal computer, from which all commands are passed to the scanner. The scanner transmits all measurements data in digital form to the computer for further processing.

Procedure

Estimation of Sennoside B from Capsule

Chromatographic conditions

The chromatographic conditions can be established by trial and error method. After stabilizing of the condition, it may keep constant during experimentation.

Stationary phase	: HPTLC precoated, silica gel 60, F_{254} (Merck)
Thickness	: 0.2 mm
Mode of application	: Band
Band width	: 8 mm
Separation technique	: Ascending
Temperature	: 25 ± 3°C
Saturation time	: 25 min. (10 min. chamber alone + 15 min. with plate)
Migration distance	: 70 mm
Measurement mode	: Absorbance/Reflectance
Slit dimension	: 6.0 × 0.30 mm
Scanning mode	: Single level
Scanning wavelength	: 308 nm
Detection TLC	: UV-Densitometric scanning

Selection of Detection Wavelength for Densitometric Evaluation

Selection of the wavelength for densitometric evaluation can be done by taking the spectrum of peak obtained from the standard Sennoside B acid through the range of 210–400 nm. The wavelength showing maximum absorbance, 308 nm was taken as the detection wavelength.

Preparation of Standard Calibration Curve

The calibration curve is prepared so that the concentration of unknown compound can be calculated. The curve is prepared by diluting the standard stock solution into a series of

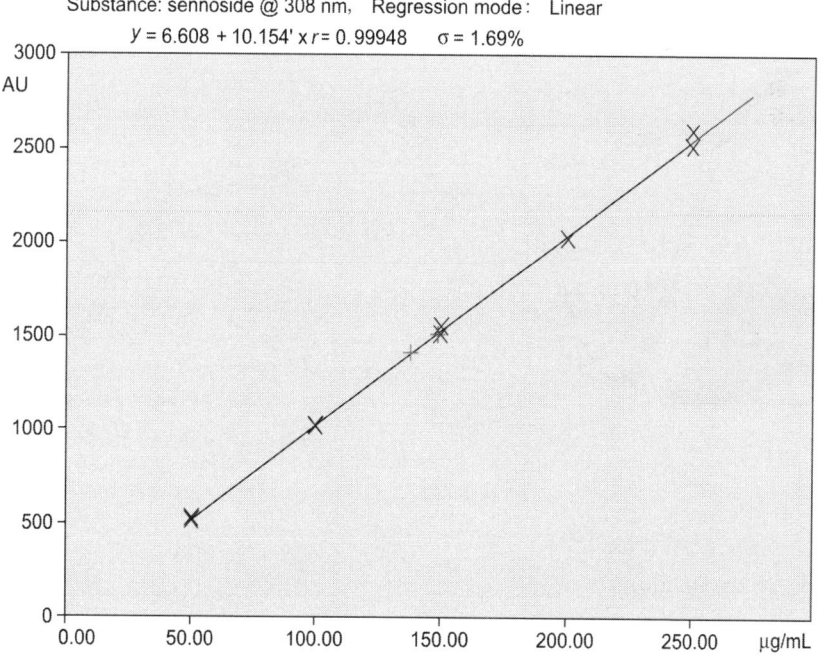

Fig. 7.11: Calibration graph for Sennoside B

264 Experimental Pharmacognosy

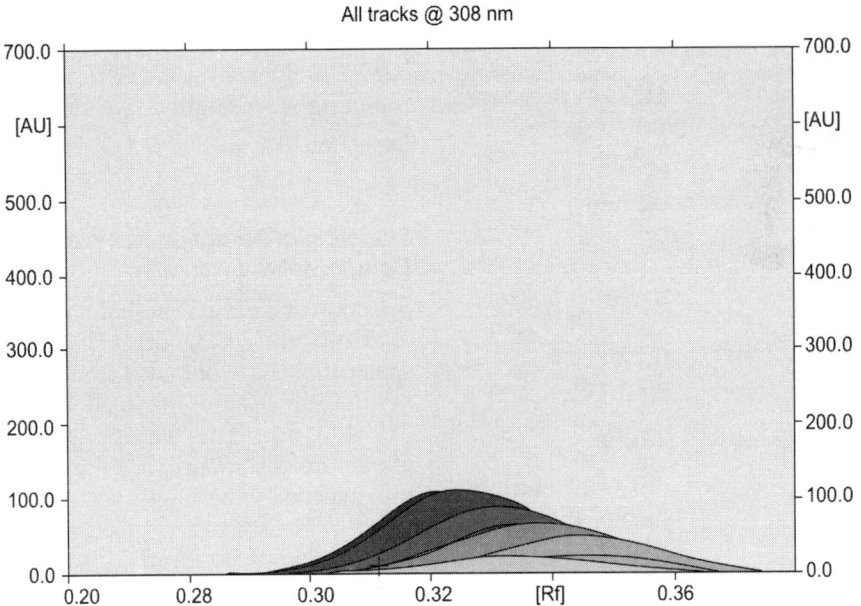

Fig. 7.12: 3D display of Sennoside B in all tracks

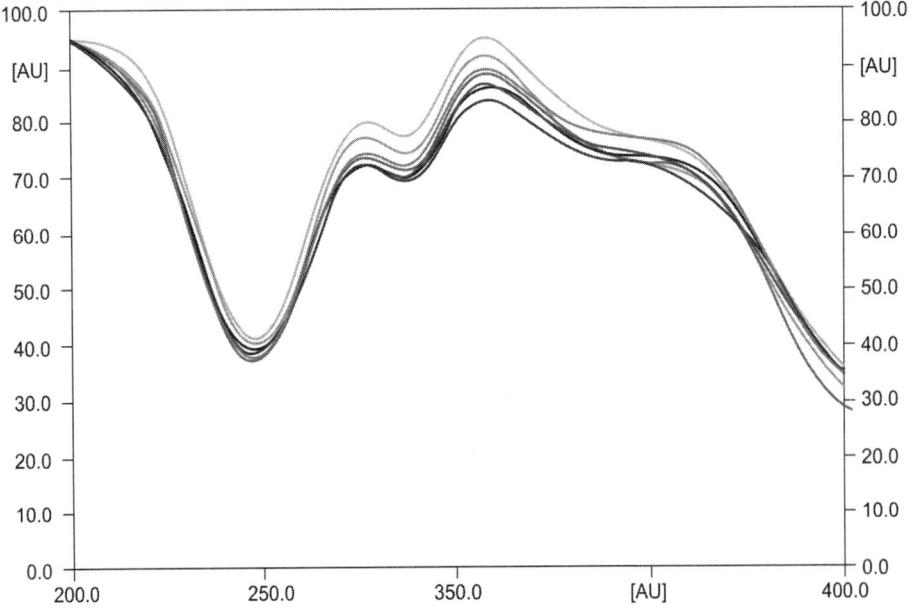

Fig. 7.13: Spectrum of Sennoside B in standard and capsule

dilution. The dilution of stock solution is done by considering the linearity range of active constituent, which is to be standardized.

Calibration curve for Sennoside Considering Area

Calibration curve for Sennoside are prepared by diluting the stock solution of Sennoside B (1 mg/ml) to 0.1 mg/ml and this solution is used in different concentration such as 0.05.... to ....0.25 mg/ml.

Sennoside B

Regression Equation via Area

$y = 6.60 + 10.15x, \quad r = 0.999, \quad \sigma = 1.69$

Estimation of Glycerrhizin from Capsule

Chromatographic Conditions

The chromatographic conditions were established by trial and error method. After stabilizing of the condition, it was kept constant during experimentation.

Stationary phase	: HPTLC precoated, Silica gel 60, F_{254} (Merck)
Thickness	: 0.2 mm
Mode of application	: Band
Band width	: 8 mm
Separation technique	: Ascending
Temperature	: $25 \pm 3°C$
Saturation time	: 25 min (10 min.chamber alone + 15 min.with plate)
Migration distance	: 70 mm
Measurment mode	: Absorbance/Reflectance
Slit dimension	: 6.0×0.30 mm
Scanning mode	: Single level
Scanning wavelength	: 257 nm
Detection TLC	: UV-densitometric scanning

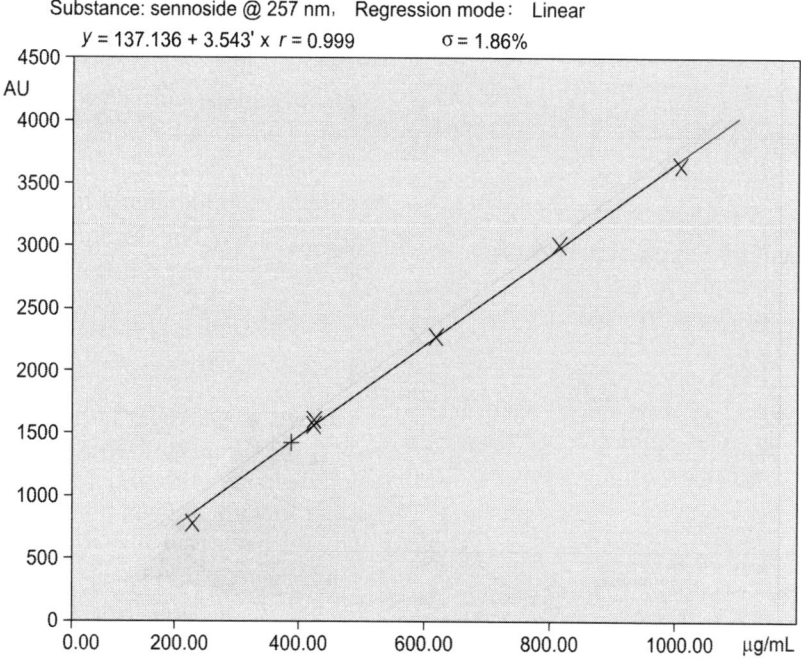

Fig. 7.14: Calibration graph for Glycerrhizin

Selection of Detection Wavelength for Densitometric Evaluation

Selection of the wavelength for densitometric evaluation was done by taking the spectrum of peak obtained from the standard Glycerrhizin acid through the range of 210-400 nm. The wavelength showing maximum absorbance, 257 nm may be taken as the detection wavelength.

Calibration Curve for Glycerrhizin Considering Area

Calibration curve for Glycerrhizin are prepared by diluting the stock solution of Glycerrhizinic acid (2 mg/ml) to 0.2 mg/ml and this solution is used in different concentration such as 0.2.... to ....1 mg/ml.

Regression Equation via area

$y = 137.1 + 3.54x$, $r = 0.999$, $\sigma = 1.86$

Chromatographic Conditions

The chromatographic conditions may be established by trial and error method. After stabilizing of the condition, it was kept constant during experimentation.

Stationary phase	: HPTLC precoated, silica gel 60, F_{254}(Merck)
Thickness	: 0.2 mm
Mode of application	: Band
Band width	: 8 mm
Separation technique	: Ascending
Temperature	: $25 \pm 3°C$
Saturation time	: 25min. (10 min chamber alone+15 min with plate)
Migration distance	: 70 mm
Measurement mode	: Absorbance/ Reflectance
Slit dimension	: 6.0×0.30 mm
Scanning mode	: Multilevel
Scanning wavelength	: 257nm and 308 nm
Detection TLC	: UV-densitometric scanning

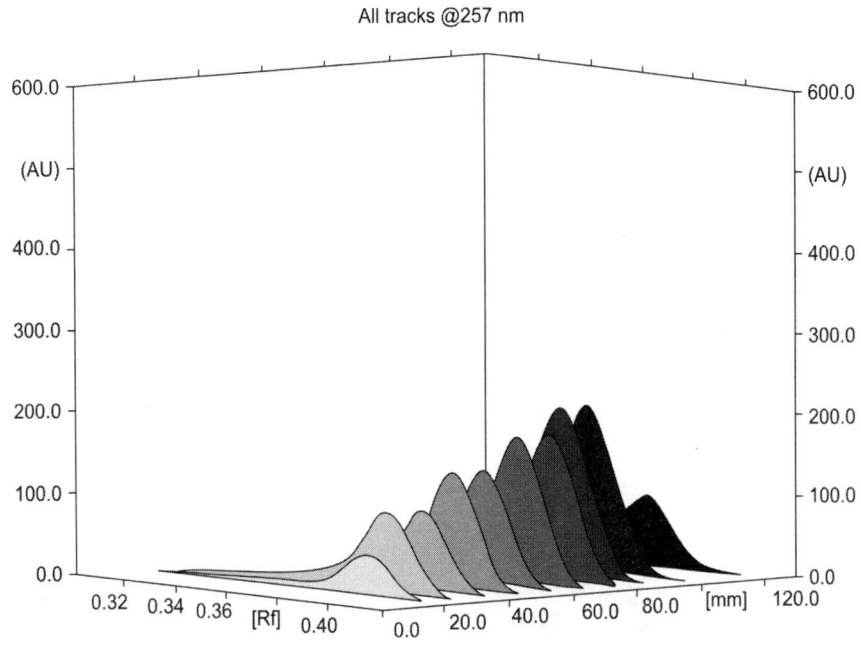

Fig. 7.15: 3D display of Glycerrhizin in all tracks

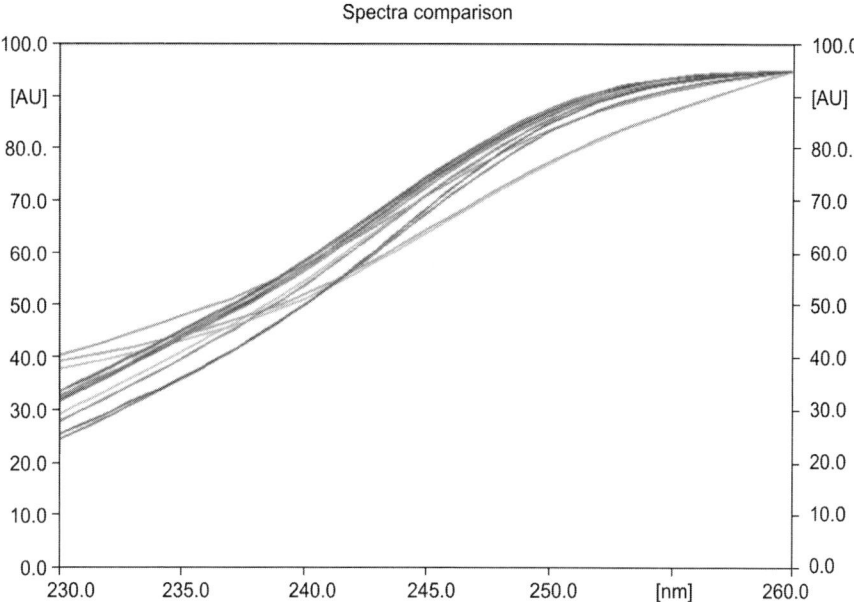

Fig. 7.16: Overlain spectrum of glycerrhizin in standard and capsule, simultaneous estimation of sennoside and glycerrhizin

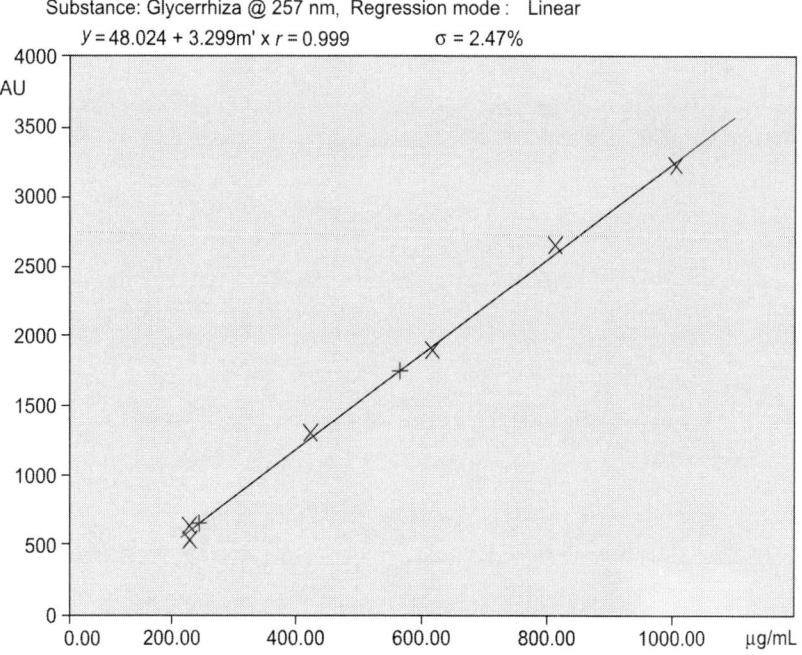

Fig. 7.17: Calibration graph for glycerrhizin in over spotting method

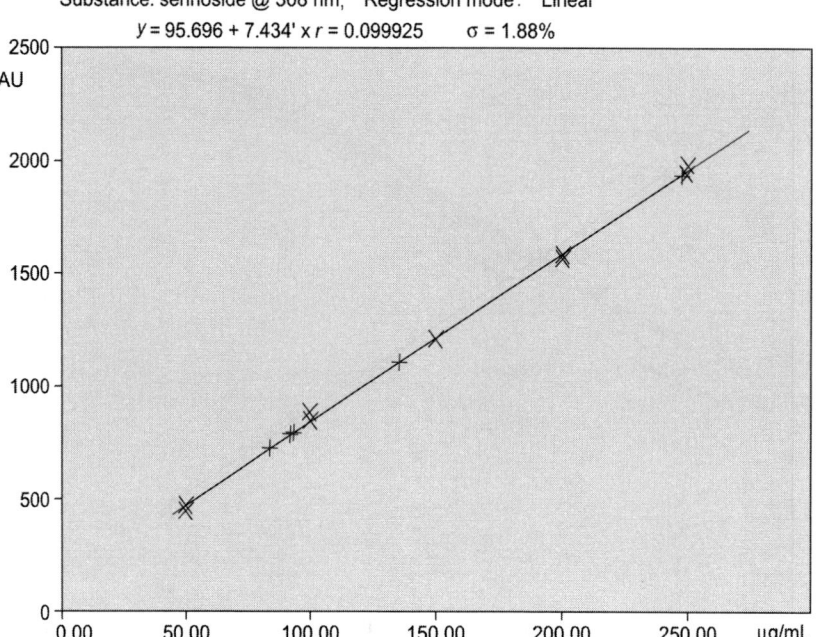

Fig. 7.18: Calibration graph for sennoside in over spotting method

Chapter 8

Stains and Reagents for Microchemical Reactions

1. **Acetic acid:** Dilute 6 ml of glacial acetic acid with 100 ml of distilled water; used for identification of cystoliths, which dissolve with effervescence.

2. **Ammoniacal solution of copper oxide (cuoxam):** Triturate 0.5 gm of copper carbonate in a mortar with 10 ml of distilled water and gradually add 10 ml of strong solution of ammonia (sp. gr. 0.880) with continued stirring; used for dissolving cellulosic materials.

3. **Aniline chloride solution:** Dissolve 2 gm aniline chloride in a mixture of 65 ml of 30 per centethyl alcohol and 15 ml distilled water and add 2 ml of conc. Hydrochloric acid. Lignified tissues are stained bright yellow.

4. **Ammonia, xN:** Solutions of any normality xN may be prepared by diluting 75 x ml of strong ammonia solution to 1000 ml with water.

5. **Ammonium chloride solution:** A 10% w/v solution of ammonium chloride in water.

6. **Ammonium thiocyanate solution:** A 10% w/v solution of ammonium thiocyanate solution.

7. **Ammonium vanadate:** Sulphuric acid solution: Dissolve 1.62 gm anhydrous ammonium vanadate in 125 ml concentrated sulphuric acid, cool and add 125 ml ice cold water. Dilute solution is used for the detecion of alkaloids, phenolic compounds and steroids.

8. **Anisaldehyde acetic acid reagent (AA):** 0.5 ml anisaldehyde mixed with 10 ml of 98% acetic acid.

9. **Antimony (III) chloride reagent ($SbCl_3$):** 20% solution of Antimony (III) chloride in Chloroform.

10. **Anisaldehyde-sulphuric acid reagent:** 0.5 ml anisaldehyde is mixed with 10 ml glacial acetic acid, followed by 85 ml methanol and 5 ml concentrated sulphuric acid in that order. The reagent has only limited stability and is no longer usable when the colour has turned to redviolet.

11. **Benedict's reagent:** 17.3 gm of sodium citrate and 10 gm of sodium carbonate are dissolved in about 75 ml of water, and filtered if necessary. Separately weigh 1.73 gm of $CuSO_4 \cdot 7H_2O$ is dissolved in about 20 ml of water and this is slowly added with stirring to alkaline citrate solution. The volume is made upto 100 ml.

12. **Barfoed's reagent:** Dissolve 13.3 gm of copper acetate in 200 ml of water and adding 1.8 ml glacial acetic acid.

13. **Bismarck brown:** Dissolve 1 gm in 100 ml of 95% of ethyl alcohol; used as a general stain for macerated material (with Schultze's).

14. **Breamer's reagent:** Dissolve 1 gm of sodium tungstate and 2 gm of sodium acetate in sufficient quantity of water to make 10 ml, yellowish to brown precipitates; indicate the presence of tannin.

15. **Bromine solution:** Dissolve 9.6 ml of bromine and 30 gm of potassium bromide in sufficient water to produce 100 ml.

16. **Chloral hydrate solution:** Dissolve 20 gm of chloral hydrate in 5 ml of water with warming and add 5 ml of glycerin.

17. **Copper sulphate solution:** A 10.0% w/v solution of copper sulphate in water.

18. **Cresol red:** Warm 50 ml of cresol red with 2.65 ml of 0.05 M sodium hydroxide and 5 ml of ethanol (90%); after solution is effected, add sufficient ethanol (20%) to produce 250 ml.

19. **Chlorinated soda solution (bleaching solution):** Dissolve 75 gm of sodium carbonate in 125 ml of distilled water; triturate 50 gm of chlorinated lime (bleaching powder) in a mortar with 75 ml of distilled water, adding it little by little. Mix the two liquids and shake occasionally for three or four hours. Filter and store, protected from light. Used for lighting highly coloured material, by warming in it and washing the tissues thoroughly.

20. **Canada balsam (as a mountant):** Heat Canada balsam on a water bath until volatile matter is removed and the residue sets to a hard mass on cooling. Dissolve residue in xylene to form a thin syrupy liquid. Used for making permanent mounts of reference slides of selected debris.

21. **Chloral hydrate solution:** Dissolve 50 gm of chloral hydrate in 20 ml of distilled water. A valuable clarifying agent for rendering tissues transparent and clear, by freeing them from most of the ergastic substances, but leaving calcium oxalate crystals unaffected.

22. **Chloral iodine:** Saturate chloral hydrate solution with iodine, leaving a few crystals undissolved; useful for detecting minute grains of starch otherwise undetectable.

23. **Iodinated zinc chloride solution:** Dissolve 20 gm of zinc chloride and 6.5 gm of potassium iodide in 10 ml of distilled water. Add 0.5 gm of iodine and shake for about fifteen minutes before filtering. Dilute if needed prior to use. Renders cellulosic walls bluish violet and lignified walls yellowish brown.

24. **Chromic acid solution:** 10 gm of Potassium Dichromate dissolved in 90 ml of dilute sulphuric acid: macerating agent similar to Schultze's.

25. **Corallin soda:** Dissolve 5 gm of corallin in 100 ml of 90% ethyl alcohol. Dissolve 25 gm of sodium carbonate in 100 ml distilled water; keep the solutions separate and mix when required, by adding 1 ml of the corallin solution to 20 ml of the aqueous sodium carbonate solution. Prepare fresh each time, as the mixture will not keep for long. Used for staining sieve plates and callus bright pink and imparts a reddish tinge to starch grains and lignified tissues.

26. **Crystal violet solution:** A 0.5% w/v solution of crystal violet in anhydrous glacial acetic acid.

27. **Cresol red solution:** Warm 0.1 gm of cresol red in a mixture of 2.65 ml of 0.1 M sodium hydroxide and 20 ml of ethanol (95 %). After solution is effected, add sufficient water to produce 100 ml.

28. **Dinitrophenyl hydrazine reagent (DNPH):** 0.1 gm of 2,4 dinitrophenyl hydrazine is dissolved in 100 ml methanol followed by the addition of 1 ml of 36% hydrochloric acid.

29. **Dragendorff's reagent:**

    Solution 1–Dissolve 0.85 gm of bismuth oxy nitrate in 40 ml of water and 10 ml of acetic acid.

    Solution 2 –Dissolve 8 gm of potassium iodide in 20 ml of water.

    Mix equal volumes of solution 1 and 2, and to 10 ml of the resultant mixture add 100 ml of water and 20 ml of acetic acid.

30. **Dragendroff's, reagent with tartaric acid:**
    solution A: 17 gm bismuth sub-nitrate and 200 gm tartaric acid in 800 ml water.
    solution B: 160 gm potassium iodide in 400 ml water.
    Stock solution: solution A and solution B
    Spray reagent: 50 ml stock solution + 500 ml water + 100 gm tartaric acid
31. **Eosin solution:** A 0.5% w/v solution of eosin in water.
32. **Eriochrome black T:** Brownish black powder having a faint, metallic sheen, soluble in alcohol, in methyl alcohol and in hot water.
33. **Eosin:** 1 percent solution in 90% ethyl alcohol; stains cellulose and aleurone grains red.
34. **Ferric chloride solution:** A percent solution ferric chloride in distilled water. Taninn containing tissues coloured bluish or greenish black.
35. **Fehling's solution:**
    a. Dissolve 69.278 gm of $CuSO_4 \cdot 5H_2O$ in water and make the volume upto 1 litre
    b. Dissolve 100 gm of sodium hydroxide and 340 gm of Sodium potassium tartarate in water and make the volume to 1 litre.
    Mix equal volumes of A and B before the experiment.
36. **Formaldehyde solution:** Formalin; (HCHO) Formaldehyde solution is a solution of formaldehyde in water with methyl alcohol added to prevent polymerization. It contains not less than 34.0% w/w and not more than 38.0% w/w of CH_2O.
37. **Formaldehyde solution (dilute):** Dilute 34 ml of formaldehyde solution with sufficient water to produce 100 ml.
38. **Folin ciocalteu reagent:** Dilute commercially available Folin-Ciocalteu reagent (2N) with an equal volume of distilled water. Transfer it in a brown bottle and store in a refrigerator (40). It should be golden in colour. Do not use it if it turns olive green.
39. **Glycerine:** Pure or diluted as required with one or two volumes of distilled water. Used as a general mountant.
40. **Haematoxylin (Delafield's):** Prepare a saturated solution of ammonia alum. To 100 ml of this add a solution of 1 gm of Haematoxylin in 6 ml of ethyl alcohol (97%). Leave the mixed solution exposed to air and light in an unstopped bottle for three or four days. Filter and add to the filtrate 25 ml of glycerine and 25 ml of methyl alcohol. Allow the solution to stand exposed to light, till it acquires a dark colour (about two months). Refilter and store as a stock solution. Dilute it 3 or 4 times volumes with distilled water. Stains cellulosic fibers blue; used only on water washed material.
41. **Hydrogen peroxide solution:** Analytical reagent grade or hydrogen peroxide solution (100 Vol.) diluted with 4 volumes of water.
42. **Hydroxylamine hydrochloride solution:** Dissolve 1 gm of hydroxylamine hydrochloride in 50 ml of water and add 50 ml of alcohol, 1 ml of bromophenol blue solution and 0.1 N sodium hydroxide until the solution becomes green.
43. **Hydrochloric acid, xN:** Solution of any normality xN may be prepared by diluting 84x ml of hydrochloric acid to 1000 ml with water.
44. **Hydrochloric acid** (1 percent w/v): Dilute 1 gm of hydrochloric acid to 100 ml with water.
45. **Hydrochloric acid, N:** Dilute 85 ml of hydrochloric acid with water to 1000 ml and standardize the solution as follows:
46. **Iodine reagent:** About 10 gm of solid iodine are spread on the bottom of the chromatography tank.
47. **Iodine water:** Mix 1 volume of decinormal iodine with 4 volumes of distilled

water. Stains starch blue, and reveals crystalloids and globoids when present in aleurone grains.

48. **Iodine and potassium iodide solution:** Dissolve 1 gm of potassium iodide in 200 ml of distilled water and 2 gm of iodine; stains lignified walls yellow and cellulosic walls blue.

49. **Lactophenol (Amman's fluid):** Phenol 20 g, lactic acid 20 g, glycerine 40 g, distilled water 20 ml Dissolve; reveals starch grains in polarised light with a well marked cross at hilum, and also minute crystals of calcium oxalate as brightly polarising points of light.

50. **Methylene blue:** A solution in 25 ml of ethyl alcohol (95%). A general stain for nucleus and bacteria.

51. **Millon's reagent:** Dissolve 1 volume of mercury in 9 volumes of fuming nitric acid, keeping the mixture well cooled during reaction. Add equal volume distilled water when cool. Stains proteins red.

52. **Mercuric chloride, 0.2 M:** Dissolve 54.30 gm of mercuric chloride in sufficient water to produce 1000 ml.

53. **Mercuric chloride solution:** A 5.0% w/v solution of mercuric chloride in water.

54. **Methyl orange solution:** Dissolve 0.1 gm of methyl orange in 80 ml of water and dilute to 100 ml with alcohol.

55. **Methyl red solution:** Dissolve 100 mg in 1.86 ml of 0.1 N sodium hydroxide and 50 ml of alcohol and dilute to 100 ml with water.

56. **Methylene blue solution:** Dissolve 150 mg of methylene blue in 100 ml of ethanol (95%) and dilute with ethanol (95%) to produce 250 ml.

57. **Molish's reagent:** Prepare two solutions in separate bottles, with ground glass stoppers:
    a. Dissolve 2 gm of α-naphthol in 95% alcohol and make upto 10 ml with alcohol (α-naphthol can be replaced by thymol or resorcinol). Store in a place protected from light. The solution can be used for only a short period.
    b. Concentrated sulphuric acid.
    Spray the plate with 10 ml solution A and 8 ml solution B respectively.

58. **Natural product reagent (natural product-polyethylene reagent):**
    Solution A: 1% ethyl acetate diphenyl-boric acid-Bethylaminoester (NP)
    Solution B: 5%ethyl acetatepolyethylene glycol 4000 (PEG)
    Spray the plate with10 ml solution A and 8ml solution B respectively.

59. **Ninhydrin reagent:** 30 mg of ninhydrin is dissolved in 10 ml of N- Butanol followed by 0.3 ml of 98% acetic acid.

60. **Nitric acid, xN:** Solutions of any normality xN may be prepared by diluting 63x ml of nitric acid to 1000 ml with water.

61. **Nitric acid dilute:** Contains approximately 10% w/w of HNO_3. Dilute 106 ml of nitric acid to 1000 ml with water.

62. **Naphthol solution**: Dissolve 10 gm of Naphthol in 100 ml of ethyl alcohol; a specific stain for detection of inulin; cells containing inulin turn deep reddish violet.

63. **Phologlucinol:** 1 gm of phloroglucinol dissolved in 100 ml of 90% ethyl alcohol; mount debris in a few drops, allow to react for a minute, draw off excess of reagent with a filter paper strip, and add a drop of conc. hydrochloric acid to the slide; lignified tissues acquire a deep purplish red colour; very effective on water washed material but not in chloral hydrate washed debris.

64. **Picric acid solution (trinitrophenol solution):** A saturated aqueous solution made by dissolving 1 gm of picric acid in 95 ml of distilled water; stains animal and insect tissues, a light to deep yellow; in a solution with ethyl alcohol, aleurone

grains and fungal hyphae are stained yellow.

65. **Potash, caustic:** A 5% aqueous solution; used to separate tenacious tissues of epidermis and also laticiferous elements and vittae, both of which are stained brown.

66. **Phenolphthalein solution:** Dissolve 0.10 gm in 80 ml of alcohol and dilute to 100 ml with water.

67. **Phosphoric acid, xN:** Solutions of any normality, xN may be prepared by diluting 49 x gm of phosphoric acid with water to 1000 ml.

68. **Dilute phosphoric acid:** Contains approximately 10% w/v of H_3PO_4. Dilute 69 ml of phosphoric acid to 1000 ml with water.

69. **Potassium chromate solution:** A 5.0% w/v solution of potassium chromate. It gives a red precipitate with silver nitrate in neutral solutions.

70. **Potassium cupri-tartrate solution:** Cupric Tatrate Alkaline Solution: Fehling's solution (A and B).
    A. **Copper solution:** Dissolve 34.66 gm of carefully selected small crystals of copper sulphate, showing no trace of efflorescence or of adhering moisture, in sufficient water to make 500 ml. Keep this solution in small, well-stoppered bottles.
    B. **Alkaline tartrate solution:** Dissolve 176 gm of sodium potassium tartrate and 77 gm of sodium hydroxide in sufficient water to produce 500 ml.
    Mix equal volumes of the solutions A and B at the time of using.

71. **Potassium dichromate solution:** A 7.0% w/v solution of potassium dichromate in water.

72. **Potassium dichromate solution 0.1N:** Weigh accurately 4.903 gm of potassium dichromate and dissolve in sufficient water to produce 1000 ml.

73. **Potassium ferrocyanide solution:** A 5.0% w/v solution of potassium ferrocyanide in water.

74. **Potassium hydrogen phthalate, 0.02 M:** Dissolve 4.084 gm of Potassium hydrogen phthalate in sufficient water to produce 1000 ml.

75. **Potassium hydroxide, xN:** Solution of any normality, xN, may be prepared by dissolving 56.11x gm of potassium hydroxide in water and diluting to 1000 ml.

76. **Potassium hydroxide solution –solution of potash:** An aqueous solution of potassium hydroxide containing 5.0% w/v of total alkali, calculated as KOH (limits, 4.75 to 5.25).

77. **Potassium iodide, M:** Dissolve 166.00 gm of potassium iodide in sufficient water to produce 1000 ml.

78. **Potassium iodide and starch solution:** Dissolve 10 gm of potassium iodide in sufficient water to produce 95 ml and add 5 ml of starch solution. Potassium Iodide and Starch solution must be freshly prepared.

79. **Potassium iodide solution:** A 10% w/v solution of potassium iodide in water.

80. **Potassium mercuric-iodide solution– Mayer's Reagent:** Add 1.36 gm of mercuric chloride dissolved in 60 ml of water to a solution of 5 gm of potassium iodide in 20 ml of water, mix and add sufficient water to produce 100 ml.

81. **Potassium mercuri-iodide solution, alkaline (Nessler's reagent):** To 3.5 gm of potassium iodide add 1.25 gm of mercuric chloride dissolved in 80 ml of water, add a cold saturated solution of mercuric chloride in water, with constant stirring until a slight red precipitate remains. Dissolve 12 gm of sodium hydroxide in the solution, add a little more of the cold saturated solution of mercuric chloride and sufficient water to produce 100 ml. Allow to stand and decant the clear liquid.

82. **Potassium permanganate solution:** A 1.0% w/v solution of potassium permanganate in water.

83. **Potassium permanganate, 0.1 N Solution:** 3.161 gm in 1000 ml
84. **Phenol red solution:** Dissolve 0.1 gm of phenol red in 2.82 ml of 0.1 M sodium hydroxide and 20 ml of ethanol (95%). After solution is effected, add sufficient water to produce 100 ml.
85. **Ruthenium red:** Dissolve 0.008 gm of ruthenium red in 10 ml of a 10% solution of lead acetate; (to be freshly prepared) used for identification of most kinds of mucilage containing tissues, which turn pink.
86. **Safranin:** A 1% solution in ethyl alcohol 50%; used to stain lignified cell walls deep red, even after clearing with choral hydrate.
87. **Schultze's maceration fluid:** Add isolated debris to 50% conc. nitric acid in a test tube and warm over water bath: add a few crystals of potassium chlorate while warming, till tissues soften; cool, wash with water thoroughly and tease out for mounting hard tissues; isolated cell structures are clearly revealed, but the structures are not useful for measurement of dimensions.
88. **Sudan red III:** Dissolve 0.01 gm of sudan red III in 5 ml of ethyl alcohol (90%) and 5 ml of pure glycerine; suberised walls of cork cells, and fatty material in cells are stained bright red.
89. **Sulphovanadic acid** (Mandelin's reagent): Triturate 1 gm of ammonium vandate with 100 ml conc. sulphuric acid. Allow the deposit to subside and use the clear liquid. This is to be prepared fresh; useful for identification of alkaloids, particularly strychnine which turns violet in the cells containing it.
90. **Sodium hydroxide, xN:** Solutions of any normality, xN may be prepared by dissolving 40 x gm of sodium hydroxide in water and diluting to 1000 ml.
91. **Sodium hydroxide solution:** A 20.0% w/v solution of sodium hydroxide in water.
92. **Sodium hydroxide solution, dilute:** A 5.0% w/v solution of sodium hydroxide in water.
93. **Starch solution:** Triturate 0.5 gm of soluble starch, with 5 ml of water and add this, with constant stirring, to sufficient water to produce about 100 ml. Boil for a few minutes, cool and filter. Solution of starch must be freshly prepared.
94. **Sulphuric acid:** When no molarity is indicated use analytical reagent grade containing about 98% w/w of sulphuric acid.
95. **Dilute sulphuric acid:** Contains approximately 10% w/w of H_2SO_4.
96. **Starch-iodate paper:** Immerse strips of filter paper in 100 ml of iodide-free starch solution containing 0.1 gm of potassium iodate. Drain and allow to dry protected from light.
97. **Thymol blue solution:** Dissolve 0.1 gm of thymol blue in 2.15 ml of 0.1 M sodium hydroxide and 20 ml of ethanol (95%). After solution is effected, add sufficient water to produce 100 ml.
98. **Vanillin phosphoric acid:**
    A. 1 gm vanillin dissolved in 100 ml of 50% of phosphoric acid.
    B. 2 parts of 24% phosphoric acid and 8 parts of 2% ethanolic vanillic acid.
    After spraying either A or B, the plate is heated for 10 minutes at 100°C and evaluated in visible or UV 365 nm.
99. **Vanillin sulphuric acid reagent:** prepare by mixing 1% w/v vanillin in ethanol (95%) and methanolic sulphuric acid (5%).
100. **Van URK reagent:** 0.2 gm of 4- dimethyl amino benzaldehyde is dissolved in 100 ml of 25% HCl with the addition of 1 drop of 10% iron (III) chloride solution.
101. **Xylenol orange solution:** Dissolve 0.1 gm of xylenol orange with 100 ml of water and filter, if necessary.

Suggested Readings

- The Ayurvedic Pharmacopoeia of India, Part I, 2nd edn, Government of India, Ministry of Health and Family Welfare, Department of Indian System of Medicine and Homeopathy, 2003.
- The Ayurvedic Pharmacopoeia of India, Part II (Formulation), Volume I, Government of India, Ministry of Health and Family Welfare, Department of Ayurveda, Yoga and Naturopathy, Unani, Siddha and Homoeopathy, New Delhi, 2008
- Arumugam, KR, *Textbook of Pharmacognosy*, Sathya Publishers, Madurai, 2003.
- Ansari SH, *Essential of Pharmacognosy*.
- Brain, KR, and Turner, TD, *The Practical Evaluation of Plrytopharmaceuticals*, Weight-Scientechnica, Bristol, 1975.
- Clarke, ECG, *Isolation and Identification of Drugs*, The Pharmaceutical Press, London, 1967.
- Gambarg, OL and Wetter, LR, *Plant Tissue Culture Methods*, National Research Council of Canada, Saskatchewan, 1975.
- Gaud, RS, Gupta, GD and Gokhale, SB, *Practical Biotechnology*, Nirali Prakashan, Pune, 2000.
- Gokhale SB, Kokate CK, "Practical of Pharmacognosy" Nirali Prakashan.
- Gupta, MK, *Textbook of Natural Products*, Pragati Prakashan, Meerut, 2009.
- Harborne JB, *Phytochemical Methods*, Chapman and Hall, London, 1973.
- Jackson BP and Snowdon, DW, *Atlas of Microscopy of Medicinal Plants; Culinary Herbs and Spices*, CBS Publishers & Distributors (P) Ltd., New Delhi, 2005.
- Kay, LA, *The Microscopical Study of Drugs*, Bailliere, Tindall and Cox, London, 1938.
- Khandelwal, KR, *Practical Pharmacognosy*, Nirali Prakashan, Pune, 2008.
- Kokate, CK, *Practical Pharmacognosy*, 5th edn, Vallabh Prakashan, Delhi, 2014.
- Kokate CK *et al*, *Pharmacognosy*, 5th edn, CBS Publishers and Distributors.
- Kumar, P, *Natural Products: A Practical Manual*, Pharma Med Press, Hyderabad, 2009.
- Miller IP, *Phytochemistry*, 1–3, Van Nostrand Reinhold Co., 1973.
- Murashige T and Skoog F, A revised medium for rapid growth and bioassays with tobacco tissue cultures. *Physiol Plant* 15(3): 473–497, 1962.
- Natori S *et al*, *Advances in Natural Products Chemistry*, Wiley, New York, 1981.
- Peach K and Tracey, MV, *Modern Methods of Plant Analysis*, I-IV, Narosa Publishing House, New Dehi, 1979.
- Pharmacopoiea of India, Govt. of India, Ministry of Health, 1955, 1966, 1985, 1996, 2007 and 2010.
- Quality Control methods for Medicinal Plant Material; World Health Organization, AITBS Publishers & Distributors Delhi.
- Quality Standards of Indian Medicinal Plants, Vol. 3.
- Ross, MSF and Brain, KR, *An Introduction, to Phytopharmacy*, Pitman Medical, Kent.

Index

A

Absorbent cotton 151
Acacia 134
Acetate rayon 154
Acid insoluble ash 57, 221, 231, 249
Acid value 41
Adhatoda vasica 202
Agar 133
Ajowan 125
Alcohal content 239
Alcohol soluble extractives 221
Alkaline reagent test 37, 218
Alkaloids 36, 45, 201, 216
Aloe 129, 149, 183, 211
Amino acids 38, 39, 200, 216
Amla 114, 223
Ammonium glycyrrhizinate 188
Aniline acetate test 39
Animal fibres 153
Anisidine value 44
Antimicrobial activity 167
Antioxidant activity 241
Arishta 236, 237, 250
Arjuna bark 111
Artemisia annua 186
Artificial regenerated fibres 154
Artificial synthetic fibres 155
Asafoetida 47, 141
Asava 240, 250
Ash value 15, 230, 248
Ashoka bark 111
Ayurvedic formulations 213

B

B5 medium 161, 164
Bada gokhru 118
Bahera 113, 224
Baljet test 36, 46, 217
Balsam of Peru 142
Balsam of Tolu 141
Barbaloin 211
Barfoed's test 217
Baudoins test 18
Benedict's test 38, 216, 239
Benzoin 47, 142
Bevan's test 18
Bial's orcinol test 39
Bioassays 18
Biuret test 38, 216
Black catechu 127, 147
Black pepper 191, 199, 248
Borntrager's test 36, 46, 217
Brahmi 122
Brown paper test 39
Brucine 45, 186

C

Caffeine 176
Calcium citrate 173
Calcium oxalate crystals 51
Calcium sennoside 179
Callus culture 166
Camera Lucida 24
Cannabis 143
Capsicum 144
Carbohydrates 38, 47, 216
Cardiac glycosides 46
Carrot combine explants 166
Cassia bark 88
Castor oil 139
Chemical evaluation 16, 148
Chemical tests 36
Chemotaxonomy 5
Chhota gokhru 117
Chitrak 124
Chromatography 16, 28, 199, 254
Chyawanprash 204, 234
Cinchona 86, 109, 148, 149, 197, 199, 201, 203
Cinnamon leaf oil 193
Circular paper chromatography 200
Citral 204
Citric acid 172
Classification 3
Clove 77, 192, 198
Cobalt-chloride test 39
Cocoa butter 138
Cod liver oil 138
Colophony 47, 143
Colorimetry 203, 204
Column chromatography 204, 255
Compound microscope 48
Coriander 82
Cotton 151
Coumarin glycosides 46
Crepe bandage 156
Culture media 160
Curcumin 178, 231
Cyanogenetic glycosides 46
Cysteine 39

D

Dashmularishtha 237
Datura 73, 149, 198
Decoction 28
Definitions 19, 20
Dhatryarista 236
Digitalis 59, 64, 109, 148
Diosgenin 182
DPPH method 241
Dragendorff's test 36
Dutch method 157

E

Ehrlich's test 45
Ellagic acid 231
Emulsion test 47
Ephedra leaf 97
Ester value 41
Ethanol 250
Eucalyptus leaves 196, 212
Eugenol 192, 193
Evaluation 7
Expression 28
Extraction methods 25, 216
Extractive value 58, 249

F

Fats 38, 40, 218
Fehling's test 38, 217
Fennel 194
Fenugreek seeds 182
Ferric chloride test 37, 217
Fibers 151
Filtration 28
Fixed oil 40, 218
Flavonoid content 244
Flavonoids 37, 217
Foam test 46
Foaming index 208

G

Gallic acid 231
Gambourg medium (B5) 161, 164
Gelatin test 37
Germination 165
Giloi 117
Ginger 80, 145, 206
GLC 33
Glycerrhiza 188, 189, 208, 260
Glycosides 18, 36, 46, 217
Goldbeater's skin test 37
Grignard's reaction 46
Guggal 121
Gum 47, 218

H

Hager's test 36
Harad 115, 202, 223
Heamolysis test 46
Heena powder 180
Herbal cream 251
Hesperidin 174
Hexose sugars 39
Hingastak churna 220, 222
Honey 135
Hot percolation 27
HPLC 31, 255
HPTLC 33, 260
Hydrodistillation 196, 197
Hydrous wool fat 139
Hydroxyl value 42
Hyoscyamus leaf 76

I

Indian squill 106
Infusion 27
Iodine value 42
Ipecac 98, 108
IR-spectroscopy 35
Isapgol 137, 209

J

Jaguar gum 133
Jalap 144, 190
Jatropha 131
Jute 151, 152

K

Kantakari 121
Kedde's test 46
Keller–Kiliani test 36, 46, 217
Kurchi bark 95
Kwath 235, 241, 244

L

Lard 140
Lawsone 180
Lead acetate test 37, 218
Leaf 10, 49
Leaf constant data 254
Legal's test 36, 46, 217
Lemon 130, 172, 173, 196, 204
Libermann Burchard test 36, 218
Liebermann's reaction 37
Linseed 139
Lipids 30, 40, 138
Liquorice 91, 109, 189, 248, 249
Loss on drying 13, 58, 221, 230
Lycopodium spore 13, 206

M

Maceration 26
Mahavasava 240
Majith 120
Mayer's test 36
Mentha piperita leaves 197
Methi 119, 209
Micrometers 24
Microscope 23, 48
Millions' test 38, 216
Molisch's test 38, 216
Monosaccharides 39
Morphine 45
Mounting of section 49
MS medium 160, 161, 164
Mucilage 47, 218
Murexide test 45
Myrobalan 148
Myrrh 47, 145

N

Natural fibres 151
Neem 128
Nicotine picarate 177

Ninhydrin test 38, 39, 216
Nirgundi 130
Non-reducing sugars 39
Nux vomica 101, 150, 186
Nylon 155

O

Oils 38
Optical microscopy 233
Optical rotation 14
Orange peel 173, 174

P

Palisade ratio 54
Paper chromatography 30, 201
Pathayadi kwatha 231
Pectin 134, 173
Percolation 26
Peroxide value 43
pH 222, 238
Phenols and phenolic compounds 37, 217, 244
Phytochemical screening 17, 215
Phytoconstituents 36, 170
Piperine 191
Plant tissue culture 159
Podophyllum 146
Potassium permanganate test 37
Potatoes 170, 171
Precipitation test 38
Proteins 38, 201, 216
Pulverization 28
Punarnava 123

Q

Quinine 203
Quinine sulphate 184

R

Rasna 119
Rauwolfia 84, 150, 199
Raymond's test 46
Refractive index 15
Resins 47, 190
Rhubarb 15, 104, 141
Rice bran oil 139

S

Salkowski test 37
Sandalwood oil 140
Saponification test 38, 43, 218, 253

Saponin glycosides   46
Saponins   217
Satavari   116, 208
Selwinoff's test   39, 107
Senna   65, 149, 179, 203, 210, 260
Shark liver oil   140
Shinoda test   37, 218
Sieving method   232
Silk   153
Simultaneous estimation   260
Sitoplodi churna   227
Solanine   171
Solubility test   38
Specific gravity   15, 40, 238
Spectroscopic methods   34
Spot test   38
Squill   106, 107
Stain test   38, 218
Staining   49
Starch   52, 136, 170
Steam distillation   27
Sterculia gum   137
Sterilization   160, 163
Steroids   36, 218
Stomata   55, 246
Strychnine   45, 186
Sudan IV test   40
Surgical dressing   156
Sutures   157

Swarna bhasma   224
Swelling index   56, 209

T

Tannic acid test   36
Tannins   37, 147, 217
Tea leaves   176
Terpenoids   36, 218
Terylene   155
Thalleoquin test   45
TLC   29, 198, 199, 214
TLC plates   175, 198
Tobacco leaves   177
Tollen's phloroglucinol test   39
Total alkaloids   250
Total ash   57, 221, 248
Total oxidation value   45
Total solid   238
Total sugar   238
Total tannin   202, 222
Tragacanth   136
Trikatu churna   220
Triphala churna   228
Trituration   28
Tryptophan   39
Tulsi   112, 205

Turmeric   125, 146
Tyrosine   39

U

Umbelliferone test   47
Unsaponifiable matter   44
UV-visible spectroscopy   34

V

Vanillin hydrochloric test   218
Vasaka   70, 108, 109, 115, 181, 202
Vein islet   56, 254
Vesication   28
Vicose rayon   154
Vinca   68, 186
Vitali morin test   45
Vitamin C   204
Volatile oil   18, 39, 194, 196, 197, 218, 212

W

Wagner's test   36
Water soluble ash   57, 231
Water soluble extractives   221
Withania somnifera   189, 248
Wool   153

X

Xanthoprotein test   38